D0065434

PSYCHOSOCIAL ASPECTS
OF TERMINAL CARE

Psychosocial Aspects of Terminal Care

EDITED BY

Bernard Schoenberg,
Arthur C. Carr, David Peretz,
and Austin H. Kutscher

With the editorial assistance of
LILLIAN G. KUTSCHER

COLUMBIA UNIVERSITY PRESS
New York and London 1972

Copyright © 1972 Columbia University Press
ISBN: 0-231-03614-0
Library of Congress Catalog Card Number: 73-184747
Printed in the United States of America

FOREWORD

For too many years it was difficult to discern any major interest in the psychosocial aspects of terminal care among the majority of those serving in the health professions. Concerning even the general problem of response to loss and its associated emotional reactions, whether experienced by sufferers or those bereaved, there was little discussion among our co-workers. About a decade ago, however, signs of a deep and penetrating concern and uneasiness began to surface within the new generation of students entering the professions. At that time a group of first-year medical students to whom I was lecturing on maturity and aging listened with an intensity and silence far exceeding that elicited by those other discussions and demonstrations of topics generally held by psychiatrists and psychoanalysts to be the major sources of anxiety. That class, and every class since, has responded in this way to discussions of the reactions of the dying patient, his family, his friends, society, and the physician.

Today within the professions of psychiatry and psychoanalysis we realize that perhaps our greatest failure in theory and practice has been the failure to face directly the cardinal anxiety of man, his concern over his own existence. The pendulum has now swung, and as professionals dedicated to the understanding and the compassionate care of those known to be terminally ill, we are ready to examine our own anxieties and fears. Nor are we alone in this readiness to examine the issues of grief and anxiety and the paralyzing inhibitions or excesses which accompany this inevitable human stress. It is clear that throughout this country and elsewhere many others are as deeply concerned and are channeling their energies and talents toward more compassionate treatment of the dying. The endeavor which follows in this volume is a testimonial to that reality.

Lawrence C. Kolb

One of the nursing journals has pointed out fairly recently that the aim of both nurses and physicians is to allow people to live as full a life as possible. Medicine fulfills this aim by analyzing the cause of the patient's difficulties, by attempting to restore the integrity of the faulty organ, replacing it, supplementing its function, correcting its defect, or compensating for its lack of efficiency.

The aim of nursing, however, is altogether different. Nursing does not aim at restoring the patient's biologic integrity, but is directed to helping the patient to live as fully as possible. This may mean that nurses assist the patient to carry out the prescribed regime, but beyond this it can also mean that the goal of nursing is to help the patient reach out for a plenitude of being that is always possible in spite of biological limitations against which medicine is helpless.

These aims apply just as much to terminal care as they do to preventive, curative, or restorative care. The aim is still to help the patient and his family to find a plenitude of being. The efforts of the physician and the nurse continue to complement each other. Our problem is that we still have much to learn in how to reach these goals. Only our joint explorations will bring us closer to them.

Mary Crawford

Dying patients are cared for by many different kinds of people in a university medical center: physicians, nurses, social workers, chaplains, practical nurses, ward aides, a host of technical assistants, students of the health professions, nutritionists, and many others. During periods when they are not hospitalized still others are involved: outpatient department personnel, the community agencies, such as the Visiting Nurse Association, Cancer Care, the Department of Welfare, nursing homes, local ministers, and physicians. When family equilibrium is threatened by anticipated death, children may show emotional disturbances which are manifest at school, and these require the understanding of still others: teachers, school counselors, psychologists, family service agencies. More severe disturbances require the intervention of a psychiatrist or pediatrician.

Does the care of the patient end with his death, or do we extend the concept of care to the bereaved family? We know that the inability to resolve grief in childhood or adulthood may result in severe emotional disturbance. We know that the incidences of somatic and emotional disturbances among the bereaved are much higher than among the normal population. The mortality rates among bereaved family members are also higher than in control groups.

A university health center, broadly committed as it must be to the practice of and training in comprehensive medical care, is faced with all the complex problems relating to the physical and psychosocial care of the dying patient. Comprehensive care requires the utilization of specialists from a number of different disciplines as well as from an integrated health care team. This necessitates a reappraisal of our teaching models and our teaching content so that students from a variety of health education programs may learn to overcome disciplinary parochialism and professional boundaries in order to function together— always with the welfare of the patient and his family as the primary goal.

Death and dying traditionally have been taboo topics, sorely neglected by society and health educators. It is essential that the psychosocial aspects of terminal care be included in the curriculum of all health professional students. In addition, related topics, such as euthanasia, organ transplant, the prolongation of life through artificial means, the definition of death, and so forth, should be discussed openly with hospital personnel and students. We recognize that steps in this direction are long overdue. Personnel, such as nurses, ward aides, house officers involved in the daily care and support of the terminal patients, are themselves frequently under severe and prolonged emotional stress. In order to sustain their morale and enable them to function effectively we must institutionalize methods to provide emotional support and opportunities to discuss their feelings with others.

We recognize the needs for a new clinical specialist to supplement and complement the activities of the physician, nurse, and dentist in almost every area of health practice. In the area of terminal care we may consider the training of a specialist, the psychiatric nurse, social worker, psychologist, or perhaps an entirely new category of worker as yet unnamed, whose function it would be to coordinate the efforts of the health care team and the various social and community agencies. This latter worker would also assist the family in coping with the imminent crises and adaptation to loss.

If the initial investigation of increased mortality and physical and mental illness among the bereaved is substantiated, should we not consider a preventive health program during the first year of bereavement? Should we not consider an approach to the dying which emphasizes that they live each remaining day fully and as free as possible from unnecessary anxiety and fear? Perhaps a "life conference" with a bringing together of all concerned with each dying patient, personnel, family, and even the patient himself, to discuss the problems involved would provide a forum for beneficial ventilation.

The most pressing problem at present is that we live in a society where death is considered unnatural. Society itself must be re-educated to regard death as a natural phase of living. Thereby, we could reduce the fear and the denial, the avoidance and the repression—all of which create the problems and deficiencies that exist today in the psychosocial care of the terminally ill.

Douglas Damrosch

PREFACE

Advances in science and technology have had in recent years a profound impact on health care in this country. In addition, an enlightened and expectant population has made increasing demands for improvements in the quality and distribution of health services. New legislation on federal, state, and municipal levels and increased participation in pre-paid health insurance plans have led to greater utilization of scarce health resources.

In an attempt to accommodate to these multiple pressures, health care is slowly being reorganized, and with this come new opportunities as well as new dangers. An important challenge is that a reorganization of our health care system may lead to further dehumanization of care and a dilution of the one-to-one relationship between patient and health professional which has been an essential component in providing care to the sick.

There is an increasing interest in the quality of life in our society as well as the quality of care in the health professions. There is a pressing need for re-evaluation of the psychosocial components of care in all illness and especially in terminal conditions. This book represents an effort of members of the health professions and occupations to examine and explore in depth the psychosocial aspects of terminal care. It is the hope of the editors that this multidisciplinary approach will help to humanize and dignify the care of the dying and the bereaved. It is written for the students and practitioners of all the health disciplines.

We express our gratitude to the Foundation of Thanatology for financial support and encouragement in the preparation of this book.

The authors wish to acknowledge the dedicated efforts of the following: Professors Helen Pettit, Elsa Poslusny, Constance Cleary, M. Ursula Brady, Roberta Spagnola, Mr. Edward Wray and Mrs. Anne O'Donnell of the Department of Nursing of the College of Physicians and Surgeons, Columbia University; and Miss Ann Calderwood, Miss Elaine Finnberg, Mrs. Ruthann Zanis, Mrs. Betty Loshin, and Mrs. Priscilla Hawkins, working in behalf of the Foundation of Thanatology.

This volume was compiled under the sponsorship of the Foundation of Thanatology.

The Editors

CONTENTS

Education

Bernard Schoenberg and Arthur C. Carr

EDUCATING THE HEALTH PROFESSIONAL IN THE PSYCHOSOCIAL CARE OF THE TERMINALLY ILL

One of the most difficult tasks confronting educators in the health professions is that of training students in the care of the terminally ill. In the more limited sense, this task may be conceived primarily as the training of physicians and nurses. In the ideal sense of *psychosocial* care not only of the patient but of his family as well, the task obviously also includes the training of social workers, clergy, and aides, as well as other professional and paraprofessional personnel. Nevertheless, whether evaluated from either the more limited goal of medical and nursing school curricula, or in terms of a broader multidisciplinary approach to the problem, the inadequate education in the management of the terminally ill probably represents one of the greatest failures in professional education today.

Typical of the evidence to support this conclusion are the results of surveys recently conducted by the Foundation of Thanatology.

In a survey of current activities and programs in medical school curricula, questionnaires were sent to the deans and to the chairmen of four departments (Medicine, Surgery, Pediatrics, Psychiatry) of sixty-eight medical schools throughout the country. Replies were received from at least one of the five representatives in all medical schools surveyed, with distribution as indicated:

Deans (29); Medicine (24); Surgery (22); Pediatrics (28); and Psychiatry (36). Although a more complete report of this and other surveys will appear elsewhere, the following facts emerge:

1. Almost half the respondents (48.1%) report that the requirements for the diagnosis of death are not included formally in their medical school curriculum.

2. Over one-third of the respondents report that the physician's responsibility in regard to the care of the bereaved-to-be (38.1%) or of the bereaved (39.1%) is not included in the medical student's curriculum.

3. Concerning their own satisfaction with their teaching efforts to prepare medical students to care for the dying patient, almost two-thirds (62.9%) report feeling either only *somewhat pleased* or *displeased,* while one-quarter (25.7%) report being *displeased.*

4. In spite of their reported dissatisfaction, only about one-third (31.5%) indicate that they plan to make any curriculum changes with regard to the care of the dying patient.

The following tabulations are the results concerning the particular departmental policies and practices:

	Medicine	Surgery	Pediatrics	Psychiatry
Department does not regularly assign students to care for patients suffering from a condition that may lead to death.	9.1%	8.7%	0%	78.1%
Department does not have a policy which defines the division of responsibility among the physician, nurse, social service worker, and the chaplain who are caring for the dying patient.	85.7%	82.6%	78.3%	93.8%

Students are rarely or never asked questions about the spe-

	Medicine	Surgery	Pediatrics	Psychiatry
cific care of dying patients in examinations.	71.5%	82.6%	84.0%	66.7%
Department does not require reading pertaining to caring for dying patients.	81.8%	95.7%	76.9%	66.7%
Department does not have a specific person who teaches the care of the dying patient.	81.8%	95.5%	50.0%	63.6%

Department does not specifically prepare medical students to understand and deal with:

	Medicine	Surgery	Pediatrics	Psychiatry
a. the patient's emotional response to dying	33.3%	56.5%	34.6%	24.2%
b. the role of denial in the dying patient	33.3%	73.9%	44.0%	18.8%
c. the process of patient's separation or disengagement from others	55.0%	77.3%	50.0%	28.1%
d. the dying patient's grief	50.0%	63.6%	52.2%	18.8%
e. the family's anticipatory grief and mourning	55.0%	60.9%	23.1%	28.1%
f. the hospital personnel's emotional reaction to the patient	38.1%	69.6%	28.0%	25.0%

	Medicine	Surgery	Pediatrics	Psychiatry
Department does not discuss with students controversial issues that are currently connected with the care of a dying patient, i.e., euthanasia, definitions of death, ethics of organ transplantations, addiction of terminal patients to narcotics.	17.4%	8.7%	37.0%	21.2%

Tentative evidence suggests that department chairmen and deans may be more optimistic than is warranted, since students from two medical schools as diverse in geographical location as the far West and the East report less encouraging views. Considering the replies of students at the end of their final years, for example, rather consistent patterns emerge for both schools:

1. Almost two-thirds (64.5%, 72.2%) report that requirements for

the diagnosis of death had not been included formally in their medical curriculum.

2. Over half of the students report the opinion that sufficient consideration in the curriculum was not given to physician's responsibility in regard to the care of the bereaved-to-be (75.0%, 66.7%) or of the bereaved (78.1%, 61.1%).

3. Concerning their satisfaction with the school's teaching efforts to prepare them to care for the dying patient and his family, almost three-quarters (74.2%, 66.6%) report feeling either only *somewhat pleased* or *displeased,* while about one-third (35.5%, 33.3%) report being *displeased*.

4. About two-thirds (64.3%, 72.2%) feel it desirable that the school make curriculum changes with respect to teaching the student how to care for the dying patient.

Consistent with department chairmen replies, students indicate that:

They are rarely asked questions on examinations about the specific care of dying patients (96.9%, 100%).

They are generally not required to do any reading with regard to caring for dying patients (93.1%, 66.7%).

There is not a specific person who teaches "care of the dying patient" (64.5%, 100%).

Students generally feel that no department conducts discussion with students concerning controversial issues that are currently connected with the care of dying patients, that is, euthanasia (67.7%, 41.2%), definitions of death (58.1%, 52.9%), ethics of organ transplantation (71.0%, 47.1%), addiction of terminal patients to narcotics (41.9%, 58.8%).

In treating the dying patient, the following percentages of students report that they are not encouraged to pursue such activities as:

a.	talking with chaplain	90.3	100
b.	talking with social worker	51.6	70.6
c.	talking with the nurse	50.0	88.2
d.	talking with the family	45.2	47.1
e.	discussing social, financial, and family problems with the patient	61.3	68.8

Results of a similar survey of the deans of ninety-seven nursing schools support the impression that nursing schools probably are much more concerned, both theoretically and in a practical way, with training students to handle and console dying patients and the bereaved than are medical schools. This conclusion emerges in several ways:

1. In regard to the curriculum itself, only 12.4% of the nursing school deans indicate that the requirements for the determination of death are not included formally in the nursing curriculum, while 48.1% of medical school respondents reported similarly about the medical school curriculum.

2. Nursing schools report almost universally that the nurses' responsibility in regard to the care of the dying patient, the bereaved-to-be, and of the bereaved is included in the nursing curriculum (100%, 96.9%, and 97.0% respectively).

Concerning their own satisfaction with their teaching efforts to prepare nursing students to care for the dying patient, only 3.2% report feeling really *displeased*. Nevertheless over half (54.4%) report plans to make curriculum changes with regard to the care of the dying patient. Thus, while medical school staff report much greater dissatisfaction with their own curricula, many fewer anticipate anything being done or changed about it.

Similar to reporting departments of medicine, a large percentage regularly assign students to care for terminally ill patients (89.4%).

Similar to most medical school departments, most nursing schools do not have a policy which defines the division of responsibility among the physician, nurse, social service worker, and the chaplain who are caring for the dying patient (91.5%).

Nursing schools place much greater emphasis than medical schools on examination questions and required professional readings on the care of the dying patient and his family. Of nursing schools, 90.1% report that at least *sometimes* students are asked questions on examinations about the care of dying patients and their families, while they universally report required professional reading for students pertaining to this area.

Similar to medical departments, nursing schools frequently do not have a specific person who teaches "the care of the dying patient" (72.0%).

Nevertheless, nursing schools almost universally report specifically preparing students (nursing) to understand and deal with:

a. the patient's emotional response to dying	100%
b. the use of denial by the dying patient	98.0%
c. the process of the patient's separation	93.8%
d. the dying patient's grief	96.9%
e. the family's anticipatory grief and mourning	99.0%
f. the hospital personnel's emotional reaction to the patient	94.7%

Nursing schools universally report that there is discussion with students concerning controversial issues that are currently connected with the care of dying patients, for example, euthanasia, definitions of death, ethics of organ transplantation, and addiction of terminal patients to narcotics.

In spite of the optimistic picture that arises from the reports of nursing school deans, there is much evidence and opinion to suggest that the aims and hopes of the deans are not fully realized in their students' self-perceptions and achievements. Relevant to locally gathered data, a survey of 56 third and fourth year nursing school students indicated that:

1. Of the students, 61.8% report that the requirements for the determination of death had not as yet been included formally in their curriculum.

2. A substantial percentage reported that the nurses' responsibility to the care of the dying patient, the bereaved-to-be, and the bereaved, was not as yet included in their curriculum (37.5%, 82.2%, and 60.0% respectively).

3. Concerning their satisfactions with the teaching efforts to prepare them to care for the dying patient, 43.6% of the students report themselves as only *somewhat satisfied,* 14.5% report feeling actually *dissatisfied,* and 70.9% feel it desirable that the school make curriculum changes with respect to teaching the student how to care for the dying patient.

No further documentation is needed to support the impression that there is a large discrepancy between what would be seen as ideal training for the health professional in the care of the terminally ill and what is actually the past and present reality. Whether evidence is derived from educational practices as reported either by educator or student, from observations of current hospital practices, or from reports either of dying patients or of their relatives, the consistent picture is one reflecting the inadequacy of training in and provision of the psychosocial care of the terminally ill.

The extent of the present failures, however, is not difficult to understand when consideration is given to the multiple forces which prevent more successful education in this area. Basic to our failures in the education of care of the terminally ill is the fact that American society in its preoccupation with perpetual youth, beauty, sexuality, and strength has typically disguised, avoided, denied, and embellished death. Eissler (1) has described "the supreme effort" to deny death that is characteristic of our present American culture. Ross (2) believes the fear of death in the United States is especially great "because people rarely see death. They can avoid it. Death becomes an almost mechanical operation— nice, clean, and sterile—something that takes place in a modern hospital. The universal fear of death in this country extends itself to physicians and nurses." Ross (3), Feifel (4), and others have described the institutional barriers they confronted in doing investigations with terminal patients and the anxiety of hospital personnel in such settings, where workers generally receive meager support in caring for dying patients and minimal opportunity to deal with their own emotional reactions to death.

Until recently, minimal attention was paid to the psychosocial care of the dying patient during training of the various health professionals who we know tend to place great emphasis on preservation of life and generally view a patient's death as a personal failure. Avoiding issues related to death is related to prized institutional values of success and to maintaining self-esteem. With the inevitable death of a patient, the usual gratifications of success are absent. In his identification with the patient, the worker may re-experience childhood fears of separation, abandonment, and injury, as well as the consequent feelings of anxiety, grief, and depression. Feelings of helplessness and ineffectuality commonly result in anger toward the patient, soon followed by guilt and emotional withdrawal. The helpless patient frequently places the practitioner in the parental role, a position which some fear and which others exploit by maintaining the patient in a helpless, dependent position.

With the modern trend in medical care toward a division of labor in caring for the patient, withdrawal by delegating responsibilities to others becomes an easy matter. Recent scientific advances, such as advanced surgical techniques, chemotherapy, radiotherapy, pain relieving surgical procedures, new analgesics and narcotics, antiemetic drugs, psychopharmacological agents, and others, allow health personnel to maintain the attitude that they can combat death and are doing something important for the patient. An orientation to activity and tasks frequently allows the physician and nurse to withdraw emotionally from the patient. The end result of the withdrawal process is the disruption of continuous care, adding to the patient's feelings of loneliness and isolation. The disengagement of hospital personnel from the patient may also serve to protect them against feelings of loss and the consequent feeling of grief. On another level, the withdrawal is also related to the individual's inability to face the inevitability of his own death.

Since a fundamental goal of medical care is to prolong life and gain power over death, the avoidance and denial of death among health personnel is not surprising. Health personnel frequently enter the health professions in an effort to master their own fears concerning death. Feifel *et al.* (5) report results which indicate that although physicians think less about death than do two control groups of patients and one of nonprofessionals, they are more afraid of death than either of the control groups. From his observations, Feifel developed the hypothesis that one of the major factors influencing certain physicians to enter medicine is to master their own above-average fears of death.

In discussing career decisions of medical students, Webster (6) notes that a significant factor influencing the choice and idealization of a medical career is experience with illness either in oneself or his family. The medical career may be viewed in terms of the knowledge and power to overcome illness and relieve suffering. Paradoxically, this ideal may be associated with the failures of a physician to cure a given case in one family, as well as the physician's success in other instances. In an extensive longitudinal study of individual medical students, Horowitz (7) noted that some students included in the study indicated that illness in a family member affected their decision to study medicine, very likely motivated by an attempt to regain feelings of control and mastery and unconsciously to fulfill a wish to rescue the family member.

Although we all rationally realize that death is inevitable, the health practitioner, unlike others, is frequently confronted with this as a certainty. It is of interest that the health professional student's encounter with the "first patient," the cadaver, is rarely mentioned in the literature. In the anatomy laboratory the cadaver is, of course, nameless; is exposed for dissection only when a particular organ or area is to be examined; and is frequently the object of humor or horror stories. The student's initial emotional reaction to his "first patient," a dead body, is rarely discussed.

Professional training ordinarily takes place at a time in life (late and post-adolescence) when feelings of uncertainty are readily displaced onto death. Usually, this anxiety is quickly repressed by college students and they report only rare or occasional thoughts about it. While other college students are coping with anxiety related to death by repression and denial, however, the medical, nursing, and chaplaincy student is repeatedly confronted with death as a fact of everyday life. He is expected to deal with problems related to dying and to remain emotionally accessible to the severely ill or dying patient.

In a recent survey of Freshmen medical students at Tufts University School of Medicine (8), students were asked to rank fifteen specific situations that they were expected to deal with in their first year, according to the anxiety they anticipated in the situation. At the end of the year they were asked to repeat the procedure. The two most anxiety-provoking situations dealt with death: discussing a fatal illness with a patient and telling a relative that a patient had died. Faculty predictions about anxiety-provoking situations estimated accurately the students' anxiety related to the discussion of fatal illness and death. The investigators concluded that early discussions and instruction concerning such issues might benefit the student.

Some students cope with the problem only by becoming inaccessible to the terminal patient and to their own emotions. Emotional withdrawal, avoidance, and isolation with emphasis on tasks and ward rituals become the means of decreasing anxiety. In order to maintain stability, the student soon realizes that the hospital social system offers many opportunities to escape from the difficult task by physical and emotional withdrawal. A defense which enables the student to avoid reality is costly, in that it induces guilt and shame and removes him from many sources of professional gratification.

Other reactions can be as detrimental as avoidance and withdrawal, for example the young physician and nurse responding with outrage at death as an enemy to be fought and conquered. Others may express excessive optimism, thus preventing the patient and family members from experiencing anticipatory grief. Some physicians and medical students may maintain too exclusive an involvement with the patient, thus omitting other personnel and preventing an integrated staff approach to the problem. Unfortunately, a student's early experience becomes the prototype for later relationships with patients. The major challenge for the educator at this time is to maintain the student's openness and to prevent emotional withdrawal. By "openness" we mean a way of reacting to the environment by permitting maximum contact with feelings and allowing a high degree of involvement with the environment. Only under conditions in which an atmosphere is provided in which the student feels free to express his anxiety and is supported in dealing with his feelings of grief and depression by appropriate role models can the student be expected to learn to provide the optimal in care for his dying patient and the family. Some educators, notably Ross (9), Saunders (10), and Hackett (11), have demonstrated that it is possible to maintain student and staff accessibility in working with terminal patients, illustrating that no untoward effects result from dealing with death candidly.

The task of managing the dying patient is sufficiently formidable as to require that it be a shared responsibility. The complex decisions concerning when or what to tell the patient, mutilating or disfiguring surgical intervention, programs for rehabilitation, outpatient treatment and decisions regarding euthanasia require the knowledge and experience of specialists from a number of different disciplines, working in a team approach. One suggested approach is the utilization of a specialist in terminal care—perhaps a psychologist, psychiatric nurse, or social worker—who could assume responsibility for integrating the diverse efforts to provide "continuity of care." When the patient returned home, the specialist could assume responsibility for enlisting the efforts of community agencies and outpatient hospital facilities to provide physical care and emotional support for the patient and his family.

Many university and teaching hospitals hold "death conferences" when a patient dies in order to determine if any additional efforts could have been expended in order to prolong the life of the individual patient. An appropriate parallel would be a "life conference" preceding death to determine what steps should be taken to assist the patient, family, and hospital personnel in managing the painful feelings of grief, guilt, depression, anxiety, and anger.

Teaching the psychosocial care of the dying patient has been largely avoided in the health professions. Greater education efforts are required of all in the health professions in order to help the dying patient to maintain his dignity and self esteem, gain pleasure and gratification in his daily life, and approach death with as much truth as he and his family can tolerate.

Strauss (12), in discussing reforms needed in providing terminal care, suggested:

First, training for giving terminal care should be greatly amplified and deepened in schools of medicine and nursing. Current training equips these professionals principally for restricted technical aspects of dealing with dying and death. The psychological, social and organizational aspects of dying are either considered secondary or are neglected. In consequence, most of the behavior of physicians and nurses toward dying patients is similar to that of the layman; only their more technical behaviors are professionalized. The clear implication is that curricula should include these neglected courses of terminal care. This will involve considerable turmoil; the reform we advocated goes beyond merely humanizing the curriculum a little more in order to make terminal care a bit more humane.

It appears that both the general population and the health professionals are showing a new openness and interest in death and dying. This trend coincides with a number of significant social changes— disintegration of familiar social institutions, erosion of belief in personal immortality, awareness of our political impotence, the imminent threat of death through nuclear war, dire predictions concerning overpopulation and environmental pollution, awareness of the miniscule place of the earth in the universe, and confrontation of social and moral values by American youth. While the relationship between all these changes is difficult to evaluate, it does appear that the present questioning of old assumptions offers opportunities for introducing new ideas and approaches to the education of the health professional as well as of the layman in the psychosocial care of the terminally ill.

The challenge facing the educator today is to determine what will be taught, what methods will be utilized, and who shall be prepared to provide psychosocial care for the dying patient and his family. For this purpose, there is a tremendous need for research and systematic evaluation in the area, not only insofar as the effects of our teaching on the care of the dying patient and his family, but also of the eventual effects on all health personnel.

REFERENCES

1. K. Eissler, *The Psychiatrist and the Dying Patient,* New York: International Universities Press, 1955.

2. E. Ross, quoted in *Archives of The Foundation of Thanatology, 2*:38, 1969.

3. E. Ross, *On Death and Dying,* New York: Macmillan, 1969.

4. H. Feifel, "Death" in *Taboo Topics,* edited by N. L. Farberow, New York: Atherton Press, 1963.

5. H. Feifel *et al.,* Physicians Consider Death. Proceedings 75th Annual Convention, American Psychological Association, 1967.

6. T. H. Webster, Career Decisions and Professional Self-Images of Medical Students in Teaching Psychiatry in Medical School, Washington, D.C.: American Psychiatric Association.

7. M. J. Horowitz, *Educating Tomorrow's Doctors,* New York: Appleton-Century-Crofts, 1964.

8. E. V. Saul and J. S. Kass, "Study of Anticipated Anxiety in a Medical School Setting," *Journal of Medical Education, 44*:526, 1969.

9. E. Ross, *On Death and Dying,* New York: Macmillan, 1969.

10. C. M. Saunders, "The Management of Patients in the Terminal Stage," *Cancer,* edited by R. W. Raven, London: Buterworth, 1959.

11. T. P. Hackett, "Current Approaches to the Care and Understanding of the Dying Patient," *Archives of The Foundation of Thanatology, 1*:109, 1969.

12. A. L. Strauss, "Reforms Needed in Providing Terminal Care in Hospitals," *Archives of The Foundation of Thanatology, 1*:21, 1969.

Medical Care

Henry O. Heinemann

HUMAN VALUES IN THE MEDICAL CARE OF THE TERMINALLY ILL

This paper deals with the relationship between a physician and a patient with an incurable and ultimately fatal illness. It contains but some of the thoughts a physician has accumulated over the years concerning this problem.

The questions to be raised are: First, what are the needs of the patient who is suffering from a fatal illness? Second, why is it that these needs cannot be adequately met by the facilities available in our society? And third, is it simply because the health professions are not trained to meet these needs, or is the issue more complex and are the deficiencies a reflection of attitudes in our society?

The problem can be defined by examining the first question: What are the needs of the patient with an incurable and ultimately fatal illness? Besides proper medical care, these patients need emotional support for their comfort and reassurance. Traditionally, this was not provided by physicians but by religious workers and by relatives within a strong, stable, extended family structure. In the past, physicians played a role in healing wounds and relieving suffering caused by illness, but they were not involved at the beginning of life when a child was born and at the end of life when death came. Assistance at birth was provided by midwives; assistance at the time of death was given by the clergy. With changing social patterns and improved medical skills, man's birth and death moved from his home to the more impersonal environment of a hospital and physicians replaced midwives and the clergy. This has cast upon physicians a role for which they are ill-equipped, for a relationship that had traditionally been accepted by the clergy as a sacred trust has devolved by default upon the physician.

The exclusion of the clergy at the time of death is partly due to changing attitudes toward religion. Theology, which for centuries tried to establish the meaning of life and the justification of death, failed to recognize the need for adaptation to changing requirements, and this has contributed to the lack of religious faith among many people today. Furthermore, loss of the traditional family structure because of urbanization and the restless mood of our present society has curtailed the emotional support of a fatally ill person previously given by the comfort of a familiar environment and filial loyalty typical of the family structures of rural communities of the past.

This leaves the majority of individuals without the comfort of religious belief or the help of loyal relatives as the end of life approaches. The resulting isolation and loneliness—especially of the aging ill—is the first problem to be recognized. The emotional needs of the sick, the aged, and the infirm have not changed, but the attitudes of society toward these needs have changed.

Urban life, with its limitation in living space, its hostility, indifference and "dehumanization" of interpersonal relationships, is difficult even for able-bodied individuals. For older people, especially if they are ill, it may become a never-ending nightmare. In cramped living quarters, a sick person rapidly becomes a burden to the family, and overt or suppressed hostility interwoven with guilt feelings often faces the fatally ill at home. For many, a hospital or home for the aged rather than the family home becomes the end station of life.

Before analyzing the patient's reaction to the hospital environment, let us not forget that every patient struck down by illness, whether serious or not, reacts with anxiety. Sometimes this is obvious even to the casual observer. Sometimes it is hidden and expressed in more subtle ways. In a patient with recurrent disease who is facing readmission to the hospital, fear is even more pronounced. The admission is not for cure or diagnosis but is usually necessary because of progression of the disease or complications. The admission, therefore, reinforces fears about the seriousness of the underlying illness, and each readmission raises the possibility that this might be the last time. The author remembers one patient, who, as he left the hospital, said: "Brother, am I glad to walk out of here, because if you walk into this place, you may never get out alive."

What we may conclude from this brief consideration of the first question is that the patient with a terminal illness is in need of emotional support, that such support is not available for most patients for reasons such as lack of religious faith, the social isolation of urbanized life, and the absence of a cohesive family structure. All this is exaggerated as the last days of a person's life are transferred from the home to the hospital. As the patient re-enters the hospital a complex emotional reaction sets in which has, as its major undertone, fear.

The patient's reception and subsequent treatment in the hospital lead to further anxiety. If the patient knows the hospital to which he is readmitted, the environment and its routines will be familiar but, depending upon past experiences, this may not necessarily be a comforting thought. The individuals the patient will meet—the nurses, aides, physicians, and other patients—will most likely be strangers, at least in any large urban medical center.

Depending upon the reason for readmission, the patient may be exposed to the whole gamut of technology that is part of contemporary patient care. The environment is a restless one, full of activity and rhythmic noises from cardiac monitors and respirators. Anxiety persists and new fears come up. How am I doing? What will come next? Is this the last time?

What is needed more than anything is comforting, compassion, and reassurance. This can be provided only by another human being; no drug can act as a substitute. But who is to provide this emotional support? One of the busy nurses on eight-hour shifts? One of the house officers rotating through? The private physician rushing between office, house calls and the hospital? The chances are that none of the professional staff has time—or sadly enough, the inclination or training—to provide the needed emotional support.

More important than the superficial reasons for neglect is the fact that people, even professional people, shy away from the dying. At a time when human compassion is most needed it is least available within the setting of a large modern hospital. Physicians often react to an incurable illness in one of their patients as if the illness is a personal failure and a reproach to their efforts. This may unconsciously lead the doctor to avoid the patient and his relatives. Thus the patient with inoperable cancer and his family may discover that the physician becomes remote in speech and behavior once the diagnosis is established. This does not go unrecognized, but patients are hesitant to ask questions, because unconsciously they are reluctant to receive a direct answer.

This behavior pattern of health care personnel may be a manifestation of their own fear of death. Fear of death is a very basic human emotional response, and its deep roots become apparent in the mysticism which shrouds the occurrence of death in ritualistic traditions. For example, the persistence of ritualized funeral practice speaks for itself.

Since the introduction of modern technology, the hospital has lost its aura of being a place of comfort and has instead become an establishment resembling a factory, where illnesses are taken care of, rather than human beings.

This brings us to the second question: Why can we not provide for the needs of these patients? The deficiencies are apparent, and we know that there is lack of compassion among health care personnel. Is it because these needs can be provided for only if we are prepared to alter our attitudes toward other human beings? Is it a consequence of the trend toward technical skill without a humanistic foundation? If this is correct, the inadequacies in the care of the terminally ill transcend the issue of the modern hospital and become a problem of human behavior in a technologically oriented society.

Is there promise that such changes in human behavior are possible, and what can be done to bring these changes about? No effort is made in our educational system, and even with a major effort there is no assurance that the humanistic approach to medical care can be recaptured and brought into harmonious balance with recent technological advances because there seems to be an inherent incompatibility between technology and humanistic values.

Cultivation of compassion among human beings, harnessing of seemingly excessive application of medical technology, and appropriate education of health care personnel to handle the terminally ill are some of the obvious concerns which need immediate attention if any change can be expected.

The scientific approach to medicine prevalent today has by inference no purpose other than to inquire into the nature of disease. The individual and his emotional response is irrelevant to this pursuit. To attempt to abandon the scientific approach would be folly; what is needed is a balance between method and its application to sick human beings.

Medicine, like other social institutions, has become a victim of runaway technology which leaves a gap between technological know-how and human emotional needs. We have to recognize this and try to establish a set of values appropriate for our times. The inadequacies of our care of our older citizens and the terminally ill need to be faced realistically and efforts should be made to provide such care. But this issue transcends medicine and is a reflection of men's altered attitudes toward each other and toward the ill. The need to educate health care personnel to understand the problems involved is obvious and urgent.

Let us take up the last question: Is inadequate education of health care personnel the only fault, or is the problem much more deeply rooted and related to problems of society in general?

In an attempt to answer this question, let us examine some of the trends in our society. We are living in a period of human existence which we might call the "technological revolution." Technology advances rapidly— almost exponentially, it seems—while philosophical, religious, and moral values change more slowly. Although these changes interact and affect each other, the differences in the rate of change lead to conflict situations.

What we are witnessing today is an almost frantic reaction to an awareness—but not an understanding—of such conflicts. Our civilization is on a collision course with existing values and perhaps with basic principles of nature itself. A critical question (raised by the German theologian Thielicke, among others) is: "Can man survive the threat of his own technological creation?" This question is not lifted out of some science-fiction novel; it is real, the events have arrived and engulf us with a speed that leaves us in bewilderment because the problems seem to multiply faster than we can recognize them, not to speak of designing solutions and applying them to these problems.

Let us extrapolate and apply this awareness to problems in medicine. What has happened and what is the direction we are heading for?

Understanding of transmission of disease, improved public health, and the introduction of effective measures to control infection have prolonged life, reduced infant mortality and contributed to the enormous population growth. More recently, effective immunization against illness of viral origin, the introduction of prosthetic devices, and organ transplantation have further added to the prevention of illness and survival of individuals afflicted with disease.

Medicine has followed pragmatically its mandate to treat illness, but has not assessed the consequences of its improved skills. Nor has it broadened its philosophical base and taken stock of its impact on society. Indeed, a great deal of effort is dissipated by the medical profession in maintaining and caring for a few rare but technically interesting cases. For example, the expenditure in time and manpower demanded to perform one heart transplant and maintain the individual thereafter is entirely out of proportion to the availability of medical care to the majority of the population.

What we are faced with now are not epidemics of transmittable diseases (although they still occur). What we are confronted with are problems related to population growth, environmental pollution, longevity, and the care of the aged. Indeed, the time may already have come when medicine must get involved in these issues and broaden its mandate, not only by treating individuals but also by assuming responsibility for issues confronting mankind as a group.

The pragmatic approach to life is based upon a value system which interprets as right what is successful and as wrong what fails. This approach has little patience with philosophical contemplation. The values of medicine have perforce always been pragmatic; and the values of a technologically oriented society are obviously so. We are therefore confronted with a crisis if something does not work. We live in such a crisis situation now because many aspects of our existence are not successful; they do not work and no alternatives seem to be in sight.

Historically, life has adapted its forms to a changing environment. Man with his ingenuity has introduced a new variant, because man himself is changing the environment, and at a rate which appears to exceed the environment's capacity to adjust to these man-made changes. We are faced with the dilemma that man's own creation—that is, our present technological civilization—overpowers our own value system. We are already living with this problem, but we do not care or dare to think about it.

If we apply these thoughts to medicine, we can state that modern medicine, like other facets of our life, has been invaded by rapidly advancing technology which has outstripped the capacities of man himself. What man "can do" is out of step with what man "is." As Karl Jaspers has pointed out, the technology produced by man is not inherently destructive; it is man's utilization of his own creation which threatens him. Man's choice is limited to these alternatives: Either man adapts to these new challenges or he will destroy himself by means of his own technology. What man in a technological society has to learn is that the ability to do everything does not justify doing it. These issues, however, are beyond the scope of the medical profession, and solutions to these problems cannot be expected from it alone.

Moral values carried over for almost 2,000 years by traditional religious belief are not directly applicable to the problems confronting us today, and only time will tell whether values of the Judeo-Christian religious tradition can be successfully adapted to fulfill our present needs. Yet, if we can learn to manage and adapt to the new powers created by technology we might enter a new golden era for generations to come. The trouble is that we might not survive the period of adaptation.

The lesson to be learned from this awareness is that one cannot initiate an intervention and just let things happen thereafter. The first step imposes a responsibility for the consequences which may require secondary and tertiary interventions to permit meaningful adaptation to these innovations. This responsibility is not inherent to man's nature. Man is prone to act without being able to weigh the consequences. The Wright brothers presumably hoped that all wars would become impossible if their invention—the airplane—could observe what was going on behind enemy lines! The Union Army surgeon Richard Gatling reasoned that the loss in human life could be reduced by reducing the size of armies, and that this in turn would be possible if the fire power of the individual soldier could be increased. He developed the Gatling gun, the predecessor of the machine gun. How wrong he was! Society at large has been slow to recognize the need for careful and responsible thought before adopting new inventions. A typical example in medicine now is organ transplantation. The technical know-how is here but thoughts about the ethical issues involved are just beginning to permeate through the profession.

This lack of thought about the consequences of new inventions also applies to present-day medical care in general, and to the relationship between the physician and the fatally ill. We have been able to extend life expectancy to unprecedented levels, thus increasing the incidence of slowly progressing fatal illnesses. In consequence, we need more facilities and broader knowledge of how to take care of the elderly and the fatally ill. This problem is apparent, yet it is hardly mentioned in our profession or our educational system, and little effort is made to explore the problem or to deal with it.

In his attitude toward the limited time-span of his own existence, man can ignore death and at times postpone it, but he can never escape it. In his unwillingness or inability to accept death, man unconsciously believes in his own immortality. Most human beings fear the end of life; few can accept death as a natural end to a full life or a welcome termination of suffering. Most people attempt to delay the process of aging and are unable or unwilling to accept that death is just as much a part of our existence as birth.

If the average man cannot face up to the natural course of life, why should this concern the physicians? Physicians have to be concerned because when fatal illness strikes patients turn to the physician. The patient and his relatives need help to plan the immediate future. Physicians are often reluctant to get involved in such a situation. There is probably more than one reason for this reaction. The simplest reason is that this aspect of the patient-physician relationship is very time consuming and not very rewarding.

There are other reasons which are less apparent. One, that inability to cure an illness is equated with personal failure, has been mentioned. Another is the physician's own fear of death, which is normally suppressed but may be aroused when he is confronted with a dying person.

The physician who is unwilling to get involved often avoids the issues by introducing medical procedures—new therapeutic trials, a new battery of laboratory tests, another series of x-rays—without ever taking time to discuss the real problem. Admittedly, many patients have similar attitudes —the results of a new test give reassurance, another drug will do the trick, and so on. Patient and doctor can become involved in a game of avoiding the real issues.

What should and what should not be done for a terminally ill person? Medical technology can permit life to go on to a point where its very meaning is in question. Indeed, improved skills have led the medical profession into ethical dilemmas few care to think about. In the day-to-day practice of medicine it has recently been decided that lack of central nervous system function manifested by a flat EEG can be equated with the end of meaningful life. This is of course an extreme situation relatively easy to define. There are many other situations where technical gadgetry cannot help us to define an endpoint, and where we are in need of ethical guidelines founded on sound philosophical thought. The medical profession, although intimately involved in the drama of human existence from birth to death, has had singularly shallow philosophical underpinnings. In a time of crisis like ours it becomes blatantly apparent that the medical profession still follows its mandate established by Hippocrates over 2,000 years ago to treat the patient to the best of its abilities to relieve pain and suffering. But it has not raised questions about its ultimate responsibility toward individuals and society.

The need for training of health care personnel to deal with dying patients, their relatives, and the problem of bereavement is obvious. Above all, training is needed to learn to understand death and face up to it when another human being is dying and in need of emotional support. The need is made more acute because the application of medical technology has prolonged the process of dying, making it more stressful for relatives and more expensive and troublesome for society at large. Should there be alternatives to the maximum prolongation of life? Euthanasia, of course, is one very controversial possibility that has been discussed repeatedly. Attempts to legalize euthanasia have been made in Great Britain and the United States, so far without success. Organizations have also been established that advocate giving an individual the choice of voluntarily ending his life when it has lost its value because of futile pain or suffering.

In our civilization, the medical profession is committed to maintaining life. It has never been and probably should never be asked to intentionally end a life. After all, the value of a man's existence cannot be judged by others. Who is to weigh the value of a few days of additional life? Who is to decide when the end should come? If direct euthanasia by active intervention is unacceptable, how about so-called indirect euthanasia by omitting treatment? We are all aware that this approach is often chosen by a tacit agreement between relatives and the physician.

Perhaps we should not consider euthanasia further but think more about the alternate option in which the patient with an incurable illness has a voice in determining the course of the last stage of his life. Should the patient have an opportunity to choose a dignified, peaceful death without exposure to the seemingly relentless application of medical technology? Can such an option be freely discussed with the patient? Who should take the initiative, the patient or the physician? Where should the patient be, at home or in a hospital? If alternatives to seemingly senseless prolongation of life should be made available, much more thought has to be given to this problem. But whoever is to decide will need a broader philosophical approach to life than most physicians have. Caring for the terminally ill is not a new problem. Wise and experienced physicians have handled this problem with compassion for years and some have written about it. What is new is the magnitude of the problem: Changing attitudes in interpersonal relationships; the transfer of death from the home to the hospital; and the exposure of the patient to impersonal technology rather than human compassion.

If the option of dignified death ever became freely available, changes in the attitudes and education of the medical profession would be an essential prerequisite. Our present attitudes generate resentment when a patient expresses the wish to enter the hospital on the condition that not too much should be done. Perhaps the hospital of the future should provide as an alternative a place where a patient can die a dignified death. This solution seems more realistic than to have a dying person occupy a bed in a modern hospital expensively equipped to treat curable diseases and establish difficult diagnoses.

Are we heading toward a culture where the patient can await death in specially designated facilities like those that have traditionally existed in China? Or should we adopt the tradition of the Eskimos whereby the elderly who consider themselves superfluous walk out in the cold to die? It seems unlikely that this is the future of terminal care in our civilization. But it may not be unrealistic to be prepared to offer the patient a choice of where and how he is to end his life.

We began this discussion by stressing the relationship between a patient with a fatal illness and his physician. In fact, we suggested that this relationship might even be considered a sacred trust. Yet can such a relationship realistically be established in our present society? Often the patients will meet physicians who are strangers to them as the end of life approaches; the majority of the population has no permanent physician, for reasons such as the mobility of our citizens, the consumer-oriented, fee-for-service approach to medical care, and the maldistribution between population density and physicians, to name a few.

We have not come to grips with the fundamental issues, which are philosophical, not technical. The question of who shall live cannot be answered. As long as we cherish our Judeo-Christian heritage and adhere to humanistic values we have to realize that the medical profession cannot change its mandate to maintain life, not to terminate it at will. If physicians and society cannot and should not decide who shall live and who shall die, how about the individual? Should the individual have the option to decide how to live and how to die? Should the individual's wish to die with dignity and in peace when life becomes an excessive burden be respected, and should such an end be facilitated by making fatal drugs easily available? Should such a decision by an incurably ill person be equated with suicide?

Is this a realistic option? Most of us cling to life, and the closer the end is the less likely it becomes that any individual born and raised in our society would choose to end his existence even if this choice were available.

It seems we have come full cycle. We listed as undesirable the meaningless prolongation of life and the excessive application of medical technology. We also came to the realization that most individuals will not choose elective death if the end of life is near. For the few who would choose early death above painful prolongation of life, the necessary meaningful relationship with a personal physician is rarely available.

Is this whole discussion an essay in futility or are there lessons to be learned?

What has to be done to lift the issue of death and terminal care out of its hiding place shrouded in mysticism? Physicians, other health care personnel, but above all, the public, need to be educated to face and try to understand the issues. Meanwhile, the medical profession can and should try to recapture some of the humanistic values of the past and apply them to the care of the sick to bring about a more harmonious balance between medical technology and the emotional needs of the sick, especially during that crucial period when they face the end of life.

Acknowledgment: The thoughts expressed in this general essay do not claim originality. Omission of a source, if it has occurred, is by accident, not by intention.

BIBLIOGRAPHY

Duff, S., and B. Hollingshead. *Sickness and Society.* New York: Harper & Row, 1968.

Feifel, H. (Editor). *The Meaning of Death.* New York: McGraw-Hill Book Co., 1965.

Fletcher, J. *Morals and Medicine.* Boston: Beacon Press, 1952.

Fletcher, J. *Situation Ethics.* Philadelphia: The Westminster Press, 1964.

Jaspers, K. *The Future of Mankind.* Chicago: The University of Chicago Press, 1958.

Kübler-Ross, E. *On Death and Dying.* London: The Macmillan Co., 1969.

Lister, J. "Voluntary Euthanasia." *New England Journal of Medicine, 280:*1225, 1969.

Platt, J. "What We Must Do." *Science, 166:*1115, 1969.

Schoenberg, B., A. C. Carr, D. Peretz, and A. H. Kutscher (Editors). *Loss and Grief: Psychological Management in Medical Practice.* New York: Columbia University Press, 1970.

Torrey, E. (Editor). *Ethical Issues in Medicine.* Boston: Little, Brown & Co., 1968.

Vaux, K. (Editor). *Who Shall Live?* Philadelphia: Fortress Press, 1970.

White, D. (Editor). *Dialogue in Medicine and Theology.* New York: Abingdon Press, 1967.

Winter, A. (Editor). *The Moment of Death: A Symposium.* Illinois: Charles C. Thomas, 1969.

Wolfle, D. "Dying With Dignity." *Science, 168:*1403, 1970.

Worcester, A. *The Care of the Aged, the Dying and the Dead.* 2nd Edition, Illinois: Charles C. Thomas, 1961.

Editorial: "When Do We Let the Patient Die?" *Annals of Internal Medicine, 68:*695, 1968.

Louis Lasagna

DYING AS A HUMAN EXPERIENCE

The problems of the dying patient offer a series of paradoxes. The approach of death has a hypnotic fascination for many people, yet its management has been grievously neglected by many whose concern it is. The modern scientific and technological knowledge applied to the medical needs of the seriously ill patient contrasts with the generally unsophisticated and unscientific use of psychosocial techniques. The traditional compassionate concern for the living patient contrasts with the unfeeling manner in which the patient's remains and effects are handled after death.

Most physicians, it has been said, assert that if they were terminally ill they would wish to be told. Yet, these same studies reveal that most doctors seem unwilling to grant their patients the same consideration.

Death can often be postponed to an extent barely conceivable a few decades ago, but man's last days are now likely to be spent in a lonely, mechanical, dehumanized atmosphere that is a far cry from the ambiance that obtained at a time when death was more likely to occur in the privacy and familiarity of one's home, surrounded by friends and family.

There are some reasonably formidable obstacles to ameliorating our management of the dying patient. Some of these apply to the physician, others to the patient and his family, and still others to the hospital or nursing home.

Many factors generate trouble for the physician as he tries to play a meaningful role in caring for the terminal patient. To begin with, many doctors are uncomfortable and ill at ease with terminally ill patients. Some physicians have been attracted to medicine because of the positive, dramatic things that they can do for their patients. They want to make their patients well; they want to have grateful, happy patients and grateful, happy relatives. Doctors are trained primarily for this active kind of therapeutic role, rather than for the supportive "holding" action that may be required in the case of a terminally ill patient. A doctor has often had little or no formal preparation for any of the problems that arise when a patient dies. There is little or no training even at the formal didactic level.

The contemporary physician generally does not seem to know his patients as well as some of his predecessors did. Perhaps this thought is only misplaced nostalgia. Maybe doctors have always been as busy as they are now. But so many things press on their time now, and there are so many technical feats to perform that they tend to be distracted from the interpersonal aspects of the practice of medicine. There is no intimate relationship with the patients' families today as there was decades ago. And as life has become more complicated the physician has tended to interact less and less well, more and more coolly, with other members of the hospital team, with the nurses, with the social workers, with the chaplain, and so forth. Communication lines seem to have become strung out to inordinate lengths. These, then, are a few of the things that affect the doctor. What about the patient?

Here too serious obstacles intervene: his fears about pain, death, and disfigurement; his anxieties about loneliness, about becoming helpless, about suffering a loss of dignity and a loss of control over his life and his relationships. These are compounded often by the patient's ignorance concerning just exactly what is wrong with him, and what the implications of his disease are. This ignorance is generated in part by his lack of medical background, but is also aggravated by the physician's unwillingness to take the time to discuss with him what is going on, and what the prognosis may be. (This, of course, applies no less to the acutely ill patient. Recently, in the course of a discussion relating to what nurses should be taught concerning drugs, a nursing supervisor said, "Well, one thing that might be helpful would be the kind of information that nurses should give patients when they leave the hospital. Often the house staff officer tells the patient, or the patient's family, that he is going to give the patient a prescription and that before he leaves someone should ask the nurse what it's all about.") Secrecy and downright prevarication surround the terminally ill patient and must contribute significantly to his uneasiness. The patient's religious feeling, or his lack of it, can work in different ways. Sometimes religion is the greatest boon available for such a patient, but at other times patients have acquired, as part of their religious upbringing, a concept of afterlife that provides no succor. It has been said that people who are deeply religious and those who are atheistic do the best when facing terminal illness, and that those in between are the worst off. But these are generalizations, and the role of religion and its potential benefit or harm should not be treated so glibly.

What of the friends and relatives of the sick patient? Here again there are fears, anxiety, sorrow, and separation to be coped with. Guilt surely looms large in the minds of some. Have they done everything that can be done? Do they really feel the love that they should for this individual as the terminal illness drags on with suffering that is not adequately relieved and expenses that mount to staggering proportions? How guilty do they feel about not having made more of their relationship with the patient when he was well? And they too have their hang-ups about disease and death.

Next, the institution and its deficiencies provide almost insurmountable obstacles. Hospitals tend not to face up to the problem of the dying person per se, except in some relatively trivial aspects such as constructing "critical lists" (which seem in most institutions to be generated primarily to handle the exigencies of visiting hours and special privileges for friends and relatives) or procedures for disposition of the corpse. At that level, the institution has rules, but it doesn't often concern itself with more important aspects. The people within an institution often fail to think of it as the sort of complex organismic whole with the concept of patients relating to each other, and the concept of an entity composed of doctors, nurses, chaplains, social workers, and so on.

Are there some principles concerning the approach to the dying patient upon which one could expect reasonable agreement? Is it possible to generate some unanimity of thought concerning any of them?

First, it is the eye of the beholder that determines whether one is terminally ill. If the patient looks upon himself as having a terminal illness, or the family looks upon the patient as having one, or the doctor regards him in that way, then for each of those individuals the problem of terminal illness obtains. On the other hand, there are patients or families or physicians who consciously or unconsciously, correctly or incorrectly, do not consider a specific patient's illness "terminal." In that case the implications for action are quite different. There are situations in which a patient is not terminally ill, but believes himself to be, and it is important for the physician to be aware of that fact.

Next, it would be desirable if the "taboo" aspects of death and the horror that is associated in the minds of many with the ending of life could be eliminated. With pediatric patients there are special worries with regard to their fears of separation and of mutilation, concepts that come up recurrently in discussions by pediatricians and psychiatrists about terminal illness in patients of that age group.

Most would agree that it would be desirable to diminish or alleviate the patient's feeling of being alone, of having no one to relate to, of being lost. I have a strong opinion that the physician ought not to lie in situations such as this any more than he should in his relationships with other patients. I have come to believe more and more that honesty is one of the few things in this world that is important. In any case, empirically one is often caught in the lie if one prevaricates. For example, some doctors say, "Well we'll tell it straight to the family but not to the patient." But relatives, people who love one another, have ways of communicating without saying anything. Messages are gotten across to someone you've lived with for a long time, and for whom you really care. There are all sorts of thoughts that are conveyed by the look of the mouth or the eyes or the way one walks.

There should, in general, be a working toward more lasting methods of handling anxiety than the denial that is so often the first response of the terminally ill patient to his disease. There may be people for whom denial all the way up to the end of life may be the most desirable approach, but, for many, such denial is less desirable than finding a way of coming to grips with the problem and accepting it in some way. Obviously, one has to distinguish between acceptance and despair. A move from denial to despair is a move in the wrong direction, but if we can help the patient move from denial to acceptance and a more positive attitude we are doing him a service.

The physician must be aware of a trap that he can fall into with any patient, but particularly with the terminally ill patient. The trap could be called misplaced concreteness. I refer to the over-precise diagnosis, and the over-precise prognosis. Doctors are not terribly good at making prognoses. They can sometimes predict pretty well the expected duration of life for someone who comes into the hospital just about dead, but there are many other situations where one is surprised either by how quickly a patient goes downhill or how long, contrariwise, he survives. This can be explained in all sorts of ways—the fundamental competence of the physician; his own know-how and experience; the state of the art at any particular moment in history; how much attention has been paid to the important physical and mental variables that affect prognosis; and the therapeutic modalities that are available at any moment in history. To a pharmacologist, it is always impressive to see the difficulties in tailoring drugs to the needs of specific patients, and the unpredictability of drug effects, good or bad, in many patients. Would that doctors could do better, but they often cannot be precise in their estimates as to what the impact of any given therapeutic modality will be.

An important variable in regard to prognosis lies within the psychology of the physician himself. The depressed, pessimistic physician is likely to have an approach to prognosis and the handling of patients different from that of the more optimistic kind of doctor. (This raises the question, as does the possibility of incompetence or lack of experience, of the desirability of having, more or less routinely, a second medical opinion.) There is also the sort of thing that could be called "corporate optimism," where an institution decides that it *can* do something to prolong life by assembling a kidney dialysis team, or by creating an intensive care unit, or by having a resuscitation team ready to move into action at any moment. This sort of facility can certainly affect prognosis.

How should one approach the problem of discussing a patient's diagnosis and prognosis with him? A former colleague once described this as a series of successive approximations, where one feeds a certain amount of information in a sort of probing way, looking for clues as to just how much the patient wants to know and how much further to proceed at that moment with the discussion. Most doctors feel very uneasy in handling this difficult situation, but this is an excellent way to do it, and a way that is both humane and scientific. To the extent that doctors don't know patients well they will not do this particular job well. There are hazards in terms of the doctor's own insecurity in disclosing the trouble to the family or patient, and the doctor must be aware lest he act in such a way as to make *himself* comfortable, rather than his patient or the patient's family. A lot of doctors avoid such discussions. One internist (who has been in practice for a long time) denies that he ever really had a patient who wanted to know when he was terminally ill. That statement is probably more a reflection on the doctor than on the wishes of his clientele.

It is uncontestable that we should alleviate symptoms whenever we can. Doctors can do a lot for pain or for insomnia. There are all sorts of pharmacologic and nonpharmacologic techniques that can be employed to make a patient more comfortable. There is no reason in the world why doctors should not take full advantage of their therapeutic riches. They must work actively at keeping up some sort of hope.

And then there are the problems that arise sometimes from premature publicity about scientific discoveries. Does it raise false hopes? And what is the matter with false hope? Provided that "false hope" does not dissuade people from seeking remedies that might in fact alter things for the better, there might be a lot to be said for having some sort of hope upon which to build and to help one survive. I often think that living is like a smoldering fire. You have to keep blowing on the embers to keep the fire going; when people don't work actively at living, they die. If this sounds mystical, think about the fact that we rarely know why anybody dies at a certain moment. If you ask the pathologist, the time arbiter, "Why did Mr. Smith die at 4:30 this morning?," he usually doesn't know. Students of this problem tell us that there are drops in the general mortality rate before religious holidays, or Christmas, or the World Series, or an election. Somehow some people manage to put off dying because there is something they want to see happen before they die.

It is well to reflect on the family's problems, both before death and after death. The family is going to be around after the patient goes, and we pay too little attention to how we should handle their concerns. In this regard, I remember a very intelligent and experienced resident once telling me that he was very surprised at what happened when he had told an elderly gentleman's family that the patient had terminal carcinoma. When the patient found out about this from them, he was upset because he felt that the family was not going to be able to handle the news very well, whereas he *did* feel able to handle it. The resident said, "You know, it never occurred to me that the patient should be the one to know and not the family."

Another question is that of continuity of care. This is a big problem in many aspects of medical practice, but in the care of the dying patient we have a particular responsibility to see to it that there is continuity of care, and that the patient isn't sloughed off from one person to another, moved from institution to institution, one ward to another, and so forth. He should feel that the people who look after him know what his disease is all about, what *he* is about, and what his family is about.

Then, finally, in this list of principles, doctors would all agree that anything they can do to diminish the dehumanization involved in handling things like autopsy permission would be a step in the right direction. They often display little compassion for relatives who are extremely vulnerable at that time.

What about specific challenges and research topics in this field? One important development is the idea that this area is a researchable one. Unfortunately, many physicians still feel that it is not a researchable area because there is something mysterious and "unscientific" and ungraspable about it all. It is easy to guess why this might be so. Students come into medicine because of an orientation toward "hard" science, and it's difficult to convince them of what Aristotle said: ". . . it is the mark of an educated man to look for precision in each class of things just as far as the nature of the subject admits. . . ." Freis and Williams put it another way some years ago: "A micrometer is not used to measure a football field." Young doctors particularly have to be impressed with the point that Fritz Machlup made about the study of economics some years ago, namely, that while you may not like the lack of precision in the field, and may wish that you were able to predict things with greater certainty, the fact is that every day in your life you are making decisions in regard to economics (and to sick patients) and you had better make the best decisions that you can.

It would be desirable to modify physicians' attitudes toward incurable diseases (especially "uninteresting" incurable diseases; there are some incurable diseases that rouse interest on the part of physicians and others that don't). Can we get the physician to look more carefully at his reactions to unattractive and ungrateful patients? Unfortunately, most physicians are not Christ-like, and it takes some doing for a doctor to continue to function well in a situation where the patients are demanding, complaining, and ungrateful because he is not achieving much for them. Then there is the patient who gets short shrift because his family is obnoxious, always pestering the doctor to do more, asking pointedly why the patient isn't more comfortable, and so on. A first step would be for the doctor to recognize the situations in which he ends up providing suboptimal care because of his emotional responses to these challenges.

Doctors should also search for better ways of informing patients about their illnesses, and better ways of preparing the family for eventualities. Another whole area where research is possible is in regard to the handling of the dead person. At present the corpse is often treated in a furtive, ghoulish manner, involving deception of other patients. Little attention is paid to those people who are left on the ward or in the adjoining rooms, people who have perhaps struck up a friendship with the patient prior to his death.

How could the work of all the members of the health team in the institution be optimized? What things should the nurse do? The priest? The patient's friend? His wife? His lover? His child? In certain situations the best person to discuss matters with the family will not be the doctor; it may be the nurse or the priest. A purposeful attack on these daily problems should yield important research gains.

Prejudices about such things as euthanasia and suicide must be reassessed. There is a sort of time-bound aspect to these problems, and attitudes toward them are likely to require change as time goes on. The advent of organ transplantation has made it critically important to pay attention to when life ends and when somebody can be pronounced "dead." Someone on the battlefield who throws himself on a grenade before it explodes, thus sacrificing his own life to save other people, or someone who dies in an attempt to save a person who is drowning might be branded heroic. Yet somebody who willingly wants to act as a donor, even if in so doing he terminated his own life might not be. These are sticky problems.

Can drugs such as LSD be used to produce a critical reassessment of the whole situation for the terminally ill patient? What can be done with such things as "total push" in achieving more peace of mind and more comfort? How effective are the various antidepressants and tranquilizers? Which are the best ones, and in what way do these pharmacologic agents interact with nonpharmacologic ways of handling anxiety and depression? With no preconceived notions as to whether drugs are better than nondrug maneuvers, I suspect that some patients will be prime candidates for pharmaceutical therapy and others will be prime candidates for psychotherapy.

One interesting phenomenon is the "critical list," and what hospitals are trying to accomplish by it. How good are doctors' guesses about the critical lists? Why are some patients put on it and others not? How many patients end up on the critical list who don't die, and, vice versa, how many patients are not put on it who do die?

Should there be some sort of terminal illness rounds in institutions? In talking to residents at teaching institutions, I have many times found them very defensive about this. They may tell you that when they make ordinary medical rounds they not only look at what the urinalysis showed or whether the serum alkaline phosphatase level was up or down, but that they also talk about the patient's psyche and how he's managing all his problems about his terminal illness. But by and large, the rounds tend to preoccupy themselves with all sorts of things other than those that concern us here. It is amazing to observe the patient who arrives on the ward critically ill with an undiagnosed illness. At the beginning of his hospital course he is often put close to the nurse's station. Then, as the days and the weeks roll on, the patient still remains seriously ill, still remains undiagnosed. The staff have gone through the diagnostic routines and have not come up with an answer. They begin to run out of things to do. As they begin to feel uncomfortable, uneasy, and incompetent, the patient gets moved farther and farther away from the nurse's station and ends up in a back room with the staff spending very little time going into the room.

In conclusion, there must be a distinction made between ascertainable facts and value judgments. Dwight Ingle published in *Perspectives in Biology and Medicine* (Spring, 1970) an article called "The Ethics of Biomedical Interventions." In it he stated that the principles of scientific inquiry are the best means of determining that which is and that which could be—that is, knowledge is necessary for morality—but these same principles of scientific inquiry do not suffice for determination of that which ought to be. So, there is always going to be room for individuality and concern for the person. As there is a time for sowing, so there is a time for reaping, a time for living and a time for dying. There is a time for drugs and a time for love and caring, a time for physiotherapy and a time for compassion and warmth. As I see it, the task of those of us who are interested in these problems is to combine science and art in the best proportions possible for each individual patient. Therein, I think, lies the challenge, and therein will lie the satisfaction.

Robert H. Moser

THE NEW ETHICS

We live in strange, disturbing, and wonderful times. The expanding intellectual achievements of this generation have begun to roll back the
vast rim of darkness and ignorance at a rate unprecedented in history.
We are witness to areas of human experience often wondrous yet often
terrifying, where no man of the past has ventured and of which few men
have even dreamed.

There can be no comparison of this age with any other. No one can
deny our enormous problems, our muddling, our frank blundering, our
mistakes, but we are beginning to see compassion emerge as a national
emotion. We are beginning to see concern for the welfare of molested
minorities develop on an international scale unprecedented in the history of this world. Today we are cheek-by-jowl with international
neighbors whose names were exotic entries in a Richard Halliburton
travel book in the days of our youth, or which did not exist at all. The

world has become too small; there is no place to hide from responsibility to our brother. We share each other's burden. And whether this country is embarked on a program of refractory political intransigence and economic suicide, or whether we are taking the first faltering steps toward an era of true brotherhood among men, will be the verdict of history. The stirrings may be feeble, and many of our impatient young are convinced they are too feeble. But the first stirrings of new life are always feeble, and no one has seemingly devised a technique as yet to accelerate the period of gestation.

Impressive progress has been made in social, political, economic, and scientific spheres. We have witnessed the bold intrusions by man into the unknown of near space; we have heard the scream of giant sonic aircraft as they leap continents in half a day. And we are attuned to the restless murmurings and militant shouts of forgotten peoples who have lived in socioeconomic eclipse since the first dawn.

But our immediate concern is the amazing leap forward in medical science. It is a truism that the incredible proliferation of knowledge in medicine has been breathtaking. Often it has outstripped our ability to collate it and apply it to patient care. Children still live in grinding squalor and suffer brain-damaging malnutrition in the shadow of great research centers. But the fact remains that we have approached a new plateau in our ability to diagnose and treat the diseases of man. Unfortunately, the machinery needed to apply it, on a broad, meaningful scale, often exceeds the capability of medicine alone. With our newfound tools we have new-found responsibility. As never before, physicians are obliged to remain current in medicine. Time must be taken to sort out what is important and valuable in the new information so that we may digest it and apply it to our patients. It is a difficult task. And as we shall see, there are occasions when many of us look upon our glistening arsenal of diagnostic and therapeutic weapons with some ambivalence; with a fleeting twinge of nostalgia for former days when things were more simple, when one could find legitimate refuge in ignorance or lack of a means with which to cope with some formidable, apparently hopeless clinical situation. But it is indeed a fleeting twinge. We thrive on the power of our new capability to defeat disease; what was formidable and hopeless yesterday may be curable today, if we have done our homework.

These thoughts lead directly to a consideration of the "new ethics"

—the new ethics of dying, if you will—a recent inheritance conferred upon us by the remarkable resuscitative innovations of modern medicine. The shifting, perhaps slightly tattered image of the physician in the public eye continues to evoke much thought and comment. When the tumult subsides, one thing will not have changed since the first aboriginal mother took her dying child to the village shaman: the status of the physician as life and death decisionmaker. Of his many roles, this role has always been the most difficult for the physician. And today it is even more agonizing. He faces a whole new constellation of philosophic dilemmas that would shake the equanimity of an Osler. How far to pursue the diagnosis? How long to continue treatment? How much energy to invest in the dying at the expense of the living?

How did we get into this situation? It began a long time ago, when we decided to become doctors. We fell heir to an ageless vendetta. To the physician, death is the enemy—the implacable ultimate foe—the symbol of failure, ever lurking in the wings, ever hovering near the critically ill patient. The missed diagnosis, the resistant microorganisms, the hidden malignancy, the irreversible degenerative lesion—all represent familiar catacombs. As physicians we accepted commitment to the lifelong conflict. Every instinct, drive and desire—every intellectual and emotional sinew has been trained to defeat death.

But there is now a new dimension. Our engineers and technologists have provided us with machines that have prodded and crowded Death onto a strange, unfamiliar terrain. The delicate yet definable border between life and death that existed in the past now has new, ill-defined interfaces with philosophy and ethics. We are denied a simple physiological endpoint for death. What morality applies in choosing live donors for organ transplantation? When is the donor of an unpaired organ dead? Must we designate some arbitrary waiting period before removing critical organs that are becoming ischemic? Is it a violation of Hippocratic ethic to dialyse or infuse mannitol into the patient dying from a head injury just to preserve his kidneys for graft purposes? Dare we remove vital organs from a patient who is not judged, by all criteria, to be totally and irrevocably dead? Who will make the decision? Just what is our obligation to potential donors and potential recipients, for example, the mother of three who just happens to be the most compatible donor for a fourth child with end-stage kidney disease?

The challenge is to define death in the modern context. Keep in mind that we have pacemakers to stimulate the heart that otherwise would remain an inert lump of muscle. We have positive pressure breathing devices to force oxygen into alveoli that otherwise would not accept oxygen and transmit it to blood. We have the capabilities to perform periodic hemo- and peritoneal dialysis to cleanse blood of impurities that otherwise would poison the patient when the kidneys fail. We can supply nutrients by veins, tube, and enterostomy to sustain life for prolonged periods.

So—when is the patient dead?

At a recent symposium (and recently there have been many as men wrestle with their consciences in this strange new arena), a learned physician-scholar attempted to provide "Rules for Death: In patients with irreversible brain trauma." The rules were: (a) bilateral fixed dilation of pupils; (b) complete absence of reflexes both natural and in response to pain; (c) complete absence of spontaneous respiration within minutes after mechanical respiration has been stopped; (d) failing blood pressure, necessitating increasing amounts of vasopressor drugs; (e) a flat encephalogram. Obviously, each of these criteria is vulnerable to attack. We have heard of rare patients with barbiturate intoxication who have flat EEGs for twenty hours, and then recover. One is reminded of the grisly cartoon which appeared during the recent cardiac transplant competition of the old fellow asleep on a Houston bus, wearing a sign which said, "I am only asleep."

So the debate continues. For the most part, some resolution has been forthcoming, and rational, albeit arbitrary guidelines have been established in most institutions involved in transplantation. But the issue is far from settled. There have been columns of prose, often elegant, but mostly tedious, in both medical and lay literature debating the role of clergyman, lawmaker, judge, and family members in the life-death decision, but as indicated earlier, the weight cannot be lifted from the sagging, often reluctant shoulders of the physician.

Each of us must derive his own personal philosophy in consonance with his own background, intellectual conviction, and emotional maturity. Each of us must decide alone what death is, and how far he is to go in prolonging survival.

I can only relate my own sentiments, not asking anyone to share them. For me, comfort and dignity in death are terribly important. Admittedly, the age of a patient is an incalculable fusion of chronology, psyche, and tissue senescence. It cannot be judged arbitrarily, but it is a factor in decisionmaking. It is not a violation of my personal ethic to permit the old dying patient in whom a diagnosis of incurable disease has long since been established to die without the pandemonium of futile, last-minute heroics in pain-free dignity.

With children, it is far more difficult. The leukemic children I have known, loved, labored with, wept over, and watched die, as I stood by in helpless anguish, will never cease to haunt me. There is an unfulfilled promise in youth. There is the mysterious, recuperative vitality of children. We cannot escape the taunting thought that someone somewhere may unlock the secret in the next few weeks or months. These are the factors that drive one to exhaust every rational therapeutic possibility to preserve that small life.

Nevertheless, in the presence of fatal disease, in the agonal hours, regardless of age, it is unspeakable cruelty to the patient, to the family, and to other patients who need your time, to prolong life by use of our new engines of brief survival. In the gray zones, those in between, there is no clear path. A tired platitude must be invoked: "Each case must be judged on its own merits." But in every instance, the responsible physician cannot stand aside; it is he who must make the ultimate decision.

This was impressed upon me many years ago. I happened to overhear (quite inadvertently) a fragment of a tragic telephone conversation. The speaker was the distraught mother of a little boy who had suffered a catastrophic, full-thickness burn. She was evidently aware of the hopeless prognosis. But she had been given the option of deciding whether resuscitative procedures should be continued. It was a chilling demonstration of the insecure physician "passing the buck." Here was a grieving mother in the extremity of her despair, being called upon to make a decision for which she was totally unprepared—from aspects of medical background and emotional stability. How many people have we thrust into similar, terrible crucibles of decision? How can they escape guilt, regardless of their decision? And what a cowardly defection by the physician.

The problem of organ transplantation presents an analogous situation. Needless anguish and agonizing ambivalence can be lifted from the shoulders of the family of the potential donor. They cannot be asked:

Can we stop the resuscitation and salvage the organs? This is a medical decision and, as has been indicated, it is not easy. Permission after the declaration of death is another matter.

To practice medicine in the 1970s is not easy. The contemporary physician is obliged to transcend mere mastery of conventional medical dogmas. Knowledge of pathology, physiology, diagnosis, therapeutics, and more, that sufficed in the past, more comfortable days, is not enough. Now we must come to grips with the psycho-social-spiritual aspects of human behavior as well. Our new technology, which almost seduced us away from the bedside with the wonderful new shiny toys in the laboratories, has come full cycle. We now have sophisticated therapeutic tools that enable us to prolong viability in the twilight zone between life and death for prolonged periods. So once again, we come face-to-face with the dying patient and his family but with a new set of ground rules.

The lonely decision as to when to turn off the symbolic switch rests with each of us. We who elected to assume responsibility for the sick must be prepared to accept our obligation to the dying.

Thomas P. Hackett and Ned H. Cassem

PATIENTS FACING SUDDEN CARDIAC DEATH*

Something is known of the manner in which a patient with a terminal illness adapts to the certainty of death. Less has been written about the emotional reactions of patients in acute medical emergencies when death is a strong possibility, but not a certainty. Although life-death crises are commonly seen in the practice of medicine, it is difficult to find a group of patients who face immediate death with sufficient awareness to appreciate what is happening to them or with the interest and energy to communicate their feelings to others. One exception is the cardiac emergency, especially the patient with myocardial infarction, for these patients are often alert enough to be cooperative. Furthermore, although in imminent danger of death, they have a reasonable chance of survival.

* This work was performed under contract PHS-43-67-1443 with the National Institutes of Health, Public Health Services, U.S. Department of Health, Education and Welfare.

Looking into the research possibilities offered by the cardiac patient, the investigators learned that these were diverse and stimulating. Four aspects of the work are discussed herein, each of which is connected directly with the threat of imminent death. These are: (a) the experience of being monitored; (b) the effect of witnessing cardiac arrest in another patient; (c) the effect of being the victim of arrest and being resuscitated; and, (d) the effect of being given Last Rites or the sacrament of the sick.

In 1958 the monitor pacemaker utilized in the intensive care wards had certain distracting features. To the observer, the most striking of these was its sound, an incessant, annoying peep similar to that of a newly hatched chick. Each patient was hooked up to such a machine. The front panel of the electrodyne monitor cardiac pacemaker contained an oscilloscope, across which an ECG tracing constantly moved. A red light blinked synchronously with the pulse and an audible "bleep" sounded with every heartbeat. Its function was to monitor the heart rate and provide an automatic electrical stimulus to the chest wall to prod the heart when it stopped or when its rate dropped beneath a certain level. Loose leads could also trigger off the alarm, and did so far more frequently than cardiac arrest. The alarm, in those days, was a klaxon, the sound of which galvanized the arrest team into action. It was perfectly possible for a drowsy patient to dislodge an electrode by turning over or shifting his weight, a mishap that would result in mayhem. Suddenly, his sleep would be shattered by a clanging bell and he would be jarred awake by a great jolt of electricity. Seconds later the bed would be surrounded by nurses and doctors ready to pound on his chest and to open it, should that be necessary. More than once the pounding commenced before the team noticed that the patient was alert and quite well except for a loose lead.

The investigators, disturbed by these facts, developed a vigorous set of objections to this form of treatment. The basic thought was that the noise along with the constant visual confrontation of the ECG, plus the continuous threat of gratuitous shocking, would serve to drive a large portion of the patient population into delirium or psychosis. Moreover, it was predicted that the instrument, even with its life-saving potential, would frighten some people to death. Nonetheless, the machine and patients furnished an ideal, almost laboratory setting in which to study life-and-death stress. The investigators set out to prove that the cardiologists were so caught up by the gadget they had created to pace the heart that they had lost sight of the heart's owner.

It was planned to interview and follow every patient who entered the Intensive Care Ward and was attached to a monitor cardiac pacemaker. In the course of twelve months nineteen cases were examined. Of the nineteen patients, selected solely because they required the monitor cardiac pacemaker, fourteen were males and five were females. They ranged in age from forty-six to eighty-two with a mean age of sixty-six and a median age of sixty-eight. They remained in the unit an average of 3.8 days and none died.

As the material began to accumulate it became evident that the investigators' original reservations regarding the machine were unfounded. Although 26 per cent of the sample were confused and intermittently delirious as had been expected, only one of the nineteen was frightened and complained spontaneously of being made nervous by the machine. The rest denied the presence of fear, apprehension, or depression in relation both to the pacemaker and to their heart trouble. In other words, only a single patient behaved in the predicted manner; the remainder denied being frightened. Some may have done so because they truly had no fear, but the others used denial as a defense.

For the purpose of this study, "denial" is defined as the conscious or unconscious, partial or total repudiation of the meaning of an illness in order to allay anxiety and to minimize emotional stress. The eighteen patients described as using denial by no means presented this defense in identical ways. Some rationalized their fears, others avoided talking or thinking of their health, while the remainder concentrated upon minor worries, such as hemorrhoids, in an attempt to displace the more serious condition from consciousness. Despite the variety of methods employed to deny, two distinct patterns emerged, distinguished by the degree of rigidity with which the patient maintained this defense. The term *Major Denial* is used to describe those patients who stated unequivocally and unremittingly that they experienced no anxiety as a result of their illness or during their time on the monitor pacemaker. Twelve major deniers (63 per cent) were found in this sample. The term *Partial Denial* applies to those patients who initially denied being frightened by their illness or the machinery of survival, but who eventually admitted concern. Six patients (32 per cent) comprised the partial denier group.

There are characteristics particular to each group. The major denier demonstrates a life-long pattern of minimizing danger and of under-reacting to threatening situations. He rarely consults physicians for even the most serious of illnesses and is staunchly fatalistic. Throughout the course of his experience on the pacemaker, he maintains a persistent indifference to his fate, denies experiencing the fear of dying, and disclaims ever having been afraid. All patients in this category were brought to the hospital unconscious or by others. No major deniers came spontaneously.

The cliché was a common method of renouncing danger. Typical of the major deniers' responses was the following. A fifty-two-year-old longshoreman was asked *why* the prospect of another cardiac arrest did not bother him. "Why worry?," he replied. "If the marker's got your name on it, you've got to buy it."

The following is a typical case history of a major denier. A sixty-three-year-old salesman entered the hospital in shock with an acute myocardial infarction. After recovering consciousness he maintained an air of friendly indifference to his disease. He was most cooperative in following orders and was well-liked by his physicians. At no time did he express the least concern about his future. When questioned specifically, he disclaimed any fear of the consequences of cardiac trouble because he was certain his heart was far better than the doctors let on. He also related that it was not his custom to worry; it never had been. His wife corroborated this story. He reminisced about a World War I experience in which his vessel had been torpedoed and he found himself alone, floating on a piece of flotsam in the South Atlantic. Asked if that worried him, he replied, "Why should it? After all, I was in one of the main shipping lanes and was bound to be picked up." He neglected to mention that shipping lanes are a hundred miles wide; that storms are rampant and are only one of the many hazards of the sea.

The partial denier often gave the same initial impression as the major denier. He might begin by disclaiming all fear, but its presence was revealed in subsequent statements. For example, one patient began saying, "I wasn't afraid because if I'm gonna go, there is nothing I can do about it. When my number's called, I'm gonna go; why panic?" This was followed by "You've got to be alarmed a little, but why go all to pieces?" A major denier would not have acknowledged the presence of any alarm.

Typical of the partial denier is the following account. An Irish matriarch of seventy-four was admitted for an episode of asystole which was followed by a myocardial infarction. When asked about the monitor pacemaker, she at first described it as "Indeed a gorgeous piece of furniture, like a console television." She emphatically denied any fear, just as she had in speaking of her cardiac illness in general. But as the interview progressed and she remembered waking in the night and peering at the luminous tracing of the ECG, she remarked, "Oh, I'd watch it flickerin' down and flarin' up, wonderin' withir it was pointing the way to heaven or hell for these ole bones, and it made me cold and shivery." Thus she gave a vivid description of fear without exactly putting a name on it.

In summary, what was learned in this study is that most people tend to deny the fear of death from serious illness and that they succeed, or at least they appear to succeed to a greater than lesser degree. Even the four patients who required painful external pacing to maintain their heart beat did not evidence more anxiety than the others nor did they develop chronic anxiety neurosis.

When that study was concluded and written up, it was felt that the results were not completely satisfactory. The series was small and the findings were provocative, but nothing more. And, there remained more questions than answers. The investigators wondered whether or not major denial existed in the general population in the same percentage (63 per cent) as was found in the CCU. Furthermore, the value of denial was questioned—whether it protected the individual physiologically, and, for that matter, whether it actually reduced fear. It was perfectly possible for a patient to be pretending fearlessness. The investigators accepted what was told to them at face value unless there were obvious discrepancies between affect and utterance. Although the patients' responses were consistent and were cross-checked with the closest relative, the internist, and at least one nurse involved in the case, there were no objective measures to support the investigators' impression.

In the following seven years, the technology of monitoring, pacing, and defibrillating advanced markedly and the concept of coronary care

units developed. In 1967 a re-evaluation of this earlier work, under better conditions and with far more patients, was made possible by a grant.
Fifty patients, ranging in age from thirty-seven to seventy-four (mean
age of fifty-eight), comprised the sample of the new patient population
studied. All had been admitted to the coronary care unit with the diagnosis of proven or suspected myocardial infarction. Thirty-five were
males and fifteen were females. Their average time in the coronary care
unit was four and eight-tenths days. Four died during the study. Patients were selected in a random fashion. The only criterion for inclusion in the study was the ability to speak English. The majority of these
patients were in a four-bed intensive care ward, which was cramped,
windowless, cheerless, and drab. The beds were separated by heavy, re-
tractable ceiling-to-floor curtains; there was no sound proofing. Sexes
were mixed. Monitors were placed on a wall shelf above and behind the
patient's bed. This made it difficult for the patient to observe his own
oscilloscope, but easy to see his neighbor's. Constant intravenous therapy was carried out on all patients, and most had indwelling urethral
catheters. Vital signs were taken hourly or more often, invariably awak-
ening each patient.

Cardiac Monitor

Twenty-six of the fifty patients questioned were reassured by the bedside presence of the monitor. Eighteen were neutral to its presence and
six disliked it. There was a trend indicating that women respond more
positively than men to the monitor's presence. Thirty-nine did not object to the monitor's sound (three found it comforting), and eleven considered it annoying. Fourteen wanted to watch their own electrocar-
diographic tracings and made an effort to do so even though it meant
twisting about uncomfortably to look over their shoulders. Three objected to seeing their oscilloscope patterns, and the remainder were neutral to it. Sixteen patients enjoyed watching the monitor of others; this
group included five patients who did not want to observe their own.
Nearly without exception they interpreted their neighbor's tracings as
being worse than their own. Men were far more interested than women

in watching the oscilloscope. There was no apparent correlation between the patient's knowledge of the monitor's purpose and his response to its sight, sound, or presence.

The alarm accidentally sounded for nineteen patients. The fact that only five of them admitted being frightened may be the result of previous explanations of the monitor's function and anticipation of the possibility of false alarm.

Witnessing Cardiac Arrest

Eleven of the fifty witnessed a fatal cardiac arrest. Seven of these denied fear either during or after the arrest; only three admitted fear. The initial response to watching the arrest was irritability and annoyance at the patient affected. This was rapidly followed by astonishment at the efficiency of the arrest team. All who witnessed the event described the activity with remarkable clarity. Sounds and imagination must have been involved because most accounts came through as if the bed curtain had not been drawn. For example, one patient "knew the doctor was massaging the heart." Another "knew they were opening the chest." In neither case was a thoracotomy performed, and the bed curtains were pulled shut in both.

One patient was reassured by the arrest drill because the victim was an elderly woman. He mused that if they did that much for her, they would go all out for him because he was so much younger. When asked if he worried more about himself after seeing the arrest he replied, "Oh, no. She was an old lady." Although empathy for the victim was expressed by all eleven, none identified with the patient affected.

One unobtrusive measure which was taken may mean that witnessing cardiac arrest is not as benign an experience as some patients describe. This has to do with room preference for readmission. Each patient was asked whether he would prefer private or semiprivate accommodations should he return to the hospital. All ward patients, with the exception of those who had witnessed an arrest, picked the four-bed ward as their choice. Those who had viewed the arrest preferred a private room.

Survival of Cardiac Arrest

Nine of the fifty had cardiac arrest. Three died without recovering consciousness, and six survived. Only two could remember anything about the event. A male patient vaguely recalled being thumped on the chest and hearing doctors' voices. The second, a woman, was unsure whether what she reported really happened or took place in a dream. "A funny experience . . . a hand down my throat squeezing my heart . . . I felt it happening . . . but I don't know if it happened in a dream."

Two patients had nightmares immediately after their arrests. The woman dreamed of smothering in a fire and the man of being caught trying to smoke cigarettes. The fire dreams have also been reported by Druss and Kornfeld. Two others had nightmares only after they returned home. One blamed sleeping medication for her bad dreams because they stopped when her bedtime barbiturate was discontinued. The other patient complained of "troubled dreams" that stopped once she returned to work. Traumatic neuroses with chronic anxiety and emotional invalidism have not developed in the three patients who are alive at the six month follow-up interval. Two have returned to work, whereas the third remains inactive because of physical disability. One of the two who died after leaving the hospital had signs of chronic anxiety and overdependency on his wife; the other man was emotionally stable until his death.

None of the six considered themselves unique as a result of having survived a period of heart stoppage. Two regarded their arrests as the equivalent of dying, but did not elaborate on this even when urged to do so by the investigator. None of the patients reported the Lazarus Syndrome.

Receiving Last Rites

Thirty patients, twenty-two men and eight women ranging in age from thirty to seventy-four were interviewed shortly after receiving this sacrament. There was no difference in mortality between this group and a comparison population who had not been given last rites. Twenty-three admitted anxiety openly or were rated as anxious by the investigator. Sixteen expressed thoughts referable to dying or death. At least four said they were sure they were going to die on the way to the emergency ward. Twenty-six of the thirty patients responded positively to last rites. Thirteen did not qualify their favorable response while thirteen admitted to experiencing anxieties or expressed some criticism of the procedure, but remained firm in their endorsement of it. Positive responders saw the procedure as something important and reassuring. For those who were ambivalently positive, the experience clearly had frightening aspects. The response of four patients was primarily anxious or negative.

The most threatening aspect of these rites had to do with the way in which they were presented. When the priest was calm and emphasized the routine nature of the sacrament, that it was administered to everyone with heart trouble, little protest occurred. Referring to it as the sacrament of the sick rather than last rites was also helpful.

Women patients seemed to respond more positively than men, and private patients more positively than ward patients. Those whose religion was important to them in premorbid life were the best responders.

The following is a humorous example of how the last rites shouldn't be done but how the patient managed to save the day, nonetheless.

A seventy-two-year-old boiler room worker, admitted with his first myocardial infarction, said, "The priest came in and told me 'I come in a rush,' he says, 'they just called me up and told me they got you in here, so I come in to anoint you.' Whaddya mean, I says, anoint me? Anoint me for what? He says, 'For death!' He says, 'We can't be too careful . . . because anybody with a heart attack can shuffle out in no time.' You know? . . . I laughed. We joked about it for a few minutes. He told me, 'Well, it's just a matter of form, we've got to anoint everybody with a heart condition—they're liable to die right away!' So he went through all the formalities and I bid him goodbye." The patient's wife said that he was "frightened when they anointed him," but the patient denied this. Both thought, however, that the priest's presentation could have been improved. Even so, they stressed that being anointed was the most important thing. Said the patient, "Everybody seriously sick should be anointed."

In summary, the data leads us to the conclusion that individuals who face the prospect of an imminent cardiac death seem able to adapt to it in a variety of ways, most of which are reasonably effective. Even the monitor is regarded as an ally, a "mechanical guardian angel." The patients seem able to extract the positive meanings from the most bleak circumstance and to enlarge upon them while ignoring or minimizing the truly lethal implications of their condition. Given one chance in ten to survive, most people grasp that one and somehow deny or negate the nine other possibilities.

Edward Henderson

THE APPROACH TO THE PATIENT WITH AN INCURABLE DISEASE

The quality of mercy is not strained
—WILLIAM SHAKESPEARE,
The Merchant of Venice

Set forth here is a derivative and evolutionary position concerning the emotional care of those adults or children who face death. Since there are no adequate controlled studies, and perhaps no cogent reasons for performing such, these conclusions are substantiated by the experiences and observations of affiliated professional personnel at the National Cancer Institute and by many reported observations both scientific and anecdotal which seem relevant to the crisis of impending death. The author's own experience has been limited mainly to patients suffering from acute leukemia. However, since this disease ranks so prominently among causes of death in childhood, approaches to the care of its victims should provide a suitable basis for discussion.

In what Fromme has described as the "dichotomy of living," no goal is more eagerly pursued than that of perpetuation of self. Nothing, therefore, is more threatening than the loss of self or the loss of one's self-image. Judging by the thirst for "immortality" even among those whose sophistication has accepted the possibility of finite existence, it must be assumed that of the two losses, loss of self-image is apparently the more critical. Accordingly, the paramount concern in caring for the doomed or dying must be the preservation of the integrity of the patient's concept of himself. At the same time, constructive modification of this concept should be allowed and encouraged so that it might be more consistent with reality.

In the treatment of patients with acute leukemia, therapists take justifiable pride in their ability to achieve and prolong remissions from the illness. During the periods of complete remission, patients are, by definition, physically able to function as entirely normal human beings. The corollary challenge is obvious: to convince the patient, his family, his friends, and society at large that for this period of physical well-being, the patient as a whole is normal.

The following are anecdotal case histories depicting certain instances in which this concept of total care has been circumscribed, and certain others, where it has been profitably and humanely adopted.

Patient 1, a forty-three-year-old diagnosed as having acute myelocytic leukemia, successfully treated with combination drug therapy in 1965, has continued without recurrence of disease to the present writing (1970). Because of the prognosis, and his morbidity during the first months of his therapy, he sold his business. For three and one-half years, despite excellent health and excellent recommendations, he was denied any permanent employment commensurate with his capabilities because of the stigma attached to the fact that he suffered from an incurable disease. During the last six months, he has become a real-estate broker, has prospered, and is no longer a burden to his family or community.

Patient 2, a twenty-three-year-old all-American football player drafted by a major professional team, developed acute myeloblastic leukemia. Following treatment, his leukemia remitted completely for a six months' period which encompassed the professional football season. Although he was in excellent physical condition during this time, and worked out daily with his team-mates, he was not allowed to play a minute of football during the professional season. He suffered a relapse and died two months after the play-offs.

Patient 3, an eight-year-old boy, was found to have acute lympho-cytic leukemia. Appropriate therapy rapidly resulted in a complete remis-sion. Despite his normal physical and laboratory status, his parents did not allow him to participate in gym or after-school activities. Because of the as yet unsubstantiated fear of horizontal transmission of the dis-ease he was rarely allowed to associate with the children in his neigh-borhood. Deterioration in the caliber of his school work was attributed to the effects of his disease and the prescribed drug therapy.

Patient 4, a twenty-year-old youth with acute lymphocytic leukemia, achieved numerous complete remissions with various drug therapies and ultimately died four years after diagnosis. During the period of post-di-agnosis survival, he completed three years of college and married a young woman who was fully cognizant of his diagnosis and its implica-tions. He remained productive and was able to enjoy life until one month before his death.

Patient 5, was a fifteen-year-old high school honor student at the time the diagnosis of acute myelocytic leukemia was made. The patient's course was one of multiple responses and multiple relapses. His death followed graduation with many honors, including the presidency of his high school student body.

The contrasts in these patients are obvious. In the first three cases, the patient's family, friends, and society in general were incapable of responding to the diagnosis of leukemia in other than a negative fash-ion. Rationalizing with coldly practical illogic, they succeeded only in diminishing the patient's enjoyment of and contributions to society. In the latter two cases, the patients were permitted and encouraged to lead as full and happy a life as their circumstances permitted. By this honest and humane approach to the illness, the lives of these patients, and those around them, were immeasurably enriched. Preservation of life and restoration of health without rehabilitation into society are certainly suboptional achievements.

The underlying principle of care of the Leukemia Service, National Cancer Institute, is that the patient should live as normally as possible, as much as possible, and for as long as possible. This does not mean, as some might interpret it, that the superficialities of normal existence should be preserved at any cost. Rather, it means that the person with leukemia shall have, as far as is possible, the same opportunities and the same burdens as he would have had free of the malignant disease. During periods of morbidity he should be relieved of his discomfort, as should any other person; during periods of well-being his personal integrity should not be unduly assaulted. Thus, he must be allowed to face both the anxiety of reality and the solace of hope.

People caring professionally and/or personally for the dying should provide as genuine an aspect as possible. What prevents them from doing so? The greatest impediments are the latent fears in all persons concerning death, fears that are heightened by the illness and death of others. This morbid involvement increases proportionally with the closeness and degree of identification between the care giver and the patient. Various postures are assumed with the patient: denial, oversolicitousness, hyperobjectivity, and more. These reflect an inner desire to be dissociated from the reality of death. Unfortunately, but predictably, such mechanisms are cruel reminders to the patient of his apartness from those around him. Faced with such rejecting albeit often well-intentioned responses, the patient is forced to develop defenses of his own, frequently in the form of denial or secondary gain, often to the further detriment of his emotional and physical well-being.

These difficulties and the reciprocating conflicts among patients, medical staff, relatives, and well-meaning friends are brought to the forefront the moment the diagnosis is established and the appropriate extent of disclosure to the patient of the true nature of his illness is raised. Since the diagnosis, and the prognosis which it implies, are of greater relevance to the patient than to anyone else, it seems hypocritical and presumptuous to deny him full disclosure of the facts concerning his illness. However, the diagnosis of a grave illness usually catches patient, parents, and physicians alike unprepared. Too often the problem of disclosure is hastily settled by an initial hedge without a satisfactory reconciliation. Therefore, from the start, the confidence among all concerned is undermined. This is a misfortune, since the diagnosis of leukemia can be revealed to patients of almost any age in a positive and, in many cases, reassuring manner. If the range of prognoses are clearly explained (and these inevitably provide some glimmer of hope), the patient will be in a position to construct his expectations according to the resources of his own character. If he then requires support and assistance, it can be provided in a rational and appropriate fashion, particularly if his care is conducted by those cognizant and sensitive to his constant needs. To the degree that such aid is not required, the patient retains a proportionately greater degree of autonomy and self-esteem.

Those patients, who are unable or unwilling to contemplate or understand their illness are deprived of even the illusion of normality during periods of remission and health by the establishment of unrealistic attitudes and activities. The relaxation of accustomed standards of behavior and duties presents an unwelcome aura of unreality, particularly in children. To be normal, if only for a moment, is the unspoken wish of the emotionally sound invalid. If this is all that physicians, parents, or friends are able to accomplish, the patient should never be denied even that small aspect of care.

In summary, those caring for the patient with an incurable illness should: (a) provide him with knowledge as to the reasonable expectations and limitations imposed by his disease; (b) help him thoroughly and thoughtfully to obtain the greatest possible rewards from his truncated existence; (c) maintain as much as possible an emotional and social environment consistent with his pre-diagnosis status; and (d) preserve his self-esteem and self-recognition for as long as his illness permits, both by allowing and requiring of him a role and voice in the decisions of his life.

Pediatric Care

Rudolf Toch

TOO YOUNG TO DIE

In 1967 nearly 109,000 children in the United States, under fourteen years of age, died of a great many causes. The leading causes of death under one year of age were "certain diseases of early infancy," congenital anomalies, infections, and accidents. Deaths in the one to four-year-old group were attributed mainly to accidents, infections, congenital anomalies, and cancer. In the five to fourteen-year-olds the primary causes were accidents, cancer, infections, and cardiovascular-renal diseases. That accidents loomed so large in all age groups is an eloquent social comment on the way we live. And then there are the 121 older children who committed suicide and the 700 children of all ages who were murdered. These statistics should teach us a great deal about future priorities, for the fight against death has too often resulted in the funding of research projects only remotely of benefit to those who need help most.

There has been an increasing amount of interest shown in the problems generated by a child's death. Most studies are psychologically or psychiatrically oriented and touch upon death only peripherally. However, a few deal specifically with the problems consequent to death. It is interesting, but by no means surprising, to note how difficult it is for investigators to maintain objectivity about such an emotion-laden subject. Particularly when the topic of children's concepts of death is discussed, the authors' biases often emerge more clearly than the subject. The present paper is based on impressions gained and interpretations made during twenty years of experience with dying children. As attending pediatricians we understood our task to be to support these children emotionally while treating them medically rather than to conduct research on their ego-structure, subconscious, and personality. This is not to say that such research is not needed but only that a dying child is rarely a suitable object of scientific study.

Every childhood death may be viewed as a classic tragedy with every member of the cast playing a well-defined role. We shall attempt to outline some of the leading roles in this dramatis personae without attempting to be comprehensive. One technique of exploring such a topic is when the reader tries to place himself in the subject's place. The hero's role in the tragedy is played by the child. We must take into account the age of the patient, since death means nothing to the infant, while thoughts of death may preoccupy the adolescent.

For simplicity's sake we shall divide childhood into three phases: from birth to age five, from six to ten, and from age ten through adolescence. We realize that this division is arbitrary since the grouping is neither fixed nor precise. The toddler and the young child view death as a natural phenomenon and rarely are aware of their own mortality. When such a child has a fatal illness, coping with his problem is relatively simple: He needs the loving care he has always known and he must not be subject to inappropriate changes in his management so that life may go on in as normal a fashion as possible under the circumstances. There is no need for explaining the future while making the present as happy and secure as possible. Children in this age group may occasionally announce that they will die but seem singularly unaffected by such a conviction. Only when there is parental reaction of grief and distress does the child realize that there is something to be feared. How children realize that they are dying we do not know; but we try to match their matter-of-fact acceptance and go on with our daily tasks. As far as is possible, these children should be cared for at home, even at the price of frequent visits to the office or clinic. When they do have to be admitted to the hospital we do not encourage rooming-in, which has become so popular with some pediatricians. We have found that its merits are outweighed by the disruption it causes in the lives of the other children in the family.

The child from six to ten has begun to think about death and may occasionally think about his own dying. He is not likely to associate any illness he may have with the prospect of dying and will rarely ask whether he might die from his illness. Rarely does he express fear of death unless some personal experience of death in the family has brought him face-to-face with the impact of death. He is more likely to ask many questions related to the disease itself, and it behooves the physician to be skillful in his answers. We see no need for forcing information upon a child that he does not specifically request. All children's questions must be answered truthfully. Using terms which may have a specific meaning only for the physician may create an entirely erroneous picture in the mind of the child. The axiom that it does not matter what one says but what one has been understood to have said is singularly applicable when talking to children. It is essential that one use terms that one can define and that one avoid words whose meaning one cannot control. We never use the words "cancer" or "leukemia" in speaking to a child because we do not know what these words mean to him. There are terms and circumlocutions with which one can get across what one wants to say and which open the way to further understanding, rather than using some word that defies explanation and may set off a train of thought in the child which may be very different from what one intended to convey. Talking to children about illness requires skill gained through thoughtfulness and experience. It is rarely necessary to give detailed explanations to young children. The important point to communicate is that one is willing to talk and to listen and, most importantly, that the child can trust the physician. If the physician does not have the answer to a child's question, he should never lie, but rather admit that he does not know the answer. There is a great deal of nonverbal communication between child and adult, and children form opinions from the way we act. No number of cheerful lies will convince a child that all is well when he sees nothing but the long faces of his attendants and the barely controlled tears of his parents. In this age group it is singularly important to control medical discussions within his hearing because imagination will begin where comprehension fails. Again, hospitalization must be kept to a minimum and normal life encouraged. Children ought to attend school and be allowed their accustomed activities whenever possible. It becomes necessary to consider what others should be told about the child's illness. We recommend that parents be reticent in discussing their child's illness with neighbors and friends. All too often people will mention the sad plight of little Joe who is dying of cancer, only to have one of the children present impart this nugget of knowledge to little Joe the next time he is angry at him.

The most difficult problems in the management of the dying child are presented by the ten-year-and-older age group. These children have learned a great many things from sources no longer under parental control and they ponder the future as well as the present. Dealing with them is, therefore, primarily a matter of attitude rather than an easily definable technique. What was said in the previous paragraph about communications with the child applies here with some additions. Teenage children will occasionally ask specific questions about their future but more often they resemble adults in not wanting to hear what they suspect to be true. There is no justification for forcing youngsters to accept the fact of their incurable illness or impending death. The building of trust and rapport are paramount in our efforts to help the patient through a difficult time. Honesty, within the limits described earlier, is essential, but again the physician must learn to detect the true meaning of a question. Only by having or making time for leisurely conversation with the child will it be possible to answer his real questions and allay his fears. And we must be sensitive to the problems that are important to the patient although they seem rather peripheral to us. The young girl facing a pneumonectomy for what she knows to be a malignant tumor still worries about the effect the surgery may have upon her breasts and the boy embarking upon radiation therapy of his pelvis for Ewing's tumor is concerned over the effect on his generative powers. Although the principle of keeping hospitalization to a minimum holds true, adolescents may more frequently require it since home care is often difficult because of their size and more complex needs. This raises the question of where such a child should be hospitalized. Should it be on a special ward or a general pediatric ward with a mixed population presenting the whole range of childhood illnesses? We tend to favor the general pediatric ward as best suited for these youngsters unless special needs are better met in an intensive care unit. Special wards are a convenience for the medical personnel but are most traumatic psychologically for the older child. These wards may help the parents, since it gives them a chance to share their sorrow with other parents of dying children, but the patient tends to identify with other patients and, unless an elaborate system of deception is practiced, he will draw often erroneous conclusions from this association.

In this age group we must also think about the influence of religion upon the patient. Most religious education includes a consideration of death, and it is important to integrate medical management with the religious background of the child. Close cooperation between physician and clergy is always of benefit to the patient and his parents. It is important to guard against the development of any basic conflict that may weaken the child's trust in either physician or clergyman.

The parents come next in our cast. Their needs must be met early and effectively if they are to become truly supporting members. They must not be expected to act as logical, objective, and detached players. Where age is the determining factor in the management of the patient, the cause of death defines our approach to parents. When death was sudden and accidental, we must do all we can to ease the burden of guilt that oppresses the parent who can not help but think what he might have done to contribute to the death or what he could have done to prevent it. There is little comfort in saying that it was meant to be and it is blasphemous to claim that it was God's will. All one can do is let the parent talk about his feelings and point out where the train of events was taken out of his hands. Often all one can do is point out that facts, however terrible, must be accepted but that one's obligations do not stop. Showing that the husband must support his wife and vice versa, and that both are needed by the remaining children, might turn their thoughts to more constructive paths. Help from religious advisors is often more effective than that from physicians, who must be willing to step aside or limit themselves to providing sedation and an opportunity to rest in a quiet spot.

The parent who must be told that his child has a fatal illness faces a different set of problems. Guilt is again the first conscious reaction after grief has been controlled. Although it is often impossible to absolve parents from guilt in accidents, only very rarely could they have contributed significantly to an illness. Whenever possible, they should be assured *before they ask* that the illness was not caused by anything they did or did not do, that it was not something caused by inherited factors, and that they did not cause any harm by delay that may have occurred in obtaining medical care. A brief explanation of the cause of the illness should follow, and then a concise discussion of what to expect of the future.

If death is inevitable it must be so stated, but under no circumstances should the physician give an estimate of probable length of life. Actuarial tables have no place in the discussion of a specific child's lifespan. Averages are of no help to a parent when *his* child's life is concerned. It cannot be stressed too strongly that much unhappiness is caused by letting parents expect a specific lifespan. It must be accepted as a basic rule that the lifespan not be mentioned but that the time be spent in helping the parents adjust to an indefinite and open-ended future. They must be helped to live with the knowledge that death will come at some future date but that for the present they must live in a way that makes every day the best possible day and tomorrow the best possible tomorrow. They must emphasize life and not anticipate death.

This brings us to the problem of how parents should be told about fatal illness. Experts differ in this but we hold that it is cruel to impart such news gradually. People can face and handle facts much better than they can cope with foreboding innuendoes and the train of imagination such innuendoes set in motion. The setting in which bad news is told is important. The corridor or the bedside is not the proper place. Every facility caring for children who might die must have some comfortably appointed room readily available where the physician may speak to the parents in privacy and where they may be left alone to regain their composure. An attendant should be available to call on them at intervals to offer coffee and to act as messenger and guide. Ideally, a social worker experienced in helping parents cope with death and all the attending formalities should be on call, but this is more easily accomplished when a child dies of an illness on the ward than when death occurs in the emergency room after an accident.

Depending upon the child's age, we must help the parents understand what makes for a happy life for the child, emphasizing the need for love and security without sacrificing discipline. Only too often the most delightful children will be stricken with a fatal illness and one can truthfully point out that what the parents have done so far must have been eminently right and that this is no time to change either attitudes or practices. A child's life should be as normal as possible for as long as possible. Parents should be advised to refrain from talking about the illness and from constantly asking the child how he feels. A goodly dash of Christian Science is most helpful at this time to avoid the constant references to illness which so annoy children. Depending upon the patient's age, we must advise the parent what to tell relatives and friends as discussed above. What to tell the patient will trouble the parent, so we advise the parent to admit ignorance to the child and to refer all such questions to the physician.

No discussion could be complete without mentioning financial arrangements, and here the services of an experienced social worker are essential. If at all possible, parents should be assured of the best care for their child, without concern about expenses.

This is also the time to mention hope, without which life is intolerable. It is just as important to warn against false hopes as it is to point out that therapy may arrest the disease or, when the disease is incurable, that medical research may yet find better ways of treating it. Parents must be warned against trying to become physicians by reading and believing all they see and hear concerning their child's illness, but at the same time they must be assigned a definite role on the team that cares for their child. Their job is the maintenance of a happy environment and a positive and hopeful outlook. Charging them with this specific task will help overcome the feelings of helplessness and frustration that flood parents when grief and guilt have been dealt with. After the initial discussion, parents require the assurance that they can ask the physician or other members of the team anything at any time and that they will get an honest answer, that the physician will not abandon their child's care when he no longer has any effective treatment to offer, and that medical assistance is never further from them than the nearest telephone.

Parents will need intensive help when the child is actually dying. Now the compassionate relationship established during the illness helps ease the acute distress. We must not forget that patients should be permitted to die with dignity and we can save parents from much grief if we remember to observe a few simple and thoughtful rules of true medical care. The patient's room should be kept neat, confusion should be kept to a minimum; there should be as little change in personnel as possible; and help should be available promptly and kindly. If the parent so desires, a child should be permitted to die at home, providing that prompt medical support can be made available. After death has occurred, parents who have been cared for in the manner suggested here will usually consent to post-mortem examinations and often offer their cooperation for donation of organs for research or transplants. Perhaps the last service that must be rendered to the parents is some advice on how to tell the other children about their sibling's death. A direct, factual approach is much the best. Euphemisms like, "He fell asleep and did not wake up," or "God took him," must not be used because children will often interpret them literally and henceforth fear sleep or resent God.

This leads us to a brief consideration of the siblings of the child with a fatal illness. They are not likely to react to their brother's illness with as much consideration as parents may expect. They may be deeply concerned and need a great deal of reassurance, but their egocentric natures will usually dominate their relationship with the ill child. The well children must not be punished or be made to feel guilty for being well. Their rights and needs must be of as much concern to the parents as those of the patient. This explains our disapproval of rooming-in, since this procedure causes the children left at home to worry not only about the disappearance of their brother but also that of a parent. We believe that the child in the hospital gets as much attention as he needs from staff and visitors while the children at home are left worrying and wondering. For this reason, we encourage parents to bring siblings with the patient to the clinic or office for visits so that they may know the people their brother talks about, what the place is like that their brother visits so often, and have some of their fears of the unknown allayed.

The medical team may be considered as one group of players. We emphasize that it has to be a team, since no fatal illness in childhood can be managed by any one physician. Experts in many subspecialties must work with the pediatrician. However, it is essential that one physician be in charge and responsible for coordination of all medical activities. Ideally, he should also be the source of all information imparted to patient and parent, thus avoiding that devastating unkindness—the sharing with the parents the differences of opinions between physicians or, even worse, making the parents the arbiters in such a dispute. Physicians who assume the responsibility for the care of fatally ill children need to have faced the fact of death in their own lives and should have arrived at some philosophy of life that will enable them to be sources of strength and comfort to patient and parent.

The primary physician should be concerned with the feelings of all other personnel involved in the child's care and should make it his duty to help the house staff, the nurses, and others to cope with the problem a dying child presents to them. Fortunately, the death of a child no longer occurs with such frequency as to permit hospital personnel to become hardened to it. Death represents the ultimate failure to those devoted to maintaining life, and adjustment to such failure has to be learned consciously. Mature physicians can be of great help to their younger colleagues by talking freely about their feelings and the way they learned to adjust to the fact of death.

The responsibilities of the physician go beyond his professional expertise and skill. He must make a firm commitment to care for the patient not only as long as his medical armamentarium provides him with weapons to fight the disease but also, literally, until death do them part. Abandoning a patient when one runs out of medicines is malpractice. It is also cruel, since the patient will wonder why he is ignored by the man whom he had learned to trust in and depend on. For this reason, clear lines of communication and responsibility should be established at the very beginning of the care of the patient and not left to be worked out in an *ad hoc* fashion as needs arise. Since the expert care will often be available only at some distance from the child's home, it is necessary to establish close cooperation between the child's immediate physician at home and the experts in the center of special knowledge. At no time must either parent or patient be left feeling that one doctor does not know what the other doctor is doing.

The practice of using the patient or parent to carry technical information from one physician to another is unkind and must be avoided. We find ourselves too often asking, "What did Dr. X say?," and then acting on the information imparted by a layman who is neither trained nor objective enough to relay such information. A special problem for the medical team is the foreign hospital physician who is unaccustomed to our ways. He may have a language barrier as well and yet still is expected to function smoothly in a most difficult situation. When a physician is aware of this problem, he may forestall any possible difficulties that may arise from cultural and linguistic differences.

Lastly, we must mention that rarely discussed task of the physician, his obligation to make some choice as to the mode and time of his patient's death. No one will argue with the statement that a physician must do everything in his power to maintain life as long as possible. This does not mean, however, that every mechanical or electronic device known to us should be used when death is inevitable. We have elected the following guide: As long as we have any means of combatting the primary disease with any hope of success, we will use every mode of therapy available to maintain life. However, when there is no therapeutic approach of any value left, we feel that we must let the patient die as peacefully and comfortably as possible. Be it infection or hemorrhage, cardiac or respiratory arrest, we will not use extreme measures to combat it, only to let the child die the next day from the same or from another cause. We have found that parents have been uniformly grateful for this policy of maintaining comfort and permitting death to occur when there is no hope left for control of the basic disease.

Nurses, social workers, laboratory technicians, dieticians, ward maids, aides, volunteers, cleaning and housekeeping personnel, school teachers, and secretaries all become involved in the death of a child. All too often they are forgotten and nobody bothers to interpret to them what has happened, or what is happening. Each has a job to do and would do it better if someone took the time to explain what the problem is and to find out how each is coping with the fact of the dying child. We suggest that the best person for this job is the physician and the time he spends will be amply repaid by the better cooperation from, and the more effective functioning of, his co-workers. Death affects us all and we need help in coping with it. This is not to say that all the people mentioned above are only an emotional liability. Their contribution to the care of the dying child is invaluable, particularly when it is founded on a sharing of information and knowledge. Senior nurses and social workers can often assume a role of coordinator for the paramedical aspects of the complex problems facing parent and child.

There are innumerable small and large issues to be resolved, decisions to be made, and advice to be given; often the social worker or the nurse will be more knowledgeable or experienced in these matters than the physician, who should gladly accept their help. There is no room for professional pride and illusions of omnipotence at the bedside of the dying child.

Before a member of a paramedical profession can become fully effective, he must be warned against the most serious pitfall in caring for patients, namely identification. We cannot stress enough how important it is for all to retain their professional objectivity and detachment without sacrificing their compassionate and devoted care. Only the person who remains detached can render truly effective service. Every team member must be able to leave the patient in the hospital when going off duty. There is nothing callous about going dancing and enjoying oneself while a child may be dying on the ward. Simple mental hygiene demands that one learn to keep professional and private lives clearly separated. Anything less leads to loss of objectivity and the end of one's effectiveness in the care of the patient.

Once the patient is cast as the tragic hero of the drama, the role of the evil antagonist falls to the fatal disease or accident. A few thoughts about the management of a fatal illness may not be amiss. The day is past when the propriety or advisability of treating a child with an incurable disease was questioned with the pseudo-thoughtful, "Why prolong his suffering?" Every physician is committed to bringing to his patient the best in medical or surgical therapy. We have noted that it is no longer within the capacity of any one physician to cope with the complexities of a fatal disease and that a team approach is mandatory if the patient is to receive the best treatment. The structure of the team depends upon many circumstances, but it should include the child's personal physician, the medical specialists, his parents, the nurses and social workers in the hospital or clinic, and all ancillary personnel necessary. One physician must assume leadership of the team and be willing to follow the child throughout his course. Medical differences must be resolved within the medical team and not shared with the parents, who are under sufficient stress without having to worry about medical problems. A plan of medical management must be evolved and every specialist on the team must refrain from unilateral action after a consensus has been achieved. Episodic and haphazard medical care by a relay of physicians and surgeons, each exhausting his own ability to help and then passing the child on to the next expert, until the child ends up in the hands of his personal physician, who must then preside over the actual dying, is still the rule and is to be deplored.

When it suits the patient and family, a child with a specific disease may be cared for in a hospital conducting research in that particular disease. Only through such research will progress be made, but the physicians conducting such research have the awesome responsibility to insure that the child never becomes an experimental subject and that the research design be oriented toward treating the patient rather than the disease. Fortunately, within the medical profession and governmental agencies keen interest in the matter of human experimentation serves as some measure of protection for the child unfortunate enough to be stricken by a disease that excites scientific interest. While efforts are directed toward the control of the illness, no limitations should be placed on the medical investment. Ways must be found to pay for the extreme effort for every single child who may benefit from such effort. However, once the available medical tools have been exhausted another concern must supervene: how to make the remaining days tolerable for the child and family. Exhaustive laboratory tests and surgical measures have no place in palliative and terminal care. The basic concern of the team must be the child's comfort, the allaying of fear, the minimum of life-supporting measures that will not interfere with death. We must know when we are licked and must be able to give in gracefully. There comes a time in every fatal illness when we must be able to say with Hans Zinsser, "Now is death merciful. . . ."

Surgical Care

Frederic P. Herter

A SURGEON LOOKS AT
TERMINAL ILLNESS

In considering terminal illness, the surgeon inevitably focuses on cancer and the many and difficult problems related to it, almost to the exclusion of other fatal diseases. Not only is the surgeon generally the central figure in the initial attack against and the subsequent palliative management of cancer, but also his experience suggests that no other form of chronic illness presents comparable degrees of anguish and suffering.

Until recently, the word "cancer" carried such terrifying implications that it was rarely used publicly. Despite the mitigating effects of educational campaigns directed to the laity, as well as notable advances in the surgical, radiological, and chemical treatment of the disease, the specter of a lingering and painful death has not been erased to any significant degree. But there is greater willingness to talk openly about malignancy, and wider recognition exists of the fact that cures are attainable. Yet the fears evoked by cancer are unmatched by those accompanying other forms of illness. These fears are shared by doctor and patient alike, and are thereby magnified. For the patient the diagnosis is all too often a death warrant; moreover, the approach to the inevitable end is poorly defined in terms of time and symptomatology. The vagaries of cancer biology are such that no informed physicians can ever with certainty outline a time schedule for a patient with apparently incurable disease. Nor can the appearance or sequence of symptoms be projected with accuracy. The patient can be sure of one thing only: If cure is impossible, suffering will inexorably follow.

For the physician, also, there are fears. Despite his experience with the mechanics of terminal illness and death itself, all too often he shares his patient's uncertainties about the meanings of these critical events, and he grows fearful of the awesome role which may be asked of him as healer, confidant, counselor, or spiritual mentor. He may often feel inadequate to the total needs of the dying; he identifies with his patient's fear of death, yet not unnaturally seeks escape from the anguish of self-examination which this identification calls for. It is little wonder that so many doctors try to divest themselves of involvement with cancer problems, or avoid, in self-defense, that candor so necessary to the establishment of important relationships with their fated patients.

Against this background, how can the surgeon's mandate be more clearly defined?

When the surgeon accepts the care of a cancer patient as his responsibility, he must do so with total commitment and with the realization that he will be playing a pivotal role in that individual's remaining life. If he is unwilling to accept this demanding charge, he should refer the patient elsewhere even before the initial steps of care are initiated. The extent of the necessary commitment is not always evident at first confrontation. The cancer may be small, well localized, and by all superficial evidence the prognosis may appear to be favorable. Envisioned is a simple confirmatory biopsy, followed by a straightforward excisional operation. Yet, every surgeon should know that no cancer can ever be considered cured on the operating table, that even under the most hopeful auspices metastases may have already taken place, and that years of careful observation will be necessary before the patient can be considered "in the clear." With some cancers (breast and melanoma are notable examples) recurrences may not manifest themselves for as long as ten to twenty years after the primary tumor has been removed. This patient is virtually never free of some anxiety—nor should the surgeon be.

When the disease presents itself in a more advanced state, when the prognosis is guarded or clearly hopeless from the first examination, or when subsequent studies or surgical explorations reveal incurability, the magnitude of the commitment becomes more readily apparent. The surgeon is faced with the dreaded reality that his function is assuming a different and vastly more disturbing dimension. No longer the healer, his scalpel useless, he cannot abdicate his primary responsibility but must continue to guide the over-all management of his patient, nonsurgical though it may be. He will possibly advise and call into play the skills of a radiotherapist or a medical chemotherapist. There may be a concerned and trusted family physician who can share the burden of day-by-day ministrations, or a responsible family ready to provide support. More often than not, however, the surgeon remains to the patient the principle embodiment of hope, and he must continue not only to coordinate therapeutic activity but also to maintain open lines of concerned communication with patient and family until the end.

Nowhere is the "art" of medicine more pertinent than in the physician's attempt to establish a meaningful relationship with his cancer patient. The fears investing cancer, alluded to above and shared alike by doctor and patient, are such that avoidance of true and candid communication about the nature of the disease and its consequences is both natural and commonplace. There are those who honestly believe that no good purpose is served by inflicting the bold truth on the patient; likewise, there are physicians who feel that the "truth" is the only effective antidote to fear and the only grounds for communication. The majority of doctors assume an intermediate or expectant posture, preferring to avoid direct discussion about the disease unless forced to by circumstance or by the persistent and urgent demands of the patient.

The author takes issue only with the extreme points of view. To consistently deny the patient the truth is indefensible. Similarly, an absolute insistence on candid disclosure in *all* cases betrays a woeful lack of perception on the part of the physician. So many and varied are the factors determining an individual's approach to death—education, religious convictions, social attitudes, family relationships and responsibilities, age, personal vanities—that to apply a single and inflexible equation for problems of so vital a nature is not only stupid but irresponsible. Surgeons have been heard to proclaim loudly that they have never confronted a patient who "couldn't take the truth." Such a statement betrays either a limited experience with cancer patients or a reluctance to examine the impact of that "truth" on the recipient. Equally damaging, on the other hand, is the attitude occasionally expressed that "no one *really* wants to know they have cancer, much less that they are going to die from it." Of course no one welcomes this sort of fateful disclosure. Yet, certain individuals *should* know the circumstances of their illness because of personal or public responsibility, and all persons should be granted the dignity of the truth if they so request it.

Regardless of the general attitude of the physician toward this question, certain guidelines, obvious in nature but frequently neglected, should always be heeded:

1. Whatever is told the patient with respect to diagnosis or prognosis should be predicated on as extensive a knowledge of that individual and the family involved as is possible. A premature commitment can be disastrous. Even before the diagnosis is established by biopsy, exploratory surgery, or other laboratory procedures, cancer should be included in the differential possibilities presented to the patient. To exclude it deliberately from discussion is to endanger trust, for few patients confront a surgeon without this fear being uppermost in their minds. The subject can be introduced in parallel with a number of less ominous diagnostic choices, and without particular emphasis, but it is surprising how often the casual, matter-of-fact verbalization of this dreaded subject can relieve tension and fortify confidence. Moreover, this form of preliminary probing can often give important information as to the particular areas of sensitivity. At least one member of the patient's family (hopefully the most responsible one) should be included in these initial discussions with the patient; information can also be gained as to the extent of support that can be anticipated from this source. Further communication with the family will almost always transpire in the absence of the patient at a later date, and attitudes may become more clearly defined. By the time, then, that the diagnosis of cancer is finally confirmed, the surgeon should be familiar enough with his patient's circumstances and emotional strengths to be able to make a wise decision regarding the necessary degree of disclosure.

2. It goes without saying that the best relationship attainable between

physician and patient is one that is based on honesty. It is the author's strong feeling that wherever possible candor should be employed in discussing the diagnosis. Nothing is more difficult than to project and implement a course of anti-cancer therapy without the understanding and confidence of the patient. We have all had experience with game-playing, and it is generally agreed that this is the most emotionally taxing activity in all of medicine. Some patients demand it—they do not ask questions, and their survival appears to depend on the avoidance of overt expressions of candor. It is almost as if their disease could be wished away by silence or the substitution of other diagnoses. The physician has no choice but to honor their desire for evasion and join the charade. The truth must never be forced on a reluctant recipient, and there are occasional instances in which it should be deliberately withheld; the majority of cancer patients, however, are best cared for in a framework of candor.

3. When such a course is chosen, the truth should rarely be so absolute as to eliminate hope. It is one thing to talk openly to the cancer patient about his diagnosis, another to discuss incurability or the finite limitations of his remaining life. Not only is accurate prognostication about survival difficult, if not impossible (we have all had experience with cancer patients in which our time estimates were wildly in error), but it is only infrequently that the question "How long have I got?" requires a literal answer. The element of hope is critical with most ordinary mortals, and it must be preserved even in obviously contradictory circumstances.

If the motivating principle guiding the surgeon's care of the incurable cancer victim is to relieve suffering (physical or emotional), thereby improving the "quality" of what life remains, then he must choose carefully among the various therapeutic options available, with sensitive concern to his patient's total needs. A price is exacted for most forms of medical palliation in terms of possible increased suffering or lengthened hospitalization. Surgery, radiotherapy, and chemotherapy all carry their own risks and disadvantages. It is not enough to advocate aggressive therapy "because there is nothing else to do." Each step in the care of the patient must be deliberately taken for a precise and justifiable reason, and with thoughtful balancing of possible gain as opposed to known losses. Such judgments require experience.

Clearly the state of the patient's disease is vital in determining the direction and extent of palliation. In most instances there is a time interval of variable length between the documentation of incurability and the terminal phase of the illness. It is during this period of "grace" that aggression is warranted. The patient has not yet suffered the systemic consequences of the disease, nutrition is still maintained, vital functions are unimpaired, and even major surgical procedures are feasible without undue risk. More importantly, the attitude of the patient is still one of optimism; he is receptive to, indeed eager for, any and all forms of suggested therapeutic activity.

The armamentarium of the surgeon for dealing with the manifestations of advancing cancer during this period is extensive. Cancers of the gastrointestinal tract often recur locally, with obstruction, requiring resections or simple bypass operations to restore intestinal continuity. Obstruction in the esophagus or at the gastroesophageal junction may require purely palliative procedures of great magnitude, entailing significant risk; yet such a risk is frequently justified by the abject misery accompanying the inability to eat or drink. Occasionally a recurrent lesion of the bowel will produce sufficient bleeding to make continuous hospitalization with periodic transfusion mandatory; such patients are candidates for laparotomy and excision, if the latter is feasible technically. Superficial lesions involving the integument, which may be ulcerated and infected, often require extensive excisional surgery because of pain, bleeding, or esthetically offensive characteristics. Pain severe enough to require narcotic control is a justifiable reason for surgical intervention. If resection of the responsible tumor is impossible, it may be necessary to call in the skills of a neurosurgeon, who through nerve block, section of the sensory tracts in the spinal cord, or even prefrontal lobotomy may be able to effect pain relief without concomitant loss of motor function.

Endocrine related tumors fall into a specialized category. Breast cancer metastatic to skin or bone responds in significant proportion to endocrine ablative surgery—oophorectomy, adrenalectomy, or hypophysectomy. Likewise, prostatic cancer invading pelvic structures or metastatic to bone will be benefited consistently by surgical castration. Occasionally, surgical techniques can be used to deliver chemotherapeutic agents in high concentration to isolated tumor-bearing areas of the body. The usefulness of regional perfusion for melanoma or sarcoma involving the extremities is well-recognized; continuous intra-arterial infusion of anti-cancer agents to specific metastatic sites is likewise of occasional benefit.

Nor are the therapeutic options open to the responsible physician limited to this wide spectrum of palliative surgical procedures. If specific indications for surgical intervention are not present, or if the tumor, because of its location or dissemination is not technically subject to surgical attack, either radiotherapy or chemotherapy may serve a useful function. Squamous carcinomas of the lung, esophagus, or skin respond occasionally in dramatic fashion to x-radiation; breast and cervical cancer, the most common forms of malignancy in females, likewise are radioresponsive in high percentage, and the patient may gain a long symptom-free interval from such therapy. For radioresistant cancers, or for those which are too widely seeded for effective radiotherapy, systemic chemical therapy may play an important role. Roughly 20 per cent of carcinomas arising in the large bowel undergo some degree of regression with antimetabolite (5-Fluorouracil) treatment; uterine and ovarian cancer frequently are benefited by therapy with alkylating agents. Indeed, most solid forms of cancer are reported to be chemically reactive on occasion to single or multiple combinations of chemicals. The use of estrogens, androgens, and adrenal corticosteroids has become an important adjunct in the treatment of advanced breast cancer; prostatic and ovarian cancer are likewise often responsive to hormone therapy.

Thus, there are numerous ways, both nonsurgical and surgical, in which active palliation can be offered the incurable patient. It should be re-emphasized, however, that such measures are applicable *only* in the advancing stage of the disease. There is a critical point beyond which aggressive therapy is not only dangerous but also entirely inappropriate. This point is generally recognizable; profound weakness, loss of appetite and weight, failure of one or more vital organ systems, together mark the beginning of the terminal phase of the illness. Therapy directed at the cancer itself is unavailing at this juncture. Chemotherapy or surgery may indeed hasten the march of events precipitously. Further hospitalization will be called for, and precious time at home with family shortened.

Despite these obvious considerations, "overtreatment" in the last stages of cancer is commonly observed; such thoughtless agression is an insult to intelligence and to the patient's dignity. Measures taken by the physicians in these last days must be directed solely toward physical comfort and emotional support. This does not imply abandonment—far from it. At no point in the patient's course of illness is more attention demanded, but qualitatively it is of a different sort. The doctor may feel impotent and awkward without a positive therapeutic program other than the titration of analgesic and tranquilizing medications; his natural inclination is to avoid more than cursory contact with his patient. No longer able to project hope with any conviction and forced into the position of having to utter patently false reassurances, his discomfort grows. This change oftentimes is perceptible to the patient. Honest and meaningful exchange ceases, and the patient finds himself frightened and very much alone.

It is clearly important (and a measure of the physician's sense of concern) that a communication lapse should *not* occur during this critical last period. The doctor's constancy as a friend and "listener" must be preserved. He must be ever sensitive to his patient's fears and loneliness, particularly if strong and sympathetic family support is not available; he must be available for questioning, hard though the questions are; and he must look and listen for particular needs of a personal nature. Even small and apparently trivial things assume an exaggerated importance at such a time; they must be recognized and met with concern. Skill and perception must be exercised in anticipating a perhaps unexpressed need for spiritual counsel from the clergy or emotional guidance from an experienced psychiatrist. Above all, the physician must remain aware of the vital role the patient's family can play as death approaches. If the home situation is a favorable one from the point of both physical and emotional support, every effort should be made to avoid or defer hospitalization as long as possible. The presence or absence of a concerned family physician can be the determinant factor in this regard. The patient must, however, be given the chance to enjoy the familiar comforts of his family life if it is at all feasible.

These thoughts are general in nature by intention, and express an attitude rather than a precise schedule of management. Details relating to therapy, important though they are, are of less consequence to the dying cancer patient than the humanity of his doctor. It is the quality of "caring" that above all makes the good cancer surgeon: If he can help his patients to cope with their fears, if he can help the "fighter" fight and withhold useless aggression from the resigned, if he can make life more meaningful for his patients while helping them to accept death as part of life, then he has served well.

Alfred S. Ketcham

A SURGEON'S APPROACH TO THE PATIENT WITH ADVANCED CANCER

There is little that is unique in the recommended surgical care of the patient who is dying of cancer. The indications for surgical intervention, whether of a minor or major degree, differ little from those which are indicated in the noncancer-bearing patient. The decision of most importance really is when and why one surgically intervenes in the care of the cancer patient rather than the relatively less important decision of how, or by whom this intervention is brought about. It is the surgeon, however, who most often assumes the prime responsibility of the therapeutic attempts at control of cancer and, therefore, he must be ready to direct the manner in which the terminal phases of life are monitored both from a clinical as well as a psychological standpoint.

Terminal Care

In view of the dismal attitude that too often prevails when the patient with cancer is being clinically appraised, it is mandatory that a very critical evaluation be made before a patient is deemed to be incurable and designated as requiring terminal care. When this latter categorization is made, the patient will usually receive either no specific cancer treatment or treatment which is less than conventional (curative). This, of course, usually leads to a nonrectifiable and irreversible clinical situation for which terminal care is the inevitable outcome.

The fears that many patients and physicians have of cancer may be, in part, justified in view of the known fact that approximately 350,000 Americans die each year of malignant disease. But this in no way should temper the clinician's judgment nor promote the pessimistic attitude with which the cancer patient is too often appraised both by his physician and his family.

The most common explanation offered by the patient for the fact that the tumor had grown to such a size before he brought it to the doctor's attention is, "Doctor, I was afraid it was cancer so I didn't dare come to see you." One of the more frequent explanations offered to the oncologist by the referring physician, at the time of the referral of a patient with cancer which had failed to respond to original treatment, is, "I decided to give the patient a trial on drug therapy, hoping that we could avoid the mutilation of surgery or the problems associated with therapy."

It must be emphasized that there are only two curative means of approaching most solid cancers, and the avoidance of using surgery and/or radiotherapy, whatever the explanation might be, only hastens the actual need for true terminal care. It is the experienced oncologist who is in the best position to weigh the potential curability of the patient versus the known morbidity and inevitable problems related to advancing disease in the face of which treatment has not been offered. An alarming but factual experience, which unfortunately is not unique, is told by the young surgeon who was attempting to establish himself in his medical community as an individual interested in the cancer patient. An allocated number of cancer beds in the University hospital really did not assist him in finding patients who were potentially curable, in that most patients who were referred to him were already hospital inpatients recovering from drug-induced toxicity. The remainder were being cared for in the subspecialty areas where categorical anatomical specialization made it impossible for the general surgeon to initiate his own aggressive therapeutic modality. This surgeon turned to two State hospitals where he screened all patients who were in residence with a diagnosis of cancer. After a clinical appraisal of many of these terminal care patients, twenty-eight appeared to have *in*adequate evidence of tumor-dissemination or *in*curability due to the local extent of tumor invasion. These patients were transferred to the University facility for further study. Twenty subsequently underwent surgical exploration; at the time of surgery, fourteen were found suitable for attempted curative surgical resection. Two years postoperatively, nine of these fourteen terminal care patients who had undergone aggressive therapy, were free not only of disease but also of the multitude of problems associated with terminal care.

It will be only through a program of intense patient and physician orientation that such situations can be avoided. As long as the community as a whole looks upon cancer as a disease which kills most people it attacks, they are only too willing to accept inadequate surgery or failure to undertake radiotherapy. The physician, similarly, must not allow prevailing attitudes, whether his own or those in his medical community, to interfere with known facts that are presently available concerning the therapeutic results of an aggressive approach to the cancer patient.

The Responsibility of Care

For one of many reasons, not the least being the acute shortage of physicians in most communities, few physicians willingly accept the burdensome responsibility of directing the medical care of the patient with incurable cancer. The internist's explanation is that it was not originally his patient and his schedule does not permit him to take another problem patient; the surgeon most often begs off, stating that he is too busy treating those whom he can offer an opportunity of cure; and the radiotherapist will suggest that he does not have the facilities for such patient care. Admittedly, it usually is not the specialist who is in a position to offer the best guidance in convalescent care. The patient and his family will more often find the consolation and needed medical guidance from their own family doctor. It is that physician who for many years has played an active role in the medical affairs of the family and established the rapport which is so necessary in avoiding the often-experienced, disagreeable misunderstandings that arise among uninformed family members. The family physician must, however, be able at any time to turn to the other members of the medical team for specialty guidance. Pain control must be monitored by the physician who best knows the patient and who can judge by visitation and experience the actual needs and hazards of narcotic assistance.

Many approaches fall within the realm of the surgeon's interest and abilities—the seldom-used but often dramatic pain-relieving procedure of nerve block or nerve transection; the care of the decubitus ulcer; the care of the urinary tract system; the hemostasis and debridement of the exophytic tumor; and the nutritional and respiratory support afforded through surgically-inserted intubation tubes. It is the surgeon who must be depended upon to play an active and cooperative role in these problems using the judgment afforded by experience to determine whether the effort is one of true palliation or an attempt at heroics.

Home or Hospital?

Seldom does the cancer-bearing patient find the same satisfying physical comfort, and particularly the emotional satisfaction, in the hospital environment that he does in his own home or the home of his loved ones. Assuming that the family situation allows "Grandpa to be brought home to die," home is generally where Grandpa wants to be regardless of whether it is where he gets the most astute medical care. Even if rehospitalization is intermittently necessary, the patient knows that every effort is being made toward discharging him back to his home, and his care is unquestionably facilitated by this motivation on the part of the patient toward discharge. The intermediate and sometimes most acceptable alternative to home care is the convalescent nursing facility where the economic stress of the illness might be lessened compared to the hospital. Unfortunately, the emotional impact on the patient differs little in such institutions from that of the hospital environment.

Many surgical problems (such as draining of abscesses and the treatment of elbow, buttocks, and heel bedsores, or the care of an ingrown toenail) can be handled at home. On the other hand, hospitalization will provide the best of facilities for the insertion of an esophygeal or gastric feeding tube. Unless the indications are of an emergency nature, seldom should a tracheostomy be inserted outside of the hospital environment. In addition, the breathing assistance which might be planned through the use of direct tracheal intubation can be better offered with the assistance of the anesthesia department in the hospital. While the usual abscess can be drained at home, the complications of bleeding which often ensue when a tumor abscess is unsuspectingly drained make it advisable that the hospital setting be used for such a procedure, just as this same environment provides the proper equipment and help for the care of emergencies of a major nature. It is at such times that the surgeon should take the initiative from the primary physician who has, until then, been directing the care at home. This does not mean, however, that medication orders and direct treatment should be carried on without the cooperative assistance of the referring family physician, who has come to know the patient's day-by-day problems, and who will again assume care soon after hospital discharge.

Pain Control

The use of narcotics to control discomfort, even in the immediate postoperative surgical period, should be directed by one physician who has taken the responsibility of prescribing the medication most suitable to control this particular patient's day-by-day complaints. It cannot be too often emphasized that few problems are more distressing to the patient or to the family than addiction to narcotics. Seldom is this problem necessary or advisable, if one physician has complete control of prescribed medications. It is the physician who has more often had the responsibility of caring for the cancer patient, even in the terminal episode, who tries to avoid the use of addicting medications until that time when the decision is made to use narcotics which he knows will inevitably promote the death of the patient. The addicted patient seldom dies of cancer per se but rather of pneumonia, malnutrition, or other natural courses of events that occur in the bedridden, sedated patient. The greatest innovation in medical care of the cancer patient has been the familiarity that all doctors now have with the tranquilizing agents—a familiarity which we must admit, in turn, has renewed our interest and appreciation of analgesics. Immediately following surgery on most areas of the body, comfort can be obtained through the temporary use of narcotics. However, in the cancer patient, such medication should ordinarily not be used unless it is agreed upon by the family physician. Otherwise, it is too easy for the excuse to be offered, "Well, it was started right after surgery and seemed to help the patient so much that we never really bothered to test its need."

Surgical Palliation

In most respects the surgical care of the patient with disease which has been deemed incurable differs little from that recommended for the patient who has been treated for cancer and apparently afforded a cure. The relief that may be obtained from intestinal obstruction can be as dramatic in the cancer patient as it is in the tumor-free patient. Similarly, the selected circumstance of offering surgical palliation by local tumor resection can, on occasion, be extremely dramatic in its immediate as well as its delayed palliative results. The unlimited aggressiveness of the therapist, whether it be surgeon or radiotherapist, must be exercised not only in the pretreatment and immediate post-treatment period of care but also, just as importantly, in the long-term management of the patient with anatomically and functionally disturbed mechanisms. The treatment of local recurrent disease, or a new primary lesion, must be as urgently and radically handled as if there were no significant past history of the presence of cancer.

This recommendation generally assumes that there is the potential for cure. The role that palliation or less than curative surgery plays in the treatment of the patient with locally-advanced disease, or with or without regional or distant metastases, is highly conjectural. The decision that the procedure would only be palliative in nature may well be based on the experienced judgment of the surgeon; this may be so especially when the preoperative workup has failed to demonstrate any evidence of tumor spread. It is the surgeon, generally most experienced in the treatment of the cancer patient, who is most reluctant to advise surgical intervention unless some hope for cure is anticipated. Among the possible exceptions are those few tumors which have demonstrated a remission or a stabilization of their growth pattern following removal of the primary cancer, or by the excision of the bulk of the tumor mass. Some of the ovarian and renal cancers possibly fall into this category. As previously mentioned, other exceptions might be such lesions as those causing intestinal obstruction, unremitting pain, or a malodorous, weeping, bleeding, exophytic growth which is readily accessible to scalpel excision. In these latter instances, no attempt at cancer palliation is intended, but immediate life-threatening situations can sometimes be relieved by relatively innocuous surgery and a very traumatic, painful problem which complicates the terminal episode can perhaps be avoided. This is in contrast to the lack of indications for surgical intervention when there is evidence of bilateral ureteral blockage or diffuse bilateral pulmonary inflammatory disease which can bring about the patient's death in a comparatively comfortable and atraumatic manner.

On occasion, electrocauterization, cryosurgery, or chemical debridement may prove to be a simple, inexpensive, comfortable means of relieving pain, bleeding, odor, and even tumor growth. Often such procedures can be carried out in an innocuous manner without taking significantly away, with days in the hospital, the patient's precious time with his family.

While attempts at the heroic management of the cancer patient who has been deemed incurable may seem at first glance to be indicated, it is infrequent that such procedures pay dividends. In the doctor's lounge of our cancer surgical unit there is posted a sign with the reminder, "Surgery which is not curative is seldom if ever palliative."

Who Should Know?

Seldom, if ever, is there a circumstance under which a patient should be treated for cancer without being aware of his primary problem. The patient who is so emotionally disturbed, or unstable enough to warrant consideration of operating in secrecy, is not really a suitable patient for surgery. The patient who responds most favorably to surgery is most often that patient who understands the problem that he faces and through the guidance of his medical and surgical team develops the desire and takes the necessary initiative in convalescence and rehabilitation. Similarly, it has been the experience of most surgeons that when primary or recurrent disease is to be approached from less than a curative standpoint it is the patient who understands the situation with which the physician is faced who best handles his subsequent medical problems. Nevertheless, it must be stated that uncompromisingly complete honesty with *all* patients may be unfair and irresponsible for some.

It should also be stated that there is no quicker way to lose the trust between doctor and patient than the patient's being highly suspicious that lies are being told. To lose trust in one's physician is the first step toward a rapid demise. It is apparent that what is told the patient is not nearly as important as *how* it is told. It is advisable to give the patient some hope which, in turn, allows him to grasp, realistically, at signs and symptoms that he will inevitably experience with his good and bad days. At the same time the surgeon need not place as much stress on problems which have a very unfavorable prognostic omen. The way in which the patient is handled should be one that does not, in any sense, allow him to lose confidence in his physician. Confidence is all too easily lost by the terminal patient, and the maintenance of rapport sometimes demands from the physician the greatest amount of patience and expertise.

While few children actually fear death, there appears to be little need to face the child or teenager with the total realization of failure to control his disease. Similarly, little is to be gained in overly frankly discussing a terminal situation with the elderly. If the patient is alert enough for the physician to consider having a frank discussion with him, then often it is not necessary because the insight and relative well-being of the patient generally afford him all the actual information that he wishes. Usually, a small amount of information will suffice, but if the patient desires a frank appraisal it depends upon the tact of the surgeon whether the discussion results in a patient who has "hopeful" pessimism or pessimistic solitude.

To be frankly dishonest with a coherent patient who specifically asks the question, "Is my cancer still in me and growing?," is a situation which must be individually handled depending upon the physician's familiarity with the patient. How encouraging it is to tell the patient that the tumor was removed and safely excised and now he must wait for the results of the pathology report to know how adequate was the excision. Seldom does the patient bother to ask any further questions, even though he knows that the pathology report was returned some days after the original discussion. An acceptable answer to the question as to whether ". . . all my cancer was removed?," is the hedging statement that this tumor was found to be one of those which experience has shown not to be best treated by surgery and that other means will be discussed while the patient is getting over the immediate effects of the operation. Such an explanation, in itself, will very often suffice for the patient who really doesn't want to know the actual truth.

To be evasive, or less than honest, with the mother who has school-age children, or the father who has family responsibilities, seems grossly unfair. Again, with the use of "hopeful" pessimism, there are kind ways in which to tell a patient that treatment was either unsuccessful or impractical. Yet, the physician must not hedge to the extent that the wage-bearing, responsible victim of cancer fails to realize or accept the fact that he may eventually die of his cancer. Often, he is the only individual who can do the appropriate long-range planning for his family. While such planning is not ideally undertaken under the stress of the knowledge that cancer still exists and is still growing in one's body, it is still better done then, at a time when the patient is coherent and is yet able to discuss and plan logically.

Certain further considerations come into play when the attentive husband frankly states that he does not want his wife told that she has cancer. If the patient remains for a long while in the hospital environment on a cancer service, she will soon be aware that her doctor has been less than honest and, as previously stated, this is the first step in the breakdown of the patient-doctor relationship as well as the husband-wife relationship, and also in the lack of confidence that the patient must have in herself relative to her ability to face and tolerate the medical problems associated with cancer. With the development of proper rapport between the family and physician, it is the family which often asks the doctor to assume the responsibility of telling the patient that there is a problem of serious importance. Ordinarily, the family is grateful that this is properly handled, because it is the family unit which has lived in fear that the secret will be discovered, with the result that the one they are trying to protect may come to actually feel a loss of kinship because of the prior dishonesty. Nearly every physician who has cared for terminal patients has a file of letters from family members telling of the wonderful days of love and togetherness they had while mother was dying because there was complete understanding between patient and family—that all were better able to handle the problems which presented themselves each day.

The doctor who takes it upon himself to be less than honest with the mentally alert cancer-bearing patient, who has family or financial responsibilities, is treading deeply in the realm of the Supreme Being. Although there is nothing sweeter to the ears of the physician than the words, "Thank you, Doctor, for curing me," or "Here I am Doc, it's been five years since you told my wife I was going to die," it can be almost as satisfying and heart-warming to hear the sincere and heartfelt expression of the patient, "Thank you, Doctor, for being honest and frank with me in telling me what I need to know, if I am to properly prepare for what lies ahead of me."

Other Medical Specialties

Morton M. Kligerman

A RADIOTHERAPIST'S VIEW OF THE MANAGEMENT OF THE CANCER PATIENT

The solution to the management of the cancer patient is to be found in the application of those principles which apply to the doctor-patient relationship in the treatment of any disease, independent of specialty. There cannot be an attitude which depends on a specific discipline. There can be various attitudes representing the philosophy of management of the many individuals who minister to all sick patients, not excluding the cancer patient.

Time must be taken during the initial consultation in such a way that the patient is convinced that he is the most important person at the interview. If other members of the family are in the room, they must be silent. The patient must feel confident that the physician is willing to listen as long as he, the patient, has something to say about his disease and his concerns. A thorough and unrushed examination must then follow. Although it is good medicine to make a drawing of any disease which can be so illustrated, measuring lesions and recording them in the patient's presence have the additional advantage of giving the patient a feeling of great care on the part of his physician. Time must be taken to explain to the patient the type of disease which may be present and the studies which are to be undertaken. It takes but a moment to tell the patient why the tests are being made and their importance in helping the doctor to reach a decision about his care. The patient is reassured if it is explained to him that the large battery of tests is not necessarily the result of the severity of his illness, but rather that much of medicine today deals with the exclusion of disease. Testing is one way to prove the absence of disease or, if disease is uncovered, the area which can be medically attacked.

It is best to have these conversations with the patient and his family at the same time. This gives all concerned the feeling that everything which has to be said is being said and that nothing remains for "back room" conversation. It has been found that 10 to 15 per cent of patients' families, however, do seek an additional interview with the doctor. Since, in certain groups of radiotherapy patients, a larger percentage can expect long-term survivals, it is not always that any different information need be given to the family in private. The first interview is not always the best one for full details to be given. During the first interview the patient and family are expectant and tense. The next day or the next visit is a much better time to explain more difficult matters. The patient should be told that he will probably have more questions to ask at the second visit, and that the physician will be available for additional exposition at that time.

What does one say and how does one answer the patient's questions? The first rule is that the physician must not be afraid of the patient's anger whether it be overt or turned inward in a depression. It goes without saying that the patient has the right to be angry or depressed and that the physician's role is to help him. There is nothing in clinical medicine that cannot be explained to the patient and family in lay language with simply defined medical terms. The exposition to the patient and family must be in these terms and must contain sufficient information for them to understand the disease. However, once the explanation is made and the patient and family present questions, it is best to answer the questions as briefly and simply as possible. Be certain that only the question asked is answered. A good attitude is similar to the one the parents have long found successful in answering young children's questions about sex. One doesn't go into the details of heterosexual love-making when the five-year-old asks where babies come from! While the patient must have a full explanation, choice of words is of utmost importance. Patients accept such words as "lumps," "bumps," "abnormal tissue," "new growth," "abnormal cells," and "tumor," far better than they accept the word "malignancy" or the worst word by far, "cancer." Furthermore, any word which is obviously distressing to the patient should be avoided. If the patient says directly "I know what I have, let's not use any hard words: we'll call it the thing, or the disease, or my problem," his directions should be followed.

This leads to the three sticklers as far as questions are concerned. They are one and the same question.

1. Is it malignant? (Is it cancer?)
2. What are my chances?
3. How long will my mother (father, son, daughter, brother, sister) live?

"Is it malignant?" By the time the patient asks this question, enough time should have been spent listening to him to understand how sensitive he might be to *the* word. If the physician feels that he can be direct, and especially if the outlook is good, he can simply say, "Yes, but this disease is highly manageable. Most patients do well. I see no reason why you should consider yourself different from most other patients with the same disease." If the patient appears less stable, he can be told "Well, what you have is like a malignancy (like a tumor; like a tumor with some abnormal cells) but this type of disease is usually well-managed in most patients. Why shouldn't you respond in the same way?"

"What are my chances?" There is usually only one honest way to handle this question. No one can say exactly what the individual patient's chances are. The physician can tell his patient that he can give him numbers—although he is rarely asked for them—about a whole population of individuals of the same age, sex, size, and similar genetic background suffering from the same disease in the same site and stage. But it should also be pointed out that such information is useful only for the attending physician or other consultants in deciding on which treatment is to be offered as the initial effort in the management of this particular disease. Other than that it should be explained that once the management decision is made it is 100 per cent for him because he is the most important person at that moment. Whatever happens to anyone else has nothing to do with him. He should, it is hoped, respond well to the treatment. If he fails to respond as expected, then successively alternate methods will be available to him. It is important to point out at this point that the management of his type of disease today is truly an interdisciplinary one and that successive methods are available not only across specialty lines but also within each specialty. When the patient directly asks if he is incurable—and if he is indeed incurable—he should be told the truth. However, he should also be told that there are many things to do to keep him operating at normal or near normal levels even though he has a disease from which his chances of dying are greater than dying from some other disease—which is also a possibility. Cancer is a chronic disease, and there are other chronic diseases—such as heart disease—which cause shorter patient survival than most cancers.

"How long will my mother (father, brother, sister, son, daughter) live?" This is the family's counterpart of question two. Although the explanation is similar to that above, it is often necessary to point out that this question indeed is a substitute for the real question in the minds of the family, namely, "When will my mother die?" This is an important take-off point in the re-education of both the family and the physician to the care of the patient. No one is interested in treating dead patients. If the family or physician considers the patient hopeless, the best will not be done for him.

To sustain the patient's confidence during his treatment and followup, there are several important DON'TS. First, don't blame symptoms on things not causing them. If the physician doesn't know and cannot find out by suitable examination and testing the cause for a symptom, he can make the decision that the symptom, although present, is not significant. The patient should be told that the cause of the symptom is unknown but that it is not considered an important one. Alternately, the patient can honestly be told that the symptom will be watched and re-examined at a later date to determine if serial examination elucidates the problem. Second, don't blame everything on cancer. Patients with cancer develop all of the acute and chronic diseases which patients without cancer develop. Blaming everything on cancer, and this is particularly likely to happen with those who see only a few cancer patients a year, immediately stops any activity to find out the real cause, which could be of significance. Third, don't turn a deaf ear to the repeated complaint of "pain." The patient may actually have pain and should be treated symptomatically for this. However, the cry of "pain" may be the patient's acceptable verbalization of his fear. Fourth, don't be fooled by the patient who wants the "little pill" when he really becomes bad. Few patients really want to die. Fifth, don't override the patient's denial of his disease.

Patients presenting with recurrence require the same handling as those presenting with the initial disease except that they are more uncertain about their outcome and require additional time and explanation. One helpful technique is that the interval of follow-up should be inversely proportional to the fear which the patient is expressing.

Referring physicians often commit the cardinal sin of telling the patient about the immediate and long-range harmful effects of radiotherapy. Such information, which is most often inaccurate, can interfere with the patient's acceptance of the very treatment he needs. It would be best to allow the patient to submit his concerns about radiotherapy to the radiotherapist. Usually these involve the length of time of the treatment, the manner in which it is to be given, and the consequences of the treatment. The room and the equipment that is to be used on the patient should be described or shown to the patient before he is given his first treatment.

In summary, the radiotherapist's relation to a patient with cancer is one which all patients have a right to have with any of their doctors, without regard to the disease being treated or the stage at which it is being treated.

Lester A. Bronheim

PSYCHOPHARMACOTHERAPY APPLIED TO DEATH-GRIEF SITUATIONS

Almost everyone can expect to face, in the course of a lifetime, the loss of a loved one by death. Yet because of a general cultural avoidance of this subject (from which the medical profession is not exempt), the requirements of persons facing death and grief have been largely neglected. This essay will emphasize the application of psychopharmacotherapy for meeting some of these needs.

No one expects a person facing imminent death or those close to him to behave as they would under ordinary circumstances. They are undergoing a severe derangement in the established pattern of their lives, a crisis. In response to this crisis one can expect such persons to experience, at minimum, fear and grief, appropriate and self-limiting reactions to a real and consciously recognized loss or anticipated loss. With the exception of sedatives, psychotherapeutic drugs would not be generally needed to counter such reactions.

But a crisis of this kind tends to activate underlying intrapsychic conflicts normally held in check—particularly in persons with inadequate emotional development. Thus, fear and grief often merge into anxiety and depression—reactions with symptoms similar to fear and grief but excessive to the triggering event and whose source is not consciously recognized. It is primarily to alleviate these conditions that psychopharmacotherapy is employed.

When selected and timed carefully, the use of psychotherapeutic drugs can be highly beneficial to the person undergoing anticipatory grief or mourning and to the dying patient also. By counteracting the self-absorbing tendencies of the person caught up in his own anxiety and depression, these drugs can: (a) release the patient to both give and receive the emotional support crucially needed by himself and other members of his family during this period; (b) permit the patient to work through the guilts and conflicts associated with bereavement and death and to begin to resolve the problem of how to continue life without the dead relative; and (c) enable the patient to continue his daily activity and carry out necessary functions. For the dying patient, this last may mean putting his business and family affairs in order; for the family, it may mean making funeral arrangements and settling the estate. Beyond this, preserving daily routine activity has a therapeutic value of its own for the bereaved. Having to get up, get dressed, get on with the job, etc., diverts depressive preoccupation and re-establishes the feeling of the continuity of life at a time when life seems, in a sense, to have stopped for him too.

How can the physician recognize anxiety and depression in persons enduring death or grief? He may observe any of the wide variety of symptoms usually associated with anxiety (irritability, jumpiness, diarrhea, cardiac palpitation, nausea, insomnia, or episodes of panic) or with depression (fatigue, lethargy, sleep and appetite disturbances, difficulty in concentration, psychomotor retardation, reduced libido, constipation, etc.). Moreover, although one may be prominent, anxiety and depression rarely occur alone. Anxiety can mask depression (1, 2), and depression can occur concomitant with anxiety.

But such symptoms, or a combination of them, still do not tell the physician when, or indeed whether, the transition from fear to anxiety and from grief to depression has occurred. What are the more specific ways that anxiety and depression present themselves in the death-grief situation?

One of the most common reactions is guilt. The dying patient may feel guilty over past hostile or aggressive wishes or actions which he feels are now too late to redress. He may feel guilt over being a burden to his family or over not leaving them as well provided for as he would wish. For the family, guilt may be activated by any ambivalent feeling toward the dying relative. If his illness is chronic and he has been a burden, the coming death may be anticipated with a sense of relief, causing guilt. Any real or imagined mistreatment of the dying person during life may cause guilt. A family member may feel he has been negligent with regard to the care given the patient and blame himself for the illness and the death. Such guilt feelings can extend to the mourning period and, if unresolved, further prolong and aggravate anxiety and depression.

Certain defensive reactions are seen in persons undergoing this kind of crisis, often in response to guilt feelings. Denial of impending death, even after clear evidence to the contrary has been presented, is a frequently seen reaction in both the dying patient and his family. Both family and patient may also exhibit regression to a less mature behavior due to dependency needs or repressed childhood fears of abandonment, or projection of guilt and anxiety to the physician or hospital staff as expressed in a resentful, overdemanding attitude with hints or accusations that the hospital has been negligent in treating the patient. Withdrawal and avoidance of the subject of death and of the dying patient himself are also seen (and the physician might watch himself for this attitude). Reaction formation may occur and reflect itself in an overly submissive or excessively courteous attitude toward the doctor and nurse—masking hostility or aggressiveness. An overly protective attitude toward the patient may reflect a form of compensation—a desperate attempt to make up for lost time or to redress past grievances and assuage guilt. Identification or introjection are common defenses in this situation, with members of the family taking on the deceased patient's symptoms and mannerisms. This most often occurs during bereavement but may begin during the period of terminal illness. During bereavement, depersonalization and sometimes dissociation may occur.

Such defenses, along with other general symptoms of anxiety and depression, tend to form patterns. For example, during the period of anticipatory grief initial denial may be followed by a period of self-blame and compensatory activity, which in turn may give way to reaction formation or projection of guilt to the physician or hospital, and then finally to resignation and depression. Such patterns and reactions vary enormously with individuals and are modified by age, religious and cultural background, and the underlying emotional stability of the people involved. In the case of the dying patient, his behavior will be altered by his deteriorating physical condition: his state of consciousness, degree of pain, and the effects of medication and other medical treatment.

Another symptom pattern in the bereaved is the aggravation or renewal of symptoms on each new reminder of the loss, such as the anniversary date of death. If defenses and guilts continue unresolved into the period of mourning, anxiety and depression can take their toll in more serious complication, both biological and psychological.

Substantial deterioration in health during the post-bereavement year was shown in 21 per cent and 32 per cent of unselected samples of widows in two cities (3). Another study showed a 10 per cent increase in the death rate among close relatives of deceased persons within a year after death as compared to the rate of a matched control group (4). Other studies have shown a greater incidence of cancer among the bereaved (5).

Studies of psychiatric morbidity reveal similar correlations. In a series of admissions studied in a psychiatric unit in England, ninety-four patients admitted in a two-year period developed their illness within six months of the death of a spouse or parent. Because the bereaved patient is expected to exhibit signs of fear and grief, and to some extent anxiety and depression, it can be easy for the physician to overlook the subtle changes which indicate the transition of grief to a more pathologic state. If he is alert to the possibility of such changes, he can be ready to initiate treatment, including psychotherapeutic medication, before complications become more serious and less amenable to treatment.

The bewildering variety of symptoms and the difficulty in judging when grief is merging into more serious complications pose a critical problem for the physician. When is he to intervene with medication?

Two basic criteria can be applied. Drugs should be given when there is a breakdown in life function and when the duration of symptoms is abnormally prolonged.

Any significant or prolonged breakdown in a bereaved person's routine eating, sleeping, personal hygiene, social, work, or family activity patterns should alert the physician. But this can mean different things at different times. For instance, if a man used to go bowling every week, and he has not returned to this activity during the four to six weeks of acute grief following bereavement, he would not necessarily be a candidate for drugs. However, if he has stopped shaving or going to work, or if six months or a year later he still hasn't resumed his bowling, drugs should definitely be considered.

In addition, psychotherapeutic drugs might be given on a short-term, emergency basis when symptoms become abnormally intense, as during episodes of panic or confusion which most often occur just after the bereavement and sometimes recur on the anniversary of the date of death.

Once the physician has decided that psychopharmacotherapy is needed, his next problem is to select the appropriate drug. A fairly wide choice is available.

Antianxiety Agents

Sedatives such as the barbiturates and bromides act as central nervous system depressants to directly diminish the hypothalamic functions, including the center for wakefulness. They are helpful in the management of insomnia and other sleep disturbances but are not useful as a general anxiolytic because they diminish psychomotor function and can interfere with understanding and cooperation. They should be used with caution in patients who are addiction- or suicide-prone.

Tranquilizers, in contrast to sedatives, which act in all parts of the brain including the cortical areas, act principally on the subcortical centers to produce mental relaxation and emotional calmness without sedation, hypnosis, or motor impairment.

The major tranquilizers, or neuroleptics, act at various subcortical sites but particularly on structures forming the limbic complex. They are effective in controlling symptoms of acutely and chronically disturbed psychotic patients. There is no evidence that habituation is associated with these tranquilizers. However, there is a relatively high incidence of side effects, including the extrapyramidal syndrome of rigidity, tremors, and drooling. Yet, at low enough doses to significantly reduce side effects, improvement may be due to placebo effects.

One of the first of these compounds to be used extensively is the rauwolfia group (which includes reserpine). It is less frequently used currently in favor of the phenothiazines (for example, chlorpromazine, thioridazine), butyrophenone derivatives (haloperidol), and the thioxanthenes—the most potent of which is thiothixene and all of which are more potent than the rauwolfia group. The phenothiazines are the largest group of major tranquilizers in use today.

These major tranquilizers would rarely be indicated for the majority of persons undergoing grief. The exception would be the person whose hold on reality and ego strength under normal circumstances is so fragile and tenuous that he would crumble under pressure, perhaps precipitating an acute psychosis (6). Otherwise, both their potency and high incidence of side effects indicate that the major tranquilizers be held in reserve.

The minor tranquilizers, or non-neuroleptics, act on comparatively fewer limbic areas than do the major tranquilizers. They are useful for relieving neurotic tension and anxiety rather than disturbed psychotic conditions, although they are also occasionally used as an adjunct to neuroleptic therapy. Side effects are less frequent and milder than with the major tranquilizers, and they do not produce the extrapyramidal syndrome. However, habituation, apathy, and euphoria are side effects associated with this class of drugs. The main groups of these compounds include the dial-carbonate group (for example, meprobamate), the diphenylmethane group (hydroxyzine, benactyzine), and chlordiazepoxide and such related compounds as diazepam and oxazepam. The latter group seems to be augmented indirectly by polysynaptic depression which releases muscular spasms.

These tranquilizers can be effective in relieving untoward tension, disabling anxiety, or panic states associated with anticipatory grief or bereavement. However, caution should be used with patients who show drowsiness or ataxia following medication, are addiction-prone, or who have a history of alcoholism, epilepsy, allergy, hepatic disorder, and blood dyscrasia.

Antidepressants

The psychomotor stimulants such as the amphetamines and methylphenidate combat fatigue and sedation effects, depress appetite, and elevate mood by direct central nervous system stimulation. They are used for mild psychic depression and can be effective as a temporary measure to allow depressed persons to continue with their life functions during the period of anticipatory grief and bereavement. However, chronic administration in large amounts or overdosage can produce hallucinatory psychotic episodes, paranoid delusions, and brain damage. (Some of these effects may be due to sleep deprivation rather than directly to the drug.) Also, while no true physiologic dependence occurs, these stimulants can be habituating and the physician should be aware of this possibility in patients who show increasing tension, weight loss, or paranoid ideation while on the medication.

The iminodibenzyl derivatives (imipramine, amitriptyline) are the principal pharmacological agents used in the treatment of psychotic depression and work by indirect stimulation. They act to elevate mood in patients with endogenous psychotic depression and usually show response within three to fourteen days from the onset of treatment. Effects on other kinds of depressive states are similar but it must not be forgotten that one must wait up to two weeks to see onset of improvement. Side effects are mild and tend to lessen after the first few weeks of treatment, or they can be controlled by adjusting the dose. These compounds might be selected for the bereaved patient whose grief has merged into profound or disabling depression of long duration.

Monoamine oxidase (MAO) inhibitors are psychic energizers which work bimodally by both direct and indirect stimulation. Both major groups, the hydrazines and the nonhydrazines, have nonspecific therapeutic effects and can produce euphorizing effects in nondepressed as well as depressed persons. However, their side effects are more frequent and more dangerous than those of the iminodibenzyl derivatives. Since they can potentiate a variety of drugs, including aspirin and alcohol, it is important to know what other drugs the patient is taking.

An MAO inhibitor and an iminodibenzyl derivative used in combination can lead to a syndrome characterized by restlessness, dizziness, tremulousness, muscle twitching, sweating, convulsions, hyperpyrexia, and sometimes death. This can also occur when an MAO inhibitor is replaced by an iminodibenzyl type of drug. Because of this possibility, a washout period of seven to ten days should be allowed before substitution is made, and a careful history of previous drug treatment should always be taken.

The problem of which specific type of antidepressant to use for a given patient is difficult since one type can be completely ineffective in a given patient, while another can produce dramatic improvement. Selection is thus on a highly individual basis; and the physician must be prepared to try more than one.

Combination Anxiolytics and Antidepressants

The problem of selecting the appropriate drug for a given patient is further complicated by the fact, mentioned previously, that anxiety and depression rarely occur alone. Tranquilizers and antidepressants are thus often used in combination and their separate effects as well as their possible reactions on one another must be considered.

A new class of psychotropic drugs, the dibenzoxepins, may prove to be of particular value for persons undergoing anticipatory grief or bereavement. The first of this new series to be made available commercially in the United States is doxepin HCl. This recently developed tricyclic substance combines in a single molecule both antidepressant and antianxiety activity, thus eliminating the problems of polypharmacy. Doxepin HCl has been found useful for psychoneurotic patients with prominent anxiety, prominent depression, coexisting anxiety and depression (including some types of psychotic depression), and anxiety associated with organic disease (7). The anxiolytic effect is usually evident within hours; the antidepressant effect may not be evident for three days to two weeks. Side effects are mild, even in the elderly, and often subside with continued therapy or reduction of dosage. The most frequently observed side effects have been drowsiness and anticholinergic effects. Less frequent side effects include the extrapyramidal syndrome (at high doses), hypotension, and tachycardia. No dependence and no euphoria have been reported to date. It is contraindicated in patients with glaucoma or urinary retention, and should not be used concomitantly or within two weeks of therapy with MAO inhibitors.

A study to determine the effectiveness of doxepin hydrochloride in persons undergoing anticipatory grief or bereavement is presently in the planning stages.

Dosage, for all of the psychotherapeutic agents mentioned, should be titrated up or down according to efficacy and side effects, keeping in mind that side effects often disappear with continued therapy. In the case of antidepressants, the dose should be regulated so that the patient is not overtired. Otherwise, the purpose of maintaining daily activity may be defeated.

As is true for all psychotropic drugs, there is no way to measure with precision just what drug a patient will need, when he will need it, and how much of it he will need. What the physician can do, and must do if he is to use these drugs to their optimum benefit, is to become a sensitive and astute observer of his patient. He can also utilize and encourage the observations of paramedical staff, such as nurses, who are in more frequent contact with the patient.

For all their beneficial effects, it should be kept in mind that one cannot cure by drugs alone. Emotional support, nutrition, medical treatment of any somatic effects—all these tools should be utilized. The busy physician should guard against the tendency to substitute drugs for emotional support. And he should be ready to refer the patient for psychiatric help when and if it becomes necessary.

When used as part of the total treatment of the total patient, psychopharmacotherapy can help the dying to face death and the living to go on with life.

REFERENCES

1. J. V. Verner, Jr., *Journal of the Florida Medical Association, 56:*15, January, 1969.

2. D. C. Friend, *Disorders of the Nervous System, 28:*29, 1967.

3. D. Maddison, *Archives of the Foundation of Thanatology, 2:*11, April, 1970.

4. B. Schoenberg, A. C. Carr, D. Peretz, A. H. Kutscher (Editors), *Loss and Grief: Psychological Management in Medical Practice,* New York: Columbia University Press, 1970.

5. *Ibid.*

6. C. M. Parkcs, "Recent Bereavement as a Cause of Mental Illness," *British Journal of Psychiatry, 110:*198, 1964.

7. N. Pitts, "The Clinical Evaluation of Doxepin—A New Psychotherapeutic Agent," *Psychosomatics, 10:*164, May–June, 1969.

Robert Kastenbaum

WHILE THE OLD MAN DIES: OUR CONFLICTING ATTITUDES TOWARD THE ELDERLY

What intentions do we have toward the dying elder? What do we expect of him and of ourselves? What do we fear? And how do these fears, expectations, and intentions co-exist with our general orientation toward life and death?

"Natural Death" in Old Age

"It is natural for old people to die."

This theme and its variations are frequently voiced by laymen, by professionals in the health and human sciences, and by personnel who work directly with geriatric patients. But what is really being said?

"Death is natural for the old. The more that I can persuade you (and the more you can persuade me) that death is natural for the old, then the more I can protect myself from facing the thought that death might be natural for the young.

"Let's face it, there is something reassuring about the death of an old person. It sort of makes me feel that the world is running the way it's supposed to. . . . The old person himself? Well, death is all right with him too. He has lived long enough. Too long, probably. Anyhow, chances are he doesn't realize what is happening to him, doesn't have that much awareness left. Frankly, I'd never want to get that old myself. I'd rather kick off first. . . . It's a blessing to be relieved of the misery and use-lessness of old age. . . . It is only natural for the old person to die. We should try to keep him comfortable and all that, but it is not realistic and not proper to make a big thing of his demise. Besides, we have only so much available in the way of economic and medical resources. We have to make some hard choices. Don't think I'm unsympathetic, but there are better uses for our money, energy, and skills."

Commentary

There are at least two senses in which the association of "natural death" with old age can be made legitimately. In a generalized statistical sense, it is "natural" for people to die, and those who do not die when younger will indeed perish some day. Furthermore, since more people are surviving into the retirement years than ever before, there are more deaths than ever before in the older age groups. Second, the death of an old person may strike us as natural in that *we* are not taken by surprise. *We* do not feel so shocked and upset. Our own freedom from deep disturbance is easily enough translated into the outer projection that the death itself was "natural."

Usually, however, we seem to mean something more by our assumption that it is natural for the old to die. But it is difficult to maintain the distinction between a "natural" and an "unnatural" death with any consistency. And it is far from self-evident that we could even obtain a consensus as to what constitutes a "natural" death in the first place.

Most popular, perhaps, is the implication that a "natural" death is one that is untainted by human hands (as in "unnatural" deaths by suicide or murder). But students of life-threatening behaviors propose, with plausible rationale, that *all* deaths involve some contribution from psychosocial factors (1). The distinction also assumes that the observer is in a position to know all the relevant facts leading up to the death—a condition which is rarely, if ever, satisfied. Even so, one could advance quite the opposite argument: suicide, murder (and such related fatalities as semi-arranged accidents, chronic self-injurious behavior, failure to seek medical treatment, etc.) are themselves quite "natural" in that many people engage in these behaviors every day; many "natural" conditions of human life seem to lead "naturally" to these outcomes; and regardless of the particular admixture of preterminal events, the terminal process and the death itself may be identical (for example, cardiovascular collapse from either intentional, self-accidental, or iatrogenetic administration of drugs).

There are other dimensions which might be introduced to distinguish between "natural" and "unnatural" deaths. But in this brief treatment of the subject we will offer only the position that the distinction is a vestigial one. It now masks and confuses more than it elucidates. As generally employed, the "natural" death viewpoint consists largely of a vague reference to metaphysical, moral, or theological intangibles. This is objectionable, for it introduces into the discussion a sense of authority and finality that has been merely assumed, not achieved. If one really means to imply that some deaths are "good," or "acceptable," while others are "bad," or "improper," then it would clarify communication to present these value judgments precisely as such.

The Old Must Die

From the view that it is "natural" for the aged to die, it is not difficult to "conclude" that they *ought* to die. Eavesdrop a bit on this conversation:

Industrialist: "Die they must, to make room for younger workers. With increasing automation and the everpresent threat of peace, it will be tougher and tougher to hold unemployment down, especially now that some of them are starting compulsory retirement. Just between us, I am concerned about older workers because they tend to know *too much,* and I don't fancy the size of the pension payments we will face if they persist in living for years after retirement."

Economist: "What disturbs me is the low productivity *and* low purchasing power of the the aged. Definitely a drag on the economy."

Conservationist: "We are faced with the most crucial problem that the human race has ever encountered—overpopulation—and there are all those old people using up valuable resources. Breathing, occupying space, they persist in living their unnecessary lives while we are trying to trim the birth rate. It is not enough to *prevent* birth—the prevention should be made retroactive after age, well, what do you say . . . 70? 65? 60? Die they must!"

Sociologist: "And who would miss them? Hardly anybody, according to our observations" (2).

Commentary

Admittedly, such conversations are not yet commonplace, but we would be victims of a sort of collective tunnel vision if we failed to recognize that certain major trends in our society are increasing the lethal pressures on the already low-valued aged. As just one example, the concern for overpopulation could hardly be greater in some informed quarters. It is certainly not an issue to be minimized or lightly dismissed. Is it absurd to suppose that one of these days panic-level concern about overpopulation and its impact, a background of extreme social tension, fear, and disorganization, *and* our mental preparation to accept the death of old people as "natural" (and, by implication, desirable) may bring about a new kind of "final solution"?

In this discussion we have not even mentioned more personal kinds of lethal sentiments toward the aged. As individuals we may at times desire the removal, disengagement, emasculation, or death of those older than ourselves—specific people who get in the way of our comfort or ambitions. Any student of psychodynamics could develop this picture in probing detail. How many vulnerable aged patients, residents, clients, have been the recipients of hostility that was displaced from the "helping person's" own child-parent problems?

The Beginning of the End

Up to this point we have been considering some of the attitudes which can confuse our intentions and perceptions. Now let us focus upon the main arena of action: the final environment (3). The concept of terminal care obviously requires an act of judgment or classification. Either explicitly or implicitly, we judge that a particular person has now taken on the status of a dying patient. Much of our subsequent behavior, as individuals, and as a system of individuals, is contingent upon this judgment. We tend to adopt a special set of thoughts, feelings, and behaviors when we believe ourselves to be in the presence of a dying person, or within a final environment (4).

Errors in attributing the preterminal status to a person can be made at any age level. There are also differences in the readiness to ascribe the dying status to a person which cannot easily be described as errors. Often it is difficult to determine the degree of jeopardy with which a person is confronted. The situation can be complex enough to make a variety of judgments seem more or less plausible. Since our orientation seems to depend so much upon the judgment that a person either is or is not preterminal, it is very pertinent to touch upon this judgmental process as it reveals itself in geriatrics. We will recognize some by now familiar attitudes at work in ways that can make a critical difference in the fate of aged men and women.

Consider a few recent empirical studies. Markson and Hand (5) have documented the existence of a pattern that has been suspected by a number of gerontologists. They have found that many elderly people who were admitted to a large state psychiatric facility should have been regarded as "dying" rather than "mentally ill" patients. This was especially true in the case of elders with a lower socioeconomic class background. As Markson and Hand comment, "The mental hospital . . . has no facilities truly appropriate to the care of the dying. Yet it is often used as a terminal facility, to which the old are referred because there is no place else for them to go or because there is insufficient knowledge or interest on the part of the referring agents to seek more appropriate treatment facilities."

Another study concentrated upon the most impaired patients in an all-geriatric hospital. These immobile and apparently unresponsive patients manifested such a low level behavior syndrome that ward staff tended to treat them as though they were already dead. Yet a simple "reach-out" procedure included for research purposes demonstrated that approximately half of these "living dead" were in fact capable of sentient experience and response (6). This finding was consistent with a previous study at the same facility which indicated that the great majority of preterminal geriatric patients did retain sufficient mental status to appreciate their condition (7).

Still another research team learned that more than 70 per cent of those who commit suicide in certain populations had consulted a physician within three months of their death—and almost 50 per cent had seen their physicians within a month or less of the fatal act (8). And an observational study of geriatric medical patients has suggested that a high percentage of such men and women can be seen to engage in self-injurious behavior. "Serious questions about the quality of the lives of those individuals must be raised when the incidence of self-injurious behavior is 43 per cent for men and 21 per cent for women in a one-week period. Multiplying this frequency by the many weeks which make up the many years of residence of a large number of patients is staggering to the imagination" (9).

The Markson-Hand investigation suggests that the final environment may be disguised by society. Elders who are not far away from death are denied whatever advantages there might be in having the status of a dying person. Social pressures (incorporating attitudes already noted here) have the effect of requiring the dying elder to accept a disguise. He dies, but he never was dying. Instead of dwelling in an environment that is in some way attuned to the special needs of the dying, the elder in this situation is treated as a deviant and reject. There is another message here, of course. To be aged and vulnerable is somehow equivalent to being a social failure . . . aging is a failure, and dying is a failure. It does not really matter whether this old man is mentally ill or dying. It is enough to know that he is old.

The two studies of responsiveness on the part of severely impaired and/or dying geriatric patients have another set of messages for us. We are reminded that our own expectations regarding the mental status of dying patients should not be permitted to interfere with accurate perception of the situation. Treated as though phenomenologically dead or mentally incompetent, the impaired and the vulnerable elder is thus given a lethal push from his environment. Deterioration and death may be accelerated by what perhaps should be called a "finalizing" environment. Although, most of the patients were institutionalized because of their own failing bodies, the environment tended to assume that they were already "as good as dead." Lifelike behavior was not expected, identified, or reinforced (yet the staff was not derelict in its technical duties nor unkind in its general feeling-tone toward the patients). Accurate definition of the old person as a dying patient can result in an overreaction on the part of the environment, a sort of premortem burial (as manifested, for example, by speaking about the patient in his presence as though he were not there at all).

The study of self-injurious behavior in geriatric medical patients (in a different institution from the one involved in the previous two studies) carries some of these implications further. "Could it be that within the institutional environment destructive behaviors may lead to *increased* survival potential because they provoke the much-wanted attention of nursing personnel . . . ? Is it possible that the same dynamics might be found in the home and the community as well as the institution? Might it be that the special care given an injured patient serves as a social reinforcer to increase the probability of further self-injurious behaviors? The elderly patient may feel (and be) ignored if he does not do something to draw attention to himself every week or so, yet every such action introduces a new risk factor" (10).

This latter study draws our attention to one of the most significant and under-researched topics in gerontology: How do the aged person and his environment conspire to hasten his death? We are focusing here upon people who are not in the advanced debilitated condition of those previously cited. Rather, these are elders with some degree of illness and vulnerability, but who still have a considerable range of possible "movement" in either direction, deterioration or improved functioning. In the usual sense they are not preterminal, not dying. Yet their lives are in more jeopardy than people in general. And—most relevantly—

the fragile relationship between self and environment could initiate the final downhill process at any time. Social neglect may elicit attention-seeking behavior, which itself may prove lethal. This is but one of many possible pathways to premature death in old age in which the environment plays the role of effective accomplice.

Similarly, the inquiry into physician-contacts of people who have subsequently suicided bears upon the problem of unrecognized premature death. It is not that easy to identify suicidal risk in all cases, and the available data do not tell us how many cases were, in fact, recognized and aided by physicians. But the fact remains that many opportunities to identify suicidal risk are missed—by all of us. Again, this is a problem at all age levels. The problem is especially salient in old age, however. We do not always seem to keep to mind the clear statistical evidence on increasing suicide rates with advanced age (11). And we seem to forget that the ratio between attempts and completions narrows considerably, especially for men. How could a physician (lawyer, nurse, social worker, landlord, friend, neighbor, relative) notice self-destructive trends in an old man and yet do nothing about it? Perhaps it is because we do not really believe that there can be such a thing as premature death in old age. It is all right for the aged to die. It is their task, their responsibility.

The concept of premature death in old age has been introduced and discussed elsewhere, including the view that "one might hold that any death of a young person is premature, while every old person is ripe for death . . . (but) some young people face death with equanimity and readiness (while) some elders give every indication of not being prepared to leave this life. Age per se may not be the most enlightened criterion to employ when considering the timeliness of death" (12).

Concluding Note

We have attempted to explore some of the ways in which our own attitudes toward aging and death are likely to affect our orientation toward terminal care of the aged. Much relevant material has been excluded, and we have passed by some points that tempted more extensive comment. The core problem is the one to concentrate upon: many of us have misgivings about the prospects of our own aging and death, and we have mixed feelings about people in our own lives who are aged. We are quick to project our own attitudes and expectations upon elderly men and women. This projection can exert powerful influence over the lives and deaths of the elderly as we are generally in a position of greater socioeconomic leverage. If we are convinced it is right or necessary for an old person to die, then we may be making it extraordinarily difficult for him to live. We may fail to bolster his chances of remaining in good health, we may fail to recognize when, in fact, his preterminal process has begun, and we may remain so closeted in our own assumptions that we do not bother to find out what it is that he really needs in his last hours.

And then, one of these days, there is somebody over us with all the ignorant benevolence we have taught him. . . .

REFERENCES

1. A. D. Weisman, Suicide, Death, and Life-Threatening Behavior. Presented at "Suicide Prevention in the Seventies," Phoenix, Arizona, Feb. 1, 1970; and R. Kastenbaum and R. B. Aisenberg, *The Psychology of Death,* New York, Springer: 1962.

2. B. G. Glaser, "The Social Loss of Aged Dying Patients," *Gerontologist,* 6:71–73, 1966.

3. The concept of a final environment was prefigured in Avery D. Weisman and Robert Kastenbaum, *The Psychological Autopsy: A Study of the Terminal Phase of Life,* New York: Behavioral Publications, 1968. It is taken further in *The Psychology of Death* (Kastenbaum and Aisenberg) and Robert Kastenbaum and Bunny Kastenbaum, "Hope, Survival and the Caring Environment," in E. Palmore and F. Jeffers (Eds.), *Psycho-Social Prediction of Longevity,* Lexington, Mass.: Heath, 1972.

4. As noted by many observers, including Barney G. Glaser and Anselm Strauss, *Awareness of Dying,* Chicago: Aldine, 1965; and Lawrence LeShan and Edna LeShan, "Psychotherapy and the patient with a limited life-span," *Psychiatry, 24:*318–23, 1961.

5. E. W. Markson and J. Hand, "Referral for Death: Low Status of the Aged and Referral for Psychiatric Hospitalization," *Aging and Human Development, 1,* 3, 261–72, 1970.

6. R. Kastenbaum, "Psychological Death," in L. Pearson (Ed.), *Dying and Death,* Cleveland: Western Reserve University Press, 1–27, 1969.

7. R. Kastenbaum, "The Mental Life of Dying Geriatric Patients," *Gerontologist, 7:*97–100, 1967.

8. D. E. Sanborn, G. D. Niswander, and T. M. Casey, "The Family Physician and Suicide Prevention," *American Family Physician/GP,* March 1970, 75–78.

9. R. Kastenbaum, and B. Mishara, "Premature Death and Self-Injurious Behavior in Old Age," *Geriatrics,* in press.

10. Kastenbaum and Mishara, *ibid.*

11. *Vital Statistics of the United States, 1968,* Vol. 11, Mortality, Part B, U. S. Department of Health, Education, and Welfare.

12. Kastenbaum and Mishara, "Premature Death and Self-Injurious Behavior in Old Age."

Austin H. Kutscher

THE PSYCHOSOCIAL ASPECTS OF THE ORAL CARE OF THE DYING PATIENT

In a recent review, the psychiatrist Avery Weisman suggested that "The overwhelming number of specialists in some aspect of death and dying now calls for the recognition of a new specialty, Thanatology" (1). Among the health professions which are busily acknowledging and de-lineating the psychosocial problems faced by terminal patients and their families is the profession of dentistry and its allied health personnel. Regrettably, the dental profession has been left behind other groups working toward permitting the dying patient a death free of pain and indignity.

The most direct and pertinent introduction to this subject, it would seem, is an exposition of the extraordinary importance of the mouth to the dying patient and, hence, the need for its maintenance in the best possible condition in order to permit the achievement of death *with* maximum dignity. Hence, the introduction will take the form of a discussion of the unique significance of the mouth which warrants singling it out for special interest and care (2).

The mouth is recognized as the first area of gratification and pleasure. The lips, tongue and buccal mucosa are erogenous zones of the body and throughout life are associated with pleasure. The infant's "view" of the surrounding world is determined by his early mouth relationships, usually with the mother. His developing contact with the world is enhanced by the emergence of speech patterns, generally a focus of much interest on the part of significant adults. Originally primarily a receptive organ, the mouth, through the use of both words and teeth, comes to have aggressive qualities as well. Expressions such as a "sharp," "biting," or "cutting tongue" are all indications of the common acceptance of the mouth as a weapon of attack. In the teaching of the twelve apostles, the mouth is a "snare of death." Familiar to every child who attends Sunday school is the story of the "burning coal" placed in Isaiah's mouth to cleanse him of his sins; this is a reminder also of the mouth as a site for punishment. Thus, the mouth easily becomes an area in which gratifications, punishments, and conflicts, both actual and symbolic, are expressed. Included in this context is the realization that, as strength (even to write) fails, the mouth becomes the sole remaining modality by which a dying patient can anger or please, demand, request, beg, entreat, command, or even, in the larger sense, still affect for good or ill the lives of others whom he loves or hates—through expressions ranging from heartfelt words perhaps fulfilling a lifelong desire, to a whim, or to executing such practical matters as making changes in a will.

Finally, as an erogenous area, the mouth can become the zone of displacement for other parts of the body, and the extraction of a tooth during terminal care as well as at other times, for instance, can unconsciously be viewed not only as bodily mutilation but even as death. Studies indicate that among well patients exposed to varying degrees of trauma, a larger number report conscious fear of minor dental procedures than of major surgery in other parts of the body (3). This fact should also be considered in relation to information developed later in this paper.

Oral Disturbances Accompanying
Unrelated Terminal Disease

There is little information in the scientific literature regarding oral lesions in terminal illness. This reflects the general failure of the dental profession to undertake studies in this area and the general tendency of the medical profession to ignore the plight of the mouth, rather than the absence of oral discomfort in dying patients. To the contrary, mouth soreness and pain, mouth dryness, moniliasis and other oral infections, taste disturbances including loss of taste, and mouth odor, as well as disturbances of chewing, swallowing, and speech functions are among the many extremely common sources of physical pain and discomfort as well as psychological trauma to the dying patient. Incredibly, the recognition, understanding, and management of these and other as yet unappreciated and unstudied phenomena have until recently been viewed as being of minor interest to dental and other practitioners. Decline of oral function and difficulties in maintenance of oral alimentation, two problems contributed to by reduction in salivary flow and alteration in salivary composition, are additional examples of clinical *and* psychosocial areas of concern greatly beyond mere academic interest.

For the clinical researcher, the dynamics of the dying cells (glandular, epithelial, neural, etc.) located in the mouth are equal in importance with and more easily studied than the dynamics of the same types of cells and tissues in less easily accessible areas of the body. However, research in the field of problems of the oral cavity in the broad sense remains minimal, especially in regard to basic science and psychosocial aspects of thanatology; but, self-evidently, such research should be entered upon at a quickened rate both in relation to the improved management of the entire individual (of whom these tissues are a representative sample) and in relation to the improved management of disturbances specifically involving the mouth.

Oral Disturbances Related to
Terminal Oral (Disease) Cancer

The management of problems involving the mouth in patients with terminal oral cancer has also received only the most sporadic attention from investigators. Obvious areas of importance that have scarcely been investigated at all include: the extent to which oral pain and discomfort exist in such patients and the treatment of these problems; maintenance of adequate alimentation; failure of other mouth functions, including speech, deglutition, etc.; the esthetics of exposed, cancer-bearing areas of the face, head, and neck; the emotional reactions of the patient and others to the patient's deformity; and, in particular, the intense mouth odors caused by uncontrolled cancer tissue with their resultant psychological overtones. Few studies are available for review even in regard to the utilization of narcotic and psychopharmacologic agents, although such information is undoubtedly available on an uncontrolled or clinical-impression basis.

Of crucial significance, therefore, is the role of the dental practitioner on the health team providing comprehensive care, both clinical and psychosocial, of the patient dying from oral carcinoma.

Training the Dental Practitioner
to Care for the Dying Patient

It is important at this point to consider the dental practitioner's role in caring for the mouth of patients dying of lesions or diseases elsewhere in the body for whom the mouth becomes the source of discomfort, pain, infection, and other complications.

The problem of obtaining adequate oral care for the dying patient stems in part from avoidance by the medical and nursing teams involved but in larger measure from the reluctance of the majority of dental practitioners to care for the dying patient, particularly if it entails entering the patient's sickroom. Doubtless, this problem holds true also for dental hygienists. Such findings should not be deemed unusual: studies of medical and nursing students have demonstrated that many members of these groups enter the health professions to overcome or in some instances to deny their fear of death, just as, apparently, some dental students choose dentistry rather than medicine to avoid situations in which they are confronted by or must be concerned with death. In fact, according to one study, the gradual decline in the popularity of medicine as an occupational choice during adolescence is in part a reflection of the increasing recognition that medicine is closely related to death. Hence, the choice of dentistry (or dental hygiene) may well reflect a phobic avoidance, just as the choice of a career in medicine can be viewed as a counterphobic denial. In any event, it is clear that if adequate oral care is to be provided for the dying patient, a larger reservoir of general practitioners of dentistry who are willing to undertake this service must be trained. Such training must begin with adequate psychosocial foundations as a base. The practitioner can, then, satisfactorily cope with his own anxiety feelings related to the dying patient by coming to terms with the inevitability of his own death, just as such problems must be met by the physician and the nurse if they are to function adequately in the same situations. The training of such a corps of dental practitioners and dental hygienists will require efforts similar to those which should be employed for physicians and nurses.

Logically, the first step in providing such training is the recently undertaken survey of dental schools and their curricula with a view to documenting the scarcity of training for such patient-care service, to be followed by the introduction of suitable course material into the curriculum to prepare the dental graduate for accepting his share of his profession's responsibilities in regard to the dying patient and his family. Another parallel survey has also been made of dental students to document their interest in and willingness to undertake such training. The findings can quite likely be used as a wedge to introduce the prerequisite psychosocial material into the dental curriculum and so create a greater pool of specially trained dentists who are psychosocially oriented to caring for the dying patient and professionally capable of providing the necessary care. In our personal experience, dental students almost invariably express the wish for further help and training in this area once the need for it has been suitably presented.

As further evidence of the need for more extensive training of dentists in the entire area of cancer considered above, the federal government is supporting clinical training programs in the care of cancer patients for dental students, the guidelines for grant proposals having in 1970 been broadened to include terminal care and its associated psychosocial problems. Although these programs differ in approach from school to school and are constantly being upgraded, all of them are planned around bringing the future practitioner into intimate contact with the cancer patient in a variety of situations, including diagnosis, radiotherapy, surgery, maxillo-facial prosthesis, psychiatry, and, now, finally, palliative and terminal care units.

It is likewise coming to be realized that the education of the future dental practitioner in the art and science of over-all patient management should include an understanding of a basic core of concepts relating to dying, loss, and bereavement. An appreciable number of dentists are needed to shoulder the responsibility of the profession to the terminal patient.

Some Problems, Some Causes, and Some Approaches to Solutions

That the dying patient, of his own accord, would neglect oral hygiene is a known fact. Prolonged neglect, unreversed by specific dental care, may result in further deterioration which may require extractions or other surgical procedures, thereby adding to the mutilation of the patient at a time when he can least afford it clinically and psychosocially. To the dying patient who longs for love, help, and attention and instead feels abandoned and helpless, a tooth extraction necessitated by professional neglect is inevitably perceived unconsciously as a further attack on his already depleted body. This can result only in the patient's being increasingly overwhelmed by feelings of anger, fear, guilt, futility and despondency. Contrariwise, continued appointments which can be tolerated physically can assist in preventing the progression of oral problems but, perhaps more importantly, can also give the patient the much-needed impression that others are concerned over his continued health and well-being and are still gladly willing to provide care.

Whatever the cause, treatment should be focused on the total individual rather than on the mouth alone. Patience, tolerance, and support by a dental practitioner can provide very considerable psychological uplift and comfort in addition to the benefits derived from any operative procedures performed within the mouth. In the over-all schema, it is just as important for the dentist, in his turn, to listen diligently to the patient, encourage verbal expression, and offer simple explanations in answer to questions as it is for the physician or the nurse.

A dental practitioner should, of course, be aware of his own feelings toward death, thereby preventing his emotional withdrawal from or inaccessibility to the patient. Open and direct conversation is reassuring to the patient. Frank communication by the dentist with the patient's physician, family members, and friends may yield important information for formulating the best approach, both physical and psychological, to the patient's frequently monumental oral problems. Under certain conditions when oral operative procedures are indicated or should not be avoided (as they too often are), the use of psychoactive drugs, if not already being employed, may be important adjuncts in the management of the patient even at a late stage.

The Psychogenic Component

Psychoanalytic investigators have consistently noted the significance of orality in depression. Freud (4) has compared depression (melancholia) to normal grief, recognizing that some patients have a predisposition, related to early life experience, to react with depression when confronted with the loss of loved persons or valued objects. He described the process as a regression to the oral stage of development. Accompanying a predisposition to depression is an overdependence upon an external supply of love, attention, and recognition for the maintenance of self-esteem. Usually, however, and most regrettably for the dying patient, the needed love and attention are gradually withdrawn, with a not surprising impact on the patient. In the nonmoribund but mourning individual, inability to cope with loss is also frequently manifested by symptoms in the oral cavity; comparable connotations for the dying person, who is also grieving, are not difficult to recognize.

Pain

Control of pain (5) and the patient's reaction to pain cannot be dissociated from psychosocial care of the terminally ill patient since pain has profound implications to the patient, especially when it is not controlled.

Oral discomfort and/or frank oral pain per se is a frequent complaint of the dying patient. The practitioner cannot avoid being confronted with complaints of soreness, tenderness, discomfort, and even overt pain at some stage in the care of these patients. Such pain is difficult to define because there are great differences in response to pain among patients in general and perhaps dying patients in particular— and at different times. Furthermore, the situational psychological status of the patient (for example, anxiety and depression) modulates the "innate" sensitivity of that person to pain.

Pain is a symptom associated with or a sequellae of mouth dryness, drooling, moniliasis, infection, and osteoradionecrosis (in the case of the oral cancer patient), among many other causes. It should also be emphasized that, in some cases, pain results from the intake or use of irritating agents such as foods and fluids (including those with an acid pH), alcohol and cigarettes. Dental prostheses may often also cause pain. It is obvious that the oral cancer patient is particularly prone to dental abnormalities (caries, odontogenic infections, defective fillings, and periodontal diseases) and that these conditions may be the sole source of pain or may intensify the symptoms emanating from the sources just mentioned. Oral pain (whether it be local soreness, tenderness, and discomfort; frank pain; or intractable pain) can usually be managed with approaches not dissimilar to those utilized in the management of pain and discomfort in other areas of the body—approaches which cannot be covered in detail within the context of this paper specifically, but which, it is emphasized, are heavily overlayed by profound psychosocial components.

It should be noted that when analgesics are necessary it is best to start with aspirin with or without a mild sedative. The next step is the addition of codeine, Darvon, or oral Talwin to the aspirin. When stronger narcotics are required, it is best to start with small doses and use the patient's response as the indication for dosage. Phenergan^R or Thorazine^R can potentiate the effects of the narcotic agents.

Narcotic administration, with its ultimate addiction problem, can often be avoided until the terminal stage* is reached, but thereafter it should not be withheld in the name of addiction—although interference with "communication" may pose problems of concern to all personnel involved, including the patient.

Drooling

Drooling (6) may become a serious problem for the terminal patient who can no longer wear dentures. Unesthetic and bothersome to the patient, his caretakers, and family, such drooling results from loss of intermaxillary distance as when all teeth have been removed or when existing dentures have been rendered unusable during the course of the illness (usually relatable to weight loss or tooth loss or breakdown).

Occasionally, drooling leads to highly discomforting and *disfiguring* angular stomatitis and circumoral dermatitis due to the irritating components of oral fluids and the microorganisms of the oral flora. The amelioration of such clinical and related psychosocial problems is well within the range of informed oral care.

* In the terminal oral cancer patient, when bone pain becomes intractable and all conservative measures have failed, the bone may be removed as a last resort. Often peripheral neurotomy and cranial nerve section can give excellent relief of intractable pain of oral cancer. Depending upon the site of the cancer, relief may be obtained by posterior rhizotomy of the trigeminal, the glossopharyngeal and the vagus nerves, alone or in combination. If neck pain is associated with the face pain, section of the upper cervical sensory roots can be performed at the same time. This procedure can be performed by a cryogenic technique and is to be considered only in a minute fraction of patients who suffer from absolutely intractable pain.

Odor

Nothing can be more distressing to the family of a terminal patient or to the persons caring for him than the mouth odor (7) which so frequently complicates progressively terminal oral illness—especially odor which arises from a large, fungating, necrotic tumor. The terminal patient has often lost his sense of smell. While the patient becomes tolerant and eventually unaware of odor, those in his environment do not. This alone is often the reason for transferring terminal oral cancer patients (as well as other cancer patients where oral involvement is not direct) to a nursing home or terminal care facility. The problem of odor, ultimately a cogent psychosocial problem, often is not satisfactorily controlled by the usual techniques of frequent dressing changes, liberal use of aerosol sprays, or the placement of containers of methylsalicylate about the room, and others.

Seldom do antibiotics, either systemically or topically administered, play a significant role in controlling exophytic tumor odor. However, a secondary infection in the mouth of a patient terminally ill of other causes often responds favorably to antibiotic therapy.

Side Effects of Psychopharmacological Agents

To indicate in somewhat greater detail and with greater forcefulness the problems related to the oral cavity faced by terminally ill patients, consider what is almost routinely the situation when psychopharmacological agents of the phenothiazine group are administered in the attempt to manage the patient, free him from pain and permit him dignity in death. The side effects of such psychopharmacologic agents, often the price for the psychosocial benefits accruing to their use, include intensified dryness of the mouth with its attendant discomfort superimposed on a mouth already dry due to debilitation and dehydration as well as to lack of adequate quantities of saliva and changes in its viscosity. As a result, the patient makes increasing demands for frequent small feedings of water, which are a drain upon the nursing care reserves for that patient and for the nurse's entire area of responsibility. Mouth dryness is also related to dysgeussia (an unpleasant taste in the mouth) concomitant with the dryness per se. The lack of a free flow of saliva contributes to accumulations of debris in the mouth. Compounding this problem may be the disagreeable taste of some drugs when they are secreted back in the mouth. A further sequela of prolonged mouth dryness is the superimposed need for an antimonilial agent—usually a most unpleasantly tasting drug, Mycostatin. Moniliasis may also follow the use of antibiotics employed to control infection in the mouth or elsewhere in the body. In those instances where both an antibiotic and a phenothiazine are being administered at once, superinfection by monilial organisms in the mouth is even more likely to occur and is more difficult to control.

Also to be considered as a price of the pharmacologic benefits of psychoactive agents is the resulting incoordination of the dying patient's limbs which inhibits reaching his mouth with food or liquids, as well as the incoordination of the mouth and deterioration of its functions including those of speech, eating, chewing, and deglutition.

Predominantly Psychological Oral Problems of the Moribund Patient

The helpless moribund person, confined in a hospital or sickbed environment and cared for by impersonal service attendants, develops heightened mouth senses, especially following the diminished use of his other senses. In this state, he seeks to utilize the mouth more than ever to re-establish links to a formerly secure and affectionate environment. Primitive sucking movements persist in all individuals in the form of bruxism and mouth habits. They are exaggerated during a time of separation from important love objects and forced helplessness.

Finger sucking, nail biting, object biting or sucking, an urgent need to eat or drink, a craving for sweets or foods once associated with a dependent relationship with a mothering person are all indicative of frustrated and perhaps secret needs for the security which can be derived from contact with a mothering person. The moribund individual often craves a food which links him to a cared-for time in his life; he may test the affection of those who visit him by demanding such food. The demand is often misinterpreted as hunger or a whim; yet it occurs frequently in individuals unable to tolerate solid food without severe nausea.

The awareness that death and separation from much-needed love objects are imminent may bring back the eerie and terror-filled experiences of early childhood when one is sure that he has been abandoned forever if his mother is late or stops talking to him, or actually abandons him when she is ill or dies. His suspicions are confirmed when he finds himself in the alien environment of the hospital and formerly loving contacts become tormented, anxious moments for both the visitor and the dying patient. Often the visitors and care specialists, including the dentist, may be unaware of the nonverbal communication by which they show their eagerness to leave the side of the dying person. Often good reasons, particularly easy for the dentist to come by, are introduced for cutting off contacts with the patient by the very specialists who have been given the responsibility for caring for him, as well as by members of his family. The dying person is often avoided by everyone, including nurses, and if the disease process has changed his appearance greatly, both the dying patient and his family suffer too much anguish to tolerate more than momentary contacts. The more dependent the family members were upon the strength, opinions, and services of the dying one, the less they can tolerate his changed facial appearance, demeanor, and status as well as their own rage at the deprivation they are experiencing.

Thus, the helpless, feeble, dying patient, unable to satisfactorily experience his once secure environment through his tactile, proprioceptive, auditory, and visual senses, now must rely increasingly upon mouth movements and mouth senses for contact with the external world (8) so to achieve as much as possible some sense of security and gratification. His body is rarely touched in any meaningful, affectionate way. Realistically he has primarily his mouth to retain a link with his former environment. Tranquilizers and dehydrating drugs produce severe oral dryness. Physical feebleness often makes it impossible for him to reach the carafe or glass of water. A device may have to be invented (as is available even for animals) to assist him in moistening his lips or mouth without calling for aid—since all too often the moribund patient either will not call for help or will annoy the staff by too frequent calls for help.

Physical contact with the dying person's hands, mouth, face, and hair are, in reality, vitally necessary. Catering to his mouth needs can be reassuring and provide feelings of security. Small but frequent feedings of favorite foods, some evocative of childhood (a peach, chicken soup, fresh fruit juice), not only would relieve mouth dryness, but may also revive the sense of being catered to by a mothering person at a time when panic has caused the moribund one to regress to a very early (oral) stage in life in which he feels physically and emotionally helpless.

Loss of body fat in the dying patient results in instability of his once secure dentures, and adjustment of these dentures is vital. When a narcissistic individual faces aging and death, the prospect of looking old and ugly is insupportable. Even when dying, such an individual remains vain, self-centered, and status-seeking. Rather than condemnation and neglect, such people need greater care than usual so they may look the best they can. The teeth, mouth, skin, and hair must thus be given special attention to preserve their vitality till the end.

Many patients would choose to die at home, and, if it is feasible without completely disrupting family life (especially that of the children in the home), every attempt should be made to give the patient the security and satisfaction of his family's presence. Being in his home environment may also relieve his anxiety that his illness is depleting the financial resources of his family. Oral care is one area in particular which, if the dentist is willing, can be rendered almost as fully at home as in the hospital.

The most frequently expressed complaint of the terminal patient is his feeling of being abandoned. No matter how difficult it may be, the patient's family and all his doctors, including the dentist, must continue their active roles in his life. Again, such basic oral care as the adjustment of dentures can be beneficial and highly symbolic, allowing the patient to die in greater physical comfort and more tenable emotional and psychological peace.

Coordination of
Terminal Care Management

The multiplicity of problems which develop in terminal care management, especially that for oral cancer, test the ingenuity of the dentist as well as that of the physician more than any other aspect of practice. Ideally, the management of these problems should be directed by a single responsible physician and a multidisciplinary team of physicians, dentists, nurses, clergymen, and social workers who work together regularly and have a similar approach to and philosophy of terminal-care management. Nothing is more distressing to the patient or to his family than poorly planned or loosely coordinated treatment instructions and practices.

Conclusions

It appears worthwhile to recapitulate those concepts which demand that particular attention be paid to the care of the oral cavity of the dying patient:

1. As total bodily deterioration progresses, the mouth increasingly becomes the most convenient and, later (following the loss of coordination of the hands and loss of both will and muscle strength for writing), the only mode of communication of all thoughts of and by the patient.

2. The mouth remains also perhaps the last area of gratification and satisfaction with which he is able to indulge himself or can be indulged. It serves the dying patient as his means of communication to obtain such gratification and/or such satisfactions (desired foods, desired presence of loved ones, wished for words of comfort and love, and more).

3. The mouth comes to be a very significant source of discomfort, even pain, not only in patients dying from oral cancer but also in an overwhelming number of patients dying from chronic diseases other than oral cancer (but including cancer of other portions of the body).

4. As the patient retreats further from his environment—as with-

drawal becomes the pattern of his existence—there is a continuing regression, psychiatrically speaking, to the stage of orality wherein the oral cavity becomes, as it once was, the most all-pervasive organ to the individual.

5. The mouth should be allowed to remain a prized body area to be admired and appreciated by patient and family as one of beauty and readily available to view; the entire mouth including the lips and teeth should be kept in the optimum state of esthetic repair, this concept including both the natural teeth or any prosthetic replacements—so that at least this one area can remain, if not as attractive as before, at least not a site of further disfigurement in the terminal phases of illness.

6. The importance of maintaining the dentition, including artificial dentures, in a state of function that permits alimentation is self-evident in relation to the patient's estimate of his own condition. For example, inability to eat would be equated by the patient with starvation, depletion, and a downhill, unremittingly and hopelessly terminal course. Eating also has social connotations, so that partaking of food in the company of others, free of pain or distress, becomes of psychosocial importance.

7. Loss of ability to speak clearly and distinctly frequently results from inadequate care or repair of the dentition or dentures which no longer fit. Surely, dentures ought to be in the patient's mouth rather than on the bedside table for the reasons just mentioned alone.

A cared-for mouth, whatever its state, is of enormous psychosocial importance to the patient who appreciates the impact of his appearance, any odor, as well as his speech and mouth functions upon those who care for him and those who love him. Certainly the dying patient also perceives loss of speech as representing both figuratively and actually a definitive sign of a terminal state when, in point of fact, this may actually represent nothing more than a failure to obtain proper dental care.

Summary

The importance of oral care in the schema of the psychosocial management of the terminal patient has been sketched. An attempt has been made to interpret the background of the importance of such care to the patient and his family, and, hence, the need for care efforts in this direction—as well as the need to train dentists and others for the acceptance of their role in the care of both the clinical and psychosocial problems related to the mouth of the dying patient and the impact of these considerations on family members.

REFERENCES

1. A. Weisman, "The Right Way To Die," *Psychiatric and Social Science Review*.

2. B. Schoenberg, "Psychogenic Aspects of the Burning Mouth," *New York State Dental Journal, 33:*467, 1967.

3. I. L. Janis, *Psychological Stress,* New York: Wiley and Sons, 1958.

4. B. Schoenberg, "Psychogenic Aspects of the Burning Mouth."

5. E. V. Zegarelli, A. H. Kutscher, D. W. Cohen, A. Ketcham, M. Ochoa, Jr., G. Stanton, "Maintaining the Oral and General Health of the Oral Cancer Patient (Part One)," *Oral Care for Oral Cancer Patients*, Washington, D.C.: U.S. Government Printing Office, June 1968.

6. *Ibid.*

7. E. V. Zegarelli, A. H. Kutscher, D. W. Cohen, A. Ketcham, M. Ochoa, Jr., G. Stanton, "Maintaining the Oral and General Health of the Oral Cancer Patient (Part Two)," *Oral Care for Oral Cancer Patients*, Washington, D.C.: U.S. Government Printing Office, June 1968.

8. *Ibid.*

Psychosocial Care

Jeanne Quint Benoliel

NURSING CARE FOR THE TERMINAL PATIENT: A PSYCHOSOCIAL APPROACH

The part played by nursing personnel in the provision of "terminal nursing care" is a complex one. In essence, the fundamental purposes of nursing practice have remained essentially the same as when Florence Nightingale observed that what nursing had to do was "to put the patient in the best condition for nature to act upon him" (1). In her time, communicable disease was a leading cause of death, and direct nursing care often had more to do with recovery than did medical treatments. Today infectious disease is no longer the primary killer (at least in Western societies), and chronic illness has assumed prominence both as a disabler and as the principal contributor to high death rates. Technological and social change has produced a radical shift in both the kinds and the quantities of nursing care required by the society and in the social contexts where nursing services are provided.

Current Knowledge
About Nursing Care

TERMINAL CARE—A DEFINITIONAL ISSUE

The concept of terminal care is somewhat inadequate and misleading for considering in a meaningful way the psychosocial aspects of nursing contacts with patients and potential patients. Terminal care generally refers to those patients who are defined as dying and thus are viewed in the final stages of their lives. Yet the reality is that death, near-death, or fear of death is a feature of many situations in which nursing personnel interact with patients and families although the definition of "dying patient" may not be explicit.

For our purposes there are at least four types of contacts involving nurses with persons facing death. First, there are patients definitely in need of terminal nursing care and requiring direct physical ministrations or assistance in matters of daily living. Some care is offered to individuals in their homes, but there is a definite trend toward the institutionalization of persons who need these services—and markedly so for the elderly. Between 1939 and 1965 the number of nursing homes and similar institutions rose from 1200 to 12,042 due to a growth in numbers of persons over sixty-five and to the expansion of public welfare programs (2). About 5 per cent of those over sixty-five (roughly 900,-000 persons), are seen as incapable of being self-sustaining due mainly to the combination of poverty and physical disablement (3).

The second type of contact occurs in situations where nursing personnel provide life-prolonging and sometimes intensive care to individuals who are facing the possibility of death (sometimes imminent death). Hospitals are organized primarily to promote the saving of lives, and this activity assumes critical importance on wards where rapid action can make the difference between life and death—for example, the coronary care unit. Here top priority is given to recovery-oriented, medically delegated nursing tasks, and "comfort care" is essentially relegated to a secondary position (4). There are other wards where death is a frequent visitor, but the work is less dramatic in character because the period of dying tends to be slow—a pattern that is common with cancer, cystic fibrosis, and progressive neurological disease. Often these patients are in and out of hospitals several times before they enter for the final time, or the hospital ward becomes the permanent abode when care at home is not possible. On some of these wards, there are increasing numbers of patients who are socially dead through partial or complete loss of brain activity yet are biologically alive and sometimes kept so with the assistance of life-prolonging machinery.

A third context for interaction occurs when immediate emergency care is required because of accidents or natural disasters, and the injured persons are brought into a centralized emergency-care setting for help. The demand for this type of service (essentially normal for military medical components in time of war) has grown tremendously in metropolitan areas where the accident rate is increasing due to crowded conditions and crosscultural pressures both within and between different ethnic and social groups. In the case of mass disaster, such as can occur with fires, floods, hurricanes, and earthquakes, the demand for care can sometimes be overwhelming and beyond the capabilities of the services normally available to a given community (as was demonstrated by Hurricane Camille in August of 1969). Nursing personnel in emergency wards work with the reality of unexpected and sudden death almost on a daily basis, and they are often in contact with families in psychological shock and in the early stages of grief (5).

Finally, there are numerous contacts with people who have chronic and life-threatening diseases at various stages of incapacitation and thus with different requirements for assistance in coping with the psychosocial and physical problems imposed by long-term illness. As Fox pointed out with respect to cancer, different approaches to patient care are needed when the lesion is new and still viewed as curable, when signs of metastatic progression appear, and when the terminal stage becomes apparent (6). One of the commonalities of experience during the adaptation to all chronic illness is the process of grieving, and nursing personnel are often in contact (either intermittently or continuously) with individuals and/or families undergoing this experience.

It is clear from these descriptions that the psychosocial needs of the recipients of nursing services vary a good deal and are dependent on a combination of circumstances including: a) the stage of illness (early, middle, late); b) the type of assistance that is needed (life-saving care, direct physical care, teaching-socialization, emotional support); c) the amount of time that is involved (short-term, long-term, permanent contact); and d) the social context in which care is provided (ambulatory-care, home-care, institutional care). Different patterns of dying come to be associated with different institutional settings, and the psychosocial needs of dying patients cannot easily be separated from the psychosocial needs of the medical and the nursing staffs (7).

THE GOALS OF NURSING CARE

The importance of personalized care has been identified in the writings of many prominent nurses. Over the years, efforts to establish a meaningful definition of nursing care have been influenced by the nursing profession's attempts to establish itself as independent in function from medicine. The search for independence is reflected in Henderson's definition: "The unique function of the nurse is to assist the individual, sick or well, in the performance of those activities contributing to health or its recovery (or to a peaceful death), that he would perform unaided if he had the necessary strength, will or knowledge (8)." Reiter also sees the principal contribution of nursing to be made through the direct care given to patients: "By clinical practice, I mean those personal services carried out at the patient's side—in contact with him and in behalf of him and his family" (9). Both definitions place a primary emphasis on the nursing function of intervening between the patient and the stresses imposed upon him from within and without.

Led by the pioneer contributions of Peplau, the notion of the nurse-patient relationship as the crux of nursing practice came into being when the psychiatric perspective became a persuasive force in nursing education during the postwar (World War II) mental health movement in the United States (10). The concept has been explored and expanded by a number of nurses in recent years, but the significance of the one-to-one nurse-patient relationship remains central (11). Concerning the dying patient in particular, Arteberry proposes the "therapeutic use of distance" as a concept for guiding the nurse's decisions in making the intimate physical and interpersonal contacts that are so often required when dying is prolonged (12). Aguilera suggests the usefulness of nursing interventions based on the model of crisis intervention (13).

More recently, the concept of the "therapeutic" nurse-patient relationship has been supplanted by a more existential approach that emphasizes the mutuality of human interaction (14). At the same time increasing numbers of publications are addressing themselves to the importance of patients having opportunities to communicate about their deaths as their lives are drawing to a close (15). Accepting the one-to-one nurse-patient relationship as centrally important, Blumberg and Drummond describe eight concepts or components that together comprise the nursing care of persons with long-term illness, including those who are dying: a) physical care; b) emotional support; c) observations; d) treatment; e) teaching the patient; f) counselling and working with others; g) complex correlations; and h) the economics of disability (16). An interpretation of the revised code for nurses published by the American Nurses' Association in 1968 states explicitly that for those who are terminally ill or dying "the nurse should use all the measures at her command to enable the patient to live out his days with as much comfort, dignity and freedom from anxiety and pain as possible" (17).

THE REALITY OF NURSING CARE

Despite these stated goals, there is considerable evidence that personalized nursing care during the terminal stages of illness is the exception more than the rule in practice. The reasons are many. Personalized care depends upon *continuity of contact* with at least one concerned person whereas institutional care is given by groups of individuals and the work is generally organized to minimize emotional involvements that might be disruptive to the social order. *Systematic accountability* for the psychosocial components of patient care is essentially lacking in many institutions (18). There are nurses who are quietly helping dying patients and their families cope with the social and psychological problems they encounter, but they are not in the majority. More than that, they are often frustrated in their efforts by a *lack of authority* in matters of patient care (19).

The work done in hospitals is a direct reflection of the values of society. Hence the social rewards go to nurses engaged in recovery-oriented care, the highest rewards going to those in intensive-care settings. Terminal care becomes a form of low-status work delegated to those in the lower echelons of the nursing department. Lack of an organized approach to the psychosocial aspects of nursing care in many institutions in combination with the low status accorded to terminal care produces social deprivation for some patients and a fragmentation of experience for others (20).

There is a growing body of knowledge that the psychosocial effects and concomitants of chronic and life-threatening illness seriously influence physical well-being and lead to social isolation for many individuals. The extreme in social deprivation occurs for those least able to defend themselves against the wishes of others (21). As for those who are hospitalized temporarily, what is lacking from doctors and nurses is communication that is personally relevant and care that is provided with a human touch (22). What is apparent for institutional care in general is even greater when the threat of death enters the picture.

It is clearly evident that working in a context of frequent exposure to death is emotionally taxing for the nursing staff, and withdrawal from personal involvement with patients functions as a protective mechanism. For some personnel, the psychological strain comes from almost continuous exposure to the lingering process of dying characteristic of nursing homes. For others, the stresses of work have more to do with the conflicting demands of recovery care and comfort care in settings where the loss of a patient is sometimes tantamount to personal failure, or with the threat to self-esteem posed by the behaviors of other people under stress—patients, their families, doctors, or other nurses (23). The difficulties are great when communication between the medical and nursing staffs is strained or limited, and when the doctors seldom put in an appearance (24). It is also clear that what the patient and his family have been told or not told about the possibility of death is a condition of crucial importance affecting their interactions with the nurses and other institutional workers (25).

Contributions from Research and Clinical Investigations

A number of recent publications have indicated that personalized care can be obtained in recovery-oriented settings when psychological supports are made available to the institutional staff and when medical and nursing care is well-coordinated (26). The settings in which personalized care for the dying has been most effectively operationalized in a systematic way have been hospice-type institutions modeled after the approach used by Saunders for terminal cancer patients and usually staffed by persons with an unusual commitment to service, such as those in religious orders (27). The success of these ventures appears to have been largely due to the personal commitment of highly motivated individuals with sufficient authority to influence the creation of psychosocial environments where death is not feared but accepted as a normal concomitant of the situation.

Recognition that nurses may well be the most important persons for influencing the emotional well-being of patients has been identified in several articles. Sobel sees the human-to-human interaction between the nurse and the patient on the coronary care unit as the focal point of personalized care (28). Stotsky and Dominick view the nursing supervisor as the key person affecting the patterning of social relationships in the nursing home, with staff-centered supervision producing more positive outcomes for patients than either a permissive or a dominant approach (29). Nurses have been active participants in experimental programs to develop the "therapeutic milieu," but more often than not these were instigated by other health workers, such as social workers or psychiatrists (30).

Participation by nurses themselves both in formal study and in clinical investigations relative to death has been on the increase. A recognition that nurses feel inadequate for meeting the psychosocial needs of dying patients was formally noted in an unpublished study by Bregg, Leddy, and Mackenzie in 1953 (31). In 1966 Dickinson found that nurses feel insecure in meeting the religious needs of patients, in coping with patients who are completely helpless, and in dealing with families but especially those that are anxious, hostile, or constantly asking for information (32). Using a sociological orientation, Folta found an ambivalent orientation toward death among hospital workers, it was viewed as peaceful and predictable in the abstract and with a high degree of anxiety when it became personalized (33). Smith and Quint both reported that nursing students are prepared for the physical and technical aspects of care of the dying but rather poorly for the psychosocial matters that come up in nursing practice (34).

Some recent reports show increasing attention being given to the meaning of death for those with fatal illness. Waechter found that children between the ages of six and ten, though not directly informed as to the nature of their life-threatening illness, showed considerable preoccupation with death in fantasy, feelings of loneliness and isolation, and a sense of loss of control over the forces impinging upon them (35). The temporal dimension of life-threatening disease has been described by Aspinwall and by Quint (36). A number of clinical investigations have described and analyzed the effects of nurse-patient interaction on the patients' opportunities to talk about death, to grieve, and to reach acceptance of forthcoming death (37). Lewis reports that the most difficult aspect of the care of the dying is the "relief of emotional stress" (38).

Most of the written reports about care of the dying are in the nature of case studies, but some have considered the influence of the social environment. After interviews with twenty-four patients who had been in intensive-care units for cardiac surgery, DeMeyer suggests that the environment tends to produce physical overstimulation and emotional deprivation that may not be in the best interests of patient well-being (39). Burchett reports that meaningful communication between the aged person and nursing personnel in nursing homes is influenced by a variety of factors, including the amount of physical care that is needed, the extent to which the patient has psychologically disengaged himself, the effect of the diagnosis on his ability to interact, the presence of sensory defects that interfere with communication, and the level of communication that the nurse is capable of providing (40). Anderson describes a sociotherapeutic approach to care for the geriatric elderly that produced a discharge rate three times higher than that found in other units. Designed to decrease personal isolation and to convey a sense of self-esteem, the program focused on maximizing normative living by incorporating these features: integrating the wards for men and women; holding all patients responsible for specific jobs in the ward community; promoting the right to self-determination through patient government; permitting family and friends to visit at any time; and making available to the elderly the treatment modalities employed with younger psychiatric patients (41).

Implications for Practice

It is clearly evident that the provision of personalized nursing care for patients facing death requires a systems-oriented approach to planning based on recognition that continuity as well as care must be built into the system when multiple numbers of people are concerned. A systems-oriented approach to patient care must be concerned with the psychosocial environment of the institution as a whole and depends upon interdisciplinary agreements and cooperation. Environments within institutions vary, depending on whether the principal orientation is toward recovery care or comfort care, and a systems-oriented plan must, of necessity, recognize and deal with the different kinds of psychosocial issues that confront the nursing staff in these different work settings.

Personalized care means that each patient has a) *continuity of contact* with at least one person who is interested in him as a human being; b) *opportunity for active involvement* in social living to the extent that he is able—including participation in decisions affecting how he will die; and c) *confidence and trust* in those who are providing his care. Making this type of care available to many instead of a privileged few requires that the difficulties of providing it on a day-by-day basis must be taken into account and that authority and responsibility for the psychosocial well-being of patients must be clearly defined and established.

Institutional planning for the improvement of care must be explicitly based on the typical patterns of dying characteristic of different ward settings (42). It is clear that psychosocial supports for the staff need to be built into the system, but what is needed in a geriatric setting is undoubtedly different from what is needed on an intensive-care unit. Special assistance is obviously needed on high-risk wards where death is frequent, but the pressures on the nursing personnel are not necessarily the same. In nursing homes, for instance, nursing care is closely intertwined with such ordinary and usual activities of daily living as eating, sleeping, bathing, and indulging in recreation activities for prolonged periods of time, and it has little to offer in the way of excitement or social reward. In fact, the major problem to be faced in providing personalized care in such settings has mainly to do with making work that is mundane, ordinary, and sometimes psychologically distasteful into a personally meaningful experience. In contrast, on a coronary care unit the stresses have more to do with the conflicting demands of recovery care and comfort care, and personalization of approach may well depend on the availability of two kinds of nursing specialists—experts in life-saving procedures, and those who are proficient in psychosocial aspects of patient care.

Institutional planning needs also to make provision for trouble-shooting services available to any ward or working group for assistance in coping with a disturbing problem involving death. The present pattern of heavy reliance on chaplains and interested psychiatrists (if they happen to be available) needs to be replaced with consultation services, offering a variety of resources, that are well organized and readily available. In-service education programs need to be developed and expanded to provide for counseling services and educational experiences that encompass more than a simple orientation to the technical tasks of the work to be done.

Institutional and community-wide planning for continuity of care for persons facing death means building positions into the system such that responsibility for psychosocial care is made explicit instead of implicit. It is clear that nurses form the group through which continuity and co-ordination take place in institutions for in-patient care, but assignments have typically been task-centered rather than person-centered (43). The talents of the clinical-specialist in nursing can probably have little effect on patient care until explicit authority and responsibility has been more clearly established. More than that, however, nurses who occupy such positions must be willing to assume responsibility for the well-being of patients and to participate actively in modifying the social institutions in which patient care is given.

In this regard, professional nurses may well need to face the reality that the improvement of terminal nursing care depends on their willingness to move away from the one-to-one concept of patient care to an acceptance of leadership in the creation of working climates in which collaboration by many people becomes a major goal (44). The present emphasis within nursing education on the one-to-one nurse-patient relationship as the crux of nursing practice needs to be balanced with a more realistic appraisal of the intermediary position that professional nurses hold within the system of health services, and education for all levels of nursing personnel needs to provide better preparation for coping with the work that involves dying patients and their families.

Recommendations for the Future

One reality seems certain. The improvement of terminal care requires the combined efforts of many disciplines and a critical assessment of the present systems through which patient care is provided. The changes required demand a shift in priorities from technically-oriented care to person-centered care and a reallocation of financial and human resources. A revision in the educational preparation for all of the helping professions is clearly necessary. For maximum effectiveness, it should be multidisciplinary in approach (45). To that end, schools of nursing in university medical centers have a responsibility to take leadership in the development of such programs, both to prepare basic practitioners and to provide continuing education for those already in the field.

It is clear that many registered nurses are in a position to play an important part in improving the psychosocial environments in which dying takes place. To do so, they must be willing to move out of the traditional nurse role and to accept increased responsibility for the quality of care that is offered. Any effort to bring about major changes in nursing practice must deal with the reality that nursing as an occupation occupies an intermediary position within the system. As a service, it is given by many levels of trained and untrained workers, and relatively high rates of job turnover are reported (46). Nursing is work that is performed mainly by women, the bulk of whom support and maintain a dependent nurse role and obtain their social rewards from associations with the goals and activities of medical practice (47). Despite the efforts of leaders in nursing to establish an independent function for the field, the rank-and-file within nursing see their work as secondary to being wife and mother and have little desire to extend their present responsibilities as practitioners (48). Although nurses outnumber physicians in active practice by almost double, nursing as a profession has had relatively little influence as a policy-making group in comparison to organized medicine (49).

The reality seems clear that the direction in which nursing developed was heavily influenced by its historical associations as "woman's work," low in social rewards and status when compared to the work done by men. Yet the provision of a meaningful psychosocial environment for those who are dying is not unlike that which is needed by infants. Their emotional as well as physical needs seem best to be met by persons who have an unhurried approach, a high degree of respect for the rights of the other, and a good deal of patience. Saunders commented about the needs of the dying in this way: "Personal, caring contact is the most important comfort we can give" (50). Care of this sort is marked as much by routine as by challenge, and it is difficult to offer day after day unless there are compensatory social relationships and satisfactions. It provides little in the way of public recognition, and it requires a willingness to become involved in the pain and the pleasure inherent in any meaningful human relationship.

The provision of this kind of care requires nurses and other workers skilled in the art of human interaction and willing to accept a commitment that is far from easy. It is a task that is perhaps not suited to the young but rather can best be done by men and women in their middle years—those who have developed a maturity of outlook out of personal experience with life's vicissitudes and are unafraid to face the reality of their own deaths. Special preparation would undoubtedly be required, but the notion of post-retirement or secondary careers might well be an approach worthy of consideration. Perhaps the ultimate hope of the future lies in the blossoming of what is today in human history an unrecognized and undeveloped human resource—the power and special talent of woman (51).

REFERENCES

1. Florence Nightingale, *Notes on Nursing: What It Is and What It Is Not,* Philadelphia: Lippincott, 1946, p. 75.

2. Patrick J. McGinity and Bernard A. Stotsky, *"The Patient in the Nursing Home,"* *Nursing Forum,* vol. vi, no. 3, 1967, pp. 238–40.

3. *Ibid.*, p. 240.

4. The terms "recovery care" and "comfort care" are used here to distinguish between care where recovery of the patient is still viewed as possible and care where this goal is no longer seen as a possibility (although the period required for dying may vary from minutes to weeks and even months). The perplexities of this matter for doctors and nurses are described by Barney G. Glaser and Anselm L. Strauss in *Awareness of Dying,* Chicago: Aldine, 1965, pp. 177–225.

5. David Sudnow in "Dead on Arrival," *Trans-action,* 5, November 1967, pp. 36–39, reports that age and social worth (presumed "moral character") are factors that influence the degree of life-saving care that is given in a county hospital emergency ward.

6. Jeanne E. Fox, "Reflections on Cancer Nursing," *American Journal of Nursing,* 66, June 1966, pp. 1317–19.

7. The concept of dying trajectory, built around the temporal dimension, serves as the focal point for discussion in Barney G. Glaser and Anselm L. Strauss, *Time For Dying,* Chicago: Aldine, 1968.

8. Virginia Henderson, "The Nature of Nursing," *American Journal of Nursing,* 64, August 1964, p. 63.

9. Frances Reiter, "The Nurse-Clinician," *American Journal of Nursing,* 66, February 1966, p. 274.

10. Hildegard E. Peplau, *Interpersonal Relations in Nursing,* New York: Putnam's, 1952.

11. Among these are Ida Jean Orlando, *The Dynamic Nurse-Patient Relationship,* New York: Putnam's, 1961; Ernestine Wiedenbach, *Clinical Nursing: A Helping Art,* New York: Springer, 1964; and Gertrude B. Ujhely, *Determinants of the Nurse-Patient Relationship,* New York: Springer, 1968.

12. Joan K. Arteberry, "Distance and the Dying Patient," in Betty S. Bergerson, *et al., Current Concepts in Clinical Nursing,* St. Louis: Mosby, 1967, pp. 128–36.

13. Donna Conant Aguilera, "Crisis: Death and Dying," *ANA Clinical Sessions 1968,* New York: Appleton-Century-Crofts, 1968, pp. 269–78.

14. Sister Madeline Clemence, "Existentialism: A Philosophy of Commitment," *American Journal of Nursing,* 66, March 1966, pp. 500–505; Grace Mahlum Sarosi, "A Critical Theory: The Nurse as a Fully Human Person," *Nursing Forum,* vol. vii, no. 4, 1968, pp. 349–64; and Josephine K. Craytor, "Talking with Persons Who Have Cancer," *American Journal of Nursing,* 69, April 1969, pp. 744–48.

15. Richard L. Vanden Bergh, "Let's Talk About Death—To Overcome Inhibiting Emotions," *American Journal of Nursing,* 66, January 1966, pp. 71–73; and Adriaan Verwoerdt and Ruby Wilson, "Communication with

Fatally Ill Patients—Tacit or Explicit?" *American Journal of Nursing,* 67, November 1967, pp. 2307–9, are examples.

16. Jeanne E. Blumberg and Eleanor E. Drummond, *Nursing Care of the Long-Term Patient,* New York: Springer, 1963, pp. 1–10.

17. American Nurses' Association, *Code for Nurses with Interpretive Statements.* A Report Prepared by ANA Committee on Ethical, Legal, and Professional Standards, New York: American Nurses' Association, 1968, p. 3.

18. Anselm L. Strauss, Barney G. Glaser, and Jeanne Quint, "The Nonaccountability of Terminal Care," *Hospitals,* 38, January 16, 1964, pp. 73–87.

19. According to Donna N. Ledney, "Is There a Nurse-Clinician Job in Your Future?" *RN,* 32, August 1969, p. 40, the biggest disadvantage faced by the clinical specialist in effecting changes in patient care is a lack of authority in the institutions.

20. For example, see Nancy S. Keller, "Care Without Coordination—A True Story," *Nursing Forum,* vol. vi, no. 3, 1967, pp. 280–323; and Bernard A. Stotsky and Joan R. Dominick, "Mental Patients in Nursing Homes, I, Social Deprivation and Regression." *Journal of American Geriatric Society,* 17, January 1969, pp. 33–44.

21. See Elizabeth M. Eddy, "Rites of Passage in a Total Institution," *Human Organization,* 23, Spring 1964, pp. 67–75.

22. On patients' reactions to hospitalization, the following are representative: James K. Skipper, *et al.,* "What Communication Means to Patients," *American Journal of Nursing,* 64, April, 1964, pp. 101–103; C. M. Ewell, "What Patients Really Think About Their Nursing Care," *Modern Hospital,* 109, December 1967, pp. 106–108; and Naomi M. Gowan and Miriam Morris, "Nurses' Responses to Expressed Patient Needs," *Nursing Research,* 13, Winter, 1964, pp. 69–71.

23. Pamela A. Holsclaw, "Nursing in High Risk Areas," *Nursing Forum,* vol. iv. no. 4, 1965, pp. 36–45; Donna Sharp, "Lessons From a Dying Patient," *American Journal of Nursing,* 68, July 1968, pp. 1517–20; Jeanne C. Quint, "When Patients Die: Some Nursing Problems," *The Canadian Nurse,* 63, December 1967, pp. 33–36; and Ruth Vreeland and Geraldine L. Ellis, "Stresses on the Nurse in an Intensive-Care Unit," *Journal of American Medical Associaton,* 208, April, 1969, pp. 332–34.

24. For more complete discussion, see Jeanne C. Quint, "The Dying Patient: A Difficult Nursing Problem," *Nursing Clinics of North America,* 2, Philadelphia: Saunders, December 1967, pp. 763–73.

25. The four types of awareness context (closed, suspicion, mutual pretense, and open) their properties, and the consequences for interaction are detailed in Glaser and Strauss, *Awareness of Dying.*

26. Ramona Powell Davidson, "Let's Talk About Death—To Give Care in Terminal Illness," *American Journal of Nursing,* 66, January 1966, pp. 74–75; and Robert F. Klein, *et al., Archives of Internal Medicine,* 122, August 1968, pp. 104–108.

27. Cicely Saunders, "The Last Stages of Life," *American Journal of Nursing,* 65, March 1965, pp. 70–75; and Sister M. Loyola Schwalb, "The Nurse's Role in Assisting Families of Dying Geriatric Patients to Manage Grief and Guilt," *ANA Clinical Sessions,* 1968, New York: Appleton-Century-Crofts, 1968, pp. 110–16.

28. David E. Sobel, "Personalization on the Coronary Care Unit," *American Journal of Nursing,* 69, July, 1969, pp. 1439–42.

29. Bernard A. Stotsky and Joan R. Dominick, "Mental Patients in Nursing Homes, III, Owners, Administrators and Nurses," *Journal of American Geriatric Society,* 17, January 1969, pp. 56–62.

30. Joel Vernick and Janet L. Lunceford, "Milieu Design for Adolescents with Leukemia," *American Journal of Nursing,* 67, March 1967, pp. 559–61; and Leonard E. Gottsman, "Resocialization of the Geriatric Mental Patient," *American Journal of Public Health,* 55, December 1965, pp. 1964–70.

31. Elizabeth A. Bregg, Mary C. Leddy, and Lillian G. Mackenzie, "A Study on the Nurses' Concept of Death," (unpublished study for a course at Teachers College, Columbia University, 1953).

32. Alene Ruth Dickinson, "Nurses' Perceptions of Their Care of Patients Dying with Cancer," (unpublished Ed.D. dissertation, Teachers College, Columbia University, 1966).

33. Jeannette R. Folta, "The Perception of Death," *Nursing Research,* 14, Summer 1965, pp. 232–35.

34. Helen Curtis Smith, "Care of the Dying Patient: A Comparison of Instructional Plans," (unpublished Ed.D. dissertation, Indiana University, 1965); and Jeanne C. Quint, *The Nurse and the Dying Patient,* New York: Macmillan, 1967.

35. Eugenia Helma Waechter, "Death Anxiety in Children with Fatal Illness," unpublished Ph.D. dissertation, Stanford University, 1968.

36. Mary Jo Aspinwall, "Nursing Intervention for a Patient with Myocardial Infarction," *ANA Clinical Sessions 1968,* New York: Appleton-Century-Crofts, 1968, pp. 209–16; and Jeanne C. Quint, "Mastectomy: Symbol of Cure or Warning Sign?" *GP,* 29, March 1964, pp. 119–24.

37. There are at least five such reports in *ANA Clinical Sessions 1968,* New York: Appleton-Century-Crofts, 1968.

38. Wilma N. Lewis, "A Time to Die," Nursing Forum, vol. iv, no. 1, 1965, p. 24.

39. JoAnna DeMeyer, "The Environment of the Intensive Care Unit," Nursing Forum, vol. vi, no. 3, 1967, pp. 262–72.

40. Dorothy E. Burchett, "Factors Affecting Nurse-Patient Interaction in a Geriatric Setting," ANA Regional Conferences, New York: Appleton-Century-Crofts, 1967, pp. 123–30.

41. Catherine J. Anderson, "Alienation in the Aged: Implications for Psychiatric Geriatric Nursing," ANA Regional Conferences, New York: Appleton-Century-Crofts, 1967, pp. 115–22.

42. Barney G. Glaser and Anselm L. Strauss, Time for Dying, pp. 251–59; and also Jeanne C. Quint, Anselm L. Strauss, and Barney G. Glaser, "Improving Nursing Care of the Dying," Nursing Forum, vol. vi., no. 4, 1967, pp. 368–78.

43. Basil S. Georgopoulos, "The Hospital System and Nursing: Some Basic Problems and Issues," Nursing Forum, vol. v., no. 3, 1966, p. 19.

44. The special competencies required for this type of leadership are described by Warren G. Bennis, "Post-Bureaucratic Leadership," Trans-Action, 6, July / August 1969, pp. 44–51.

45. Elisabeth Kübler-Ross, On Death and Dying, New York: Macmillan, 1969, pp. 218–39, provides persuasive evidence of the need for multidisciplinary dialogue that includes the dying patient.

46. According to Lorraine L. Hill, et al., "Is There a Correlation Between Attrition in Nursing Schools and Job Turnover in Professional Nursing?" Nursing Outlook, 11, September 1963, p. 666, the Department of Health, Education and Welfare reported turnover rates for full-time professional nurses to be 66.9 per cent in 1955 and 67 per cent in 1963.

47. William A. Glaser, "Nursing Leadership and Policy: Some Cross National Comparisons," Fred Davis (ed.), The Nursing Profession, New York: Wiley, 1966, p. 27.

48. Ibid., p. 25.

49. Facts About Nursing, New York: American Nurses' Association, 1968, p. 7, shows a total of 593,694 registered nurses actively employed in nursing in the United States in 1966 and (p. 208), 313, 559, physicians in practice during that year.

50. Cicely Saunders, "The Moment of Truth: Care of the Dying Person," in Leonard Pearson (ed.), Death and Dying, Cleveland: Case-Western Reserve University Press, 1969, p. 67.

51. So long as women consider their special competencies as inferior to

rather than different from those of men, they can probably have little effect on the society as a whole. As Phillip Goldberg, "Are Women Prejudiced Against Women?" *Trans-Action,* 5, April 1968, p. 30, points out, women consider themselves as inferior to men even in the traditionally feminine fields of work.

Avery D. Weisman

PSYCHOSOCIAL CONSIDERATIONS IN TERMINAL CARE*

Psychosocial Problems in Terminal Care

The goals of terminal care are those of medical care in general. Because the terminal patient will not recover, however, special emphasis must be placed upon the continuity, rather than the cure that medical care implies. In general, medical care has four major purposes: 1) Diagnosis; 2) Treatment; 3) Relief; and 4) Safe Conduct. The first two purposes need no further explanation. The last two are central considerations for appropriate care of a patient who will not recover. Adequate relief of

* Findings presented in this paper are based upon a study funded by the Center for Studies of Suicide Prevention, NIMH Grant No. MH15903. Project Omega is a multidisciplinary study of preterminal illness and suicide, based upon the psychological autopsy method.

pain is mandatory; almost everything else is secondary to pain relief. One of the most demoralizing fears of terminal illness is that of suffering and pain. Many people fear not only pain, but also having to ask for, and even plead for, adequate medication. The psychosocial stigma of requiring medication should not be overlooked; patients who are regarded as "good" or "cooperative" are often those who are stoical about pain and discomfort. In addition to primary pain relief, there is the element of "secondary suffering," the emotional and social isolation and disparagement that may follow inadequate control of pain. Conversely, terminal and preterminal patients find the future easier to bear when the people who will take care of them explicitly promise to relieve pain.

The goal called "Safe Conduct" is one that is an imperative for the care of terminal patients. Most patients do not need this guarantee; they will recover, following accurate diagnosis and appropriate treatment. If they are afflicted with a chronic disease, then symptomatic relief can be provided. But it is safe conduct that the doctor and other concerned professionals must promise, even pledge to those patients who are obliged to surrender their autonomy as time goes on and must yield essential control to someone else. After all, the difference between a healthy dependency and a sick victim is entirely a problem of being able to trust and to be trusted.

Although "terminal care" refers to the final weeks, days, and hours of life, it really begins at the unspecified point when the aim of treatment is no longer to cure, but to preserve life and to relieve distress as long as possible. More specifically, terminal care should begin in the preterminal period, just before the patient begins the descent until death.

A person who dies does not die only of a fatal disease. He dies as a person, someone who is significant within a distinct psychosocial context. Consequently, he encounters a series of critically significant events —we call these "Omega Points"—on the way to the final cessation of function, death. Terminal care rightfully includes members of the family, close friends and colleagues, even professionals. This is not a matter of mere compassion for the bereaved. Therapeutically, people who stand to lose the most by a patient's death may be those who can give the most and contribute to safe conduct and a dignified, harmonious exitus.

Stages of Fatal Illness

Salient psychosocial problems occur at any stage of fatal illness, and we must realize that such problems not only differ from stage to stage, but also from person to person, depending on the diagnosis, age, social and cultural resources, interpersonal affiliations and disengagements, economic independence, and ethnic customs, as well as upon physical and personal incapacity. We cannot oversimplify, nor should we overgeneralize, even though three stages of fatal illness can be outlined.

Stage I is the period from the onset of symptoms until the diagnosis is made. Few people are under medical observation when Stage I begins. But they may need family and friends to encourage them to seek help. Most of the psychosocial problems during Stage I are related to delay, denial, and postponement.

Stage II is the interval between diagnosis and the onset of terminal decline. Most treatment is given during this period, but from the psychosocial standpoint few people pass directly from a healthy state to Stage II. Furthermore, regardless of the treatment given during Stage II, the psychological problems are recognized by changes in the equilibrium of denial and acceptance. The major defensive operations are those of mitigation and displacement.

Stage III starts when active treatment is found to have diminishing value. Therapeutic emphasis gradually shifts from cure to control to symptomatic relief and nursing care. Doctors are apt to begin withdrawing during the incipient decline and to become more routine in ministrations. Patients are increasingly faced with the prospect of yielding personal control to someone else, and of coming to terms with cessation. Stage III is the sickness until death.

At each stage, the psychosocial problems of the patient's potential survivors should be anticipated. These are not only general problems of bereavement, but also highly practical issues, such as contending with the disruption of households, financial problems, critical communications, or what to tell children. Planning is both long- and short-range. Bereavement does not start at the moment of death, but at any stage when a significant person realizes that loss is inevitable and that drastic change cannot be avoided.

We are not clear about the criteria that enable us to diagnose the "high risk" family, people who are apt to develop abnormal or protracted grief responses. We know, however, that the recently bereaved are vulnerable to a variety of disorders, somatic and psychological, and that total bereavement may represent the confluence of many smaller griefs. The essence of community medicine is to prevent people from becoming primary patients themselves. So an ounce of prevention may save a much larger investment of skill and resources later on.

Psychosocial Management of Terminal Patients

Psychosocial management is intended to prevent and control "secondary suffering" from terminal illness. To do so, therapists should understand that patients may fear both annihilation and alienation, and that specific fear of dying is often less disturbing than is dread of being deserted. Dying patients may not be clinically anxious, but they will show impairment of self-esteem, endangerment, annihilation-anxiety, and alienation-anxiety. Psychotherapeutic intervention can test itself by assessing how effectively these symptoms can be controlled.

Briefly, impairment of self-esteem is expressed in feelings of worthlessness, quiet withdrawal from customary interests, unusual tendencies to mirror what the staff seems to expect. Unless specifically investigated, a busy staff may misidentify gathering depression and derogation and confuse inertness with cooperation. Terminal illness is seldom marked by excessive protests about guilt and retribution, except early in the diagnostic period, not toward the end. Feelings of worthlessness, however, may be subtly intertwined with the general sickness unto death, as in the following case:

Example (Impairment of Self-Esteem): A fifty-three-year-old man, dying of lymphosarcoma, gradually realized that his remissions were becoming fewer, and that relief of his symptoms was less complete. He followed doctor's orders completely, and cooperated in whatever was decided. He also knew that there was no alternative, other than to take medication and to be periodically transfused. For many months, he was passive and diffident in dealing with the staff and with his family, fearing that he might, unwittingly, give offense.

As he deteriorated, the patient's manner changed. He became surly, sarcastic, and recalcitrant. When his family visited, he complained constantly about his treatment, and doubted the sincerity or competence of doctors he had formerly praised. He became loud, arrogant, and dogmatic, insisting upon having his way in all matters.

In trying to fathom the patient's personality change, the psychiatrist finally realized that this man had been taken over completely by an invincible, tyrannical, and fatal disease, against which all treatment, conciliation, and struggle were unavailing.

The patient's feeling of progressive deterioration, weakness and worthlessness led him to feel that he had nothing left to bargain with. The disease was like an invader that takes over a country. The patient became its victim, and became inseparable from the disease. Therefore, he *became* the disease. His manner of pseudo-arrogance was an image of an illness that could no longer be withstood. His loss of autonomy, self-respect, and personal esteem for what mattered most were converted into the opposite. Just as he felt victimized, he sought to dominate and to make others feel worthless.

Endangerment refers to unnecessary regression, such as extreme denial, projection, magical expectations about recovery, and even hallucinatory experiences. Although few terminal patients attempt suicide, they may respond to the danger of their situation by false optimism, careless disregard of symptoms, and excessive preoccupation with peripheral problems.

Example (Endangerment): Shortly before her death, a fifty-eight-year-old woman executive started to make plans for a new business venture. She had long known about the scope and severity of her illness, carcinoma of the uterus. Now, however, although she felt very sick, she seemed to believe that everything was under control and that she had a viable future. She wanted to go back to her home town, which she left about fifteen years before, and to begin a project that was feasible only for someone who was both younger and in good health. It was significant that this woman had continued to work until progressive pain, fatigue, and disability required so much medication that executive decisions could no longer be made. Her associates continued to seek her opinions, even in her last hospitalization, but these were therapeutic gestures, intended to maintain her self-esteem in the face of growing endangerment.

Annihilation-anxiety is fear of dying and disintegration, often associated with impaired reality testing. The sense of being a victim, that is, dependency without trust, may precede overt anxiety.

Example (Annihilation-anxiety): As a rule, patients cannot directly say that they fear total disintegration, but they do reveal themselves in secondary complaints and convictions about losing their hold on reality. "This food doesn't taste right. Don't they care what they feed me any more?" "I'm just a number to these people here. Why do they want to get rid of me? Do they think I'm dying or something?" "People don't make sense. They say I'm sick, and I've got to believe them." "I'm an old woman and I wish they'd leave me alone to die in peace. But they seem to want to drive me crazy, first!"

The emphasis upon impersonality is almost diagnostic. The staff and family become "they," or "those people," just as the patient fears becoming only a number or a thing. Fear of losing sanity means fear of losing whatever makes sense and becoming nothing at all. "Doctor, I look in the mirror every morning, and see my face hanging on the bones. Everything I do goes wrong, nothing works right any more. What is becoming of me, anyway?"

Alienation-anxiety stems from fear of separation, especially separation from key supports and rewarding activities. It is important to appreciate that much of one's personality is attached to things in the world, and that we die not only *from* illnesses but also *to* many other activities that generate our sense of being alive. Alienation refers to both major and minor losses, partial griefs and total bereavement. As life slowly dwindles, women patients worry about their homes, men about their jobs. The future is an illusion.

Sometimes awareness of progressive alienation shows itself in preoccupation with trivia, as if attachment to something routine and smaller than life-size will preserve contact with the world. Loneliness and depression are more prevalent than anxiety during the terminal period.

Example (Alienation-anxiety): An eighty-year-old woman who suffered from generalized arteriosclerosis complained that her family ignored her, contrary to fact. She could not recall recent events or current conversations, but felt utterly bereft and vulnerable. She talked about people who had been dead for many years, especially about a favorite brother. She wept about problems of long ago, and on one occasion wondered why her parents had not visited her.

We have often observed that the terminal phase of a fatal illness may begin after the loss of a pet, such as a dog, cat or canary. Changes in the neighborhood, which mean that old friends move away, are apt to create alienation from everything that remains.

Appropriate management depends upon accurately monitoring the degree of denial and acceptance demonstrated by the patient. Most terminal patients show three types of denial during their illness: Type I is denial of the facts of illness; Type II is denial of the implications and extensions of illness; and Type III is denial of mortality itself. A patient who denies the diagnosis, is an example of Type I. A patient who acknowledges that he has a tumor, but ascribes his symptoms to insignificant causes unrelated to the primary diagnosis, is an example of Type II. A patient who accepts the diagnosis and progress of his illness, but talks as if he would ultimately recover and not die, is an example of Type III denial. Most terminal patients, regardless of how recently they have been diagnosed, show only denial, Type II and III. Only an occasional patient seems utterly free of denial.

Example (Type I): A forty-six-year-old man who sustained a second heart attack denied that he suspected a recurrence when the chest pain developed. In the first attack, pain had spread from his chest to the left shoulder, then down his arm to the finger tips. This time, however, the pain had stopped at his wrist. Therefore, he knew that it was not another heart attack.

Example (Type II): A seventy-two-year-old man had his left thumb amputated because of a melanoma under the nail. Several weeks later, he returned for an axillary biopsy. If the nodes were "positive," he said, this meant that all the tumor cells had been caught, much as debris might be filtered out by a drainpipe. If the nodes were "negative," this would indicate that there had been no spread and that the initial operation had removed all the tumor.

Example (Type III): A twenty-eight-year-old father was diagnosed as having Hodgkin's Disease. Within six months his four-year-old son died of acute lymphatic leukemia. It was reliably reported that the son, like so many leukemic children, was especially endearing, and that his last words were, "Tomorrow will be Christmas."

The patient did not openly grieve for his son, but early in his course blamed himself for "transmitting" sickness to the boy. He was both happy and angry about having a fatal illness—"happy" because he would not live to be a helpless old man, "angry" because nature was getting rid of him, as a superfluous misfit.

As months went on, the patient followed treatments, but reported correctly that doctors said he could go on for many years. It really didn't matter, he said, because people will always look after me. What's the use in thinking about a death that may never come. Even when his symptoms became very severe, he maintained that nature was so arbitrary that he might live to be an old man, despite his illness.

Patients fluctuate in the balance between denial and acceptance during the course of illness, but as a rule the tendency is to surrender denial and to replace it with acceptance. Unusual persistence of denial is often brought on by fear of alienation and endangerment. Efforts to encourage denial may have an opposite effect; alienation is heightened, people withdraw more and more, and communication becomes more and more remote and ritualized.

Appropriate Interventions

Given a chance, dying people are willing to talk about their plight. Militant efforts to deny and to mitigate may silence a terminal patient, but this does not mean that he has been helped toward a significant and dignified death.

Even experienced therapists find themselves withdrawing from the presence of death. Despite efforts to remain in contact, openness near the abyss may not be possible; the threat of annihilation is still too great. Faced with a terminal patient, many well-meaning people feel a natural revulsion. Some are put off by the sights and smells of disease. Others are distraught by the atmosphere of hopelessness and helplessness which infects all who are present. Nevertheless, given a modicum of persistence and courage to combat their own dismay, constructive psychosocial interventions can be honestly and realistically planned and carried out, in contrast to the customary procedure in which death is denied or the patient is subjected to vainglorious reassurances. One of the guiding principles is that global reassurance *of* the patient is seldom reassurance *for* the patient, but rather denial of the patient's singular reality.

There are no inflexible rules that do not contradict the principle that dying is an individual matter, and therefore should be individualized. Management is most appropriate when the therapist at the outset projects his imagination into the future toward the "Omega Point" and considers when, where, how, and with whom this inexorable death ought to occur. If he can make this Omega Point explicit enough, he can work backward through the successive steps necessary to achieve this goal which, simply, is an appropriate death.

Rules and Reminders for the Therapist

Accept the terminal patient according to what he would be like *without* the illness and disease. Otherwise we may fall victim to a tendency to confuse the person of the patient with the disease, lesion, or symptoms.

Make allowances for the deterioration and disability caused by illness. But this should not mean supporting regressive defenses.

Permit, encourage the patient to talk about how illness has changed him. But emphasize the person who is sick, not disease in the abstract.

Be sure that you understand the difference between disease, fatal sickness, and the sickness until death (terminality itself).

Ask about the people, possessions, and pursuits that meant the most during the patient's healthy life. This includes both factors that supported his ego ideals and self-esteem, and factors that made him feel discouraged, demoralized, or defeated.

Preservation of the highest practical communication and behavior also preserves self-esteem. This is even more important than the fact of illness itself.

Monitor your own feelings: You are not immune to denial, dissimulation, antipathy, and fears of personal annihilation. Do not be ashamed to admit that caring for the dying is, itself, exposure to endangerment. Therefore, do not hesitate to enlist the assistance of significant key persons, and other kinds of support.

Safe conduct requires acceptance, clarity, candor, compassion, and mutual accessibility.

Time your confrontations to meet what is relevant to the moment. Do not rush to talk about death or to underscore the gloomiest side of the illness, nor should you persist with empty optimism when facts no longer justify it.

Unless a patient's physical condition and state of consciousness have compromised his judgment, do not exclude him from decisions and information about illness.

While we do not allow the family to make decisions for the patient, we encourage decisions with the patient, since he will yield control to others as the illness progresses.

Do not hesitate to assess the specific changes that death will bring to the family. The optimal attitude toward the terminal situation is one of compassionate objectivity. A therapist who is stringently clinical is scarcely a therapist, but a technician. If he becomes a surrogate mourner he is not very helpful, since he displays his helplessness. The therapist remains sufficiently detached to be the intermediary between family and other professional staff, without usurping the prerogatives of either.

Help survivors to accept the inevitable death, but do not force a theory of bereavement and mourning upon anyone. In addition to bereavement, families may need help with the practical problems of readjustment to an altered life.

Recognize signs of iatrogenic distortions and psychosocial complications that the terminal situation creates. False hopes, displacement of interest to the illusory or to the trivial, withdrawal of personal concern, and premature burial are but a few signs of iatrogenic problems.

The Psychosocial Therapist

The professional credentials and field of specialization are less important for the qualified therapist than is his capacity to be there—alert, compassionate, available, and reasonably responsive to the plight. Terminal patients cannot be fractionated into special organs and problems, but there is always a strong tendency for therapists to fractionate themselves and to forfeit parts of their own responsibility. Consequently, those who undertake primary responsibility for safe conduct and appropriate psychosocial management need to assess and to correct for their own biases and distortions. Excessive despair, for example, is merely an inverted image of unrealistic expectations. If we are afraid of working in vain, then it is likely that we are working with a sense of vanity. To be significant does not mean that we are all-important or required to have magical powers. The psychosocial therapist works most effectively when he realizes that he is a significant part of the psychosocial field, and that the predominant task is to help patients die their own deaths. An appropriate death, if such things exist, is, after all, not an ideal death. Rather, an appropriate death is one that a person might choose, had he a choice.

Ruth D. Abrams

THE RESPONSIBILITY
OF SOCIAL WORK
IN TERMINAL CANCER

"Long illness is so humiliating," said a brilliant young woman dying of acute leukemia. These few words suggest the feelings of fear, frustration, anger, guilt, and rejection frequently noted in patients in the terminal stage of malignancy. When these feelings are turned inward, they frequently cause the patient to develop symptoms of depression, or, when turned outward, the relationships with significant caregivers are threatened. In addition, when outbursts of anger or despair were contrary to the patient's life style, the good image he desperately wants to leave behind is altered. These areas of potential threat to the medical personnel, the survivors-to-be, and most important, the patient, suggest that the social worker's role should be significant. Certainly the terminal cancer patient relies primarily on his physician. However, frequently the social worker can help sustain the patient's faith in the physician, family members, and himself, especially in the terminal stage when the patient often feels rejected or abandoned by the medical personnel who are responsible primarily for helping him live rather than helping him die.

The Social Worker's Area of Concern

In spite of a patient's "poor" prognosis, many of us are aware that cancer patients often live longer than is medically anticipated. How these patients adjust to their illness and how their families react play a large part in prolonging life—life that can be useful and serene. The goal of the social worker's treatment, no matter what the life expectancy may be, is to help the patient live with himself to the best of his ability and desire and, whenever possible, to soften the burden of pain and suffering which survivors-to-be often experience. Although in this presentation the focus is primarily upon the patient with terminal cancer, it is a well-known fact that frequently close family members need help from professional personnel, not only to maintain their equilibrium for the patient's sake, but also to prevent their own physical, mental, and emotional deterioration. We must not forget that members of the patient's family are part of the treatment team and thus important as caregivers.

Too frequently, the nurse, social worker, laboratory technician, and even the minister or physician tend to shield themselves when confronted by the terminal cancer patient—by silence, by changing the subject, by speedy withdrawal, or by referral of all questions to a higher authority. With increasing patient sophistication, social workers are on the spot. The patient knows we have some of the answers. We can no longer change the subject or rush to our peers or supervisors for advice without increasing the emotional stress within the patient. In essence, we can no longer expect the patient to have more courage than we ourselves possess. The social worker must have self-awareness and the knowledge to help these patients at this crisis period.

What do social workers have to believe in or accept before offering support to the patient with terminal cancer? First, that "crisis brings both danger and opportunity" (1). Second, that social workers are in a unique position to anticipate possible or probable crisis situations and therefore are useful in case finding. Third, that prevention is one of the major functions and contributions of the helping professions. Fourth, that crisis intervention is not contrary to the principles and skills of the helping professions. Fifth, that intervention can bring about change for better mental health. Sixth, that short-term therapy has a definite place and is often the treatment of choice. Seventh, that it is possible and necessary to investigate while one heals. And lastly, that neglecting to make this particular type of skill available to people in crisis may block the help they really need and want and have a right to expect.

This presentation stems from the conviction that each professional who treats a terminal cancer patient has an obligation to add to his particular skill the type of support for which the patient expresses or implies a need. Experience reinforces the observation that each crisis period in the course of a malignant condition requires a different kind of support (2).

This paper will focus on the responsibility of social workers in the face of an irreversible malignancy. The material is drawn from experience in several clinical and research projects with terminally ill cancer patients, varying in respect to economic levels, sites of lesions, and sophistication about the disease. At all times, the case work methods used were generic to the profession of social work. Although based on my experience as a social worker in medical and psychiatric settings, the content of this paper applies equally to social workers in all settings and from all the specialties of social work.

The discussion will focus on the following areas: 1) the attitudes and reactions of professional and lay personnel and the patient himself to the diagnosis of cancer, especially at the time the disease process becomes irreversible; 2) the generic skills of social work applicable to the situation created by the patient with a terminal malignancy; and 3) the responsibility of social work to the bereaved-to-be not only during the process of separation, but also throughout the period of bereavement.

The Diagnosis of Cancer: Its Significance in Treatment

Before describing findings relative to how the terminal cancer patient reacts to and copes with his diagnosis and treatment, I wish to stress that it is almost imperative in treating the cancer patient at any stage of the illness to understand one's own reactions to the diagnosis of cancer. This does not imply that each one of us needs to undergo psychotherapy to understand his own reactions. However, if one regards cancer as hopeless, that a particular site of the deteriorating disease is repulsive, or that a specific type of treatment is unacceptable, then discussion should be sought with consultants in this field.

The following example is illustrative of the need to know one's own reactions and attitudes. A young professional person, a nurse, recorded her experiences with a patient in the advanced stages of carcinoma of the breast as follows: "Every day when I entered her room, I felt a strong upsurge of feelings of guilt. I was going to live while she of my own age was about to die. I know she wanted to talk to me, but I always turned it into something light, a little joke, or into some evasive reassurance which had to fail. The patient knew and I knew. But as she saw my desperate attempt to escape and felt my anxiety, she took pity on me and kept to herself what she wanted to share with another human being—and so she died and did not bother me" (3).

Cancer Is Different

The question of whether or not patients with cancer are "different" from those with other chronic or fatal diseases has been raised. I am inclined to affirm that they are, and for two distinct reasons: The first is the constant anxiety for the patient because of the threatening fatal illness, the course of which he cannot alter. This is unlike the situation of the heart patient, who through rest and medication frequently can stabilize his illness, or the diabetic patient who controls his illness through diet and insulin. The second reason for this "difference" relates to the attitude of family members and the professional personnel charged with the cancer patient's care. The family is usually doubtful of a cure and hence remains fearful of a fatal outcome. Certainly, the professional personnel involved adopt a guarded attitude. Perhaps it is this attitude on the part of the professional personnel that so often increases apprehension and promotes mounting anxieties. In *Psychological Variables in*

Human Cancer (4), Philip West and his associate found that "highly defensive, markedly anxious, inhibited persons ran a much more rapid course from carcinoma than did the more relaxed patient." The addition of this concept that psychosomatic states affect the course of the disease adds even more authority to the necessity for further study of patients' reactions to their disease and examination of the need for thorough understanding of supportive services to control or relieve the pent-up emotions of these patients.

It is a recognized fact that the initial response to crisis is anger and rage. And what crisis could be more devastating than the threat to life! It was not unexpected to find in a research study of sixty terminal cancer patients that fifty-six—that is, 93 per cent of these patients—responded to their condition by directing anger at themselves or others. These patients appeared to have a need to find a cause for their illness (5). The illness was their fault or it was someone else's fault. In fact, all but four of these patients spontaneously assigned responsibility for having their disease to their misdeeds or those of others. Thirty-one reproached themselves. It was the venereal disease contracted years ago, a misdeed, a blow, their own negligence, or their own misconception of what cancer was that resulted in the present fatal illness. Twenty-five patients placed blame on others. This group felt that their cancer had been caused initially by inheritance or contagion, a blow dealt by their mother, father, husband, or child, overexertion in the care of a sick relative, too frequent sexual demands made upon them, or their doctor's negligence.

In addition to feelings of guilt are attitudes denoting fear that the disease is "dirty" or repellent and the feelings of inferiority and inadequacy which many patients express or imply during the course of terminal treatment. There are considerable data to support the finding that change in one's body image threatens the core of one's being and the meaning of one's life. In a study of sixty-two gynecological cancer patients, the greatest percentage (fifty-eight) were housewives having the responsibility of their homes, their husbands, and their children (6). Many represented the pivot around which the home took shape. These patients usually were not the providers for the home, rather they were the guardians. Taking from the wife or mother her normal duties presented threats to her functioning as housekeeper, wife, and mother. Sim-

ilar fears regarding maintaining a role are expressed by male patients
with cancer of the genital organs.

The mutilation which takes place at the different stages of the illness
can and does foster feelings of guilt, inferiority, and inadequacy. These
feelings frequently are harder to bear than the threat to life itself. It
would appear essential that in situations where the patient becomes unusually fearful, angry, or depressed, social workers consider how they
can help the patient with these uncomfortable feelings. Frequently, the
patient needs to have the opportunity to reveal his reactions, to understand them and to have them accepted. The patient at such times needs
support from a professional member of the team who can and will indicate either by verbal or nonverbal activity that there is nothing about
the patient's illness, the effect of treatment or his reactions to the present crisis, which cannot be understood and dealt with by the caregivers.
Through the mental health practitioner's acceptance, the patient regains
confidence in himself and in the significant caregivers in his environment.

Denial and Depression: The
Patient Is Coping

The outstanding characteristic of these patients is that they usually
are concerned about just how ill they are and often are aware that they
have reached the hopeless stage of their illness. Yet at this time the patient usually indicates an unwillingness or inability to talk about his
present situation. In the early terminal stage he uses the defense of denial
in the content of his communication, coupled with increased physical or
mental activity. In the later terminal phase the patient often withdraws
into himself with symptoms of depression. In fact, compulsive activity
and avoidance of any reference to the advance of the disease itself cause
the caregiver to assume that the patient is denying its progression. In
the later terminal stage, when the patient may be bedridden and
dependent physically for most of his care, his method of avoidance now
suggests the depressed patient who withdraws from contact with significant others and who has feelings of worthlessness and even of anger. He

may become almost mute. This avoidance and withdrawal generates the rejection of his caregivers and family members. Rejection and abandonment dominate the atmosphere between patient and caregivers. It is to be understood that often these uncomfortable, unacceptable reactions are fostered as much by the dying patient as by those around him. The important aspect of care at this time centers around whether or not to disturb the denial or the depression to which the patient is clinging. To this the social worker must be alert. She, as well as the other members of the professional team, must identify these defense devices chosen by the patient and learn how to deal with them. Most often the patient gives evidence that he wishes his defenses to be supported, to be guarded. Only when the defense or reaction is causing changes which are disturbing to the patient, *not the caregiver,* should interventive procedures be considered. Usually this intervention takes the form of telling the patient more of the truth than he is asking.

The Social Worker's Contribution
to Care

Although it is the physician, the clergyman, or a member of the patient's family, and not the social worker, who decides what each patient should know about his diagnosis and prognosis, the social worker can and should be called upon and be able to contribute much significant data in helping in this decision. With the data she has collected and by the relationships she has established, the social worker frequently is in a strategic position to offer advice in regard to what the patient knows, wants to know, and can accept about his diagnosis. The social worker may suggest who should take care of the patient's anxieties and make sure that this information is communicated and hopefully accepted. However, experience has shown that these patients usually do not present evidence of changes in personality patterns, provided they have the support they need and want. The problem of responsibility for determining whether or not to intervene with the patient's defenses should be considered not only by the clinical team, but equally by the professional personnel in other agencies and in the community outside the hospital setting. In other words, there are times when the social worker reaches out to the professional personnel, the family, friends, clergy, and community both to deepen her understanding of the patient and his needs and to translate these findings to his caregivers.

The Bereaved: Planning
for Loss

Now let us focus on the social worker's responsibility to the bereaved. This silent majority of caregivers frequently suffer from the same feelings of fear, anger, guilt, and rejection as the dying patient. Actually, the primary caregiver inevitably becomes the most rejected member of the team. His degree of rejection increases as the life of the patient is prolonged. Not only do the physician and medical personnel tend to shun the patient's family, but the patient himself frequently withdraws from those closest to him.

Attention to the primary caregiver requires first awareness and then use of the social worker's skills. In a sense, this preparatory indoctrination for final separation has implications for a plan in which effective grief work can be carried out. The need for this type of preparation for optimum recovery from loss has been highlighted by the data collected on the bereaved in the Conjugal Bereavement Study (7), Laboratory of Community Psychiatry, Harvard Medical School, and in my private practice. There is sufficient evidence to confirm recent findings by other investigators that men and women under the age of forty-five who have lost a spouse through death have a higher incidence of medical and mental ill health than the average population. In our bereavement study twenty-six out of the total sixty-nine primary subjects died of cancer. In other words, these were not sudden or unexpected deaths. There was time to prepare, possibly even to do some anticipatory grief work. Nonetheless, at thirteen months following loss, less than one-half of these widows and widowers had made a relatively good adjustment. Only four of the twenty-six survivors had been known to social service during their spouse's illness and only one of these had had regular supportive therapy, even though treatment and death took place in general hospitals with well-established and available social service departments. It might be assumed that support may have been offered by other professional individuals within or outside the medical setting, such as physicians, nurses, or community mental health workers, but the data yield little evidence that such support was regularly offered or sustained.

In addition, this study corroborates a repeated finding of other social workers in hospital settings that the bereaved rarely return for any type of emotional help from a caregiver in the setting where the patient was cared for. Formerly, it was my belief that to return to the scene of the tragedy was more than the survivor could bear. However, it is my impression, based on further study, that care of the bereaved by the social worker was discontinued not because the latter did not reach out with appropriate empathy and support but because the bereaved tended to assume that he was no longer significant once the patient had died.

This brief reference to the needs of the bereaved in the terminal care situation suggests that the preventive and interventive skills of social work should be applied to this particular population at risk. Some plan should be considered wherein one of the physicians treating the dying patient should designate a professional social worker within or outside the setting whose focus of responsibility would be to determine the needs of the bereaved-to-be, and, wherever indicated, offer ongoing preventive mental health services. In order to achieve this, the medical profession must be alerted to its responsibility not only to help the patient to live as long as possible with grace, but also to offer the same opportunity to the bereaved-to-be, so that they may live more effectively and comfortably following loss. How to develop such a program, how to make this type of plan acceptable to the physician, nurse, social worker, and even to the bereaved-to-be, is a challenge to the profession of social work.

REFERENCES

1. H. J. Parad and G. Caplan, "A Framework for Studying Families in Crisis," in *Crisis Intervention,* ed. Howard J. Parad, New York: Family Service Association of America, 1965.

2. R. D. Abrams, "The Patient with Cancer—His Changing Pattern of Communication," *New England Journal of Medicine,* February 10, 1966.

3. I. S. Wolfe, "The Magnificence of Understanding," in *Should the Patient Know the Truth,* ed. Samuel Standard and Helmut Nathan, New York: Springer Publishing Co., Inc., 1955, p. 32.

4. J. A. Generelli and F. J. Kirkner (eds.), *Psychological Variables of Cancer,* University of California Press, 1954.

5. R. D. Abrams and J. E. Finesinger, "Guilt Reactions in Patients with Cancer," *Cancer,* Vol. 6, May 1953.

6. R. D. Abrams, "Social Service and Cancer," *Journal of Obstetrics and Gynecology,* November 1945.

7. R. D. Abrams, "A Guide for the Caregivers and Families of the Cancer Patient." (In preparation.)

Care of the Family of the Patient

David Maddison and Beverley Raphael

THE FAMILY OF
THE DYING PATIENT*

The relatives of the terminally ill patient will manifest a wide variety of responses, healthy or pathological, to the bewildering situation in which they are involved. For a period of time, which may be substantial and which is almost always of indefinite duration, they live with the certain knowledge of impending major object loss, often with the continuous presence of pain and suffering, futility and helplessness. They must cope with this situation until the threatened loss becomes an actuality, when they have to face the further crisis of bereavement itself.

The dynamics involved are complex, and while many theoretical formulations are borne out by clinical experience, most of them have only a limited consensus in current research findings. Our knowledge of the

* The preparation of this paper was made possible by financial support from the Foundations Fund for Research in Psychiatry, the National Health and Medical Research Council of Australia, and the New South Wales Institute of Psychiatry.

effects of bereavement, while highlighting the scope of intervention and the perceived discrepancies between what is needed and what is able to be provided from present resources, is at best only a retrospective glimpse of the problem of the dying patient. Even with our limited current knowledge, however, the implications for medical practice, from the point of view of primary, secondary, and tertiary prevention, are extensive and obvious. Our very limitations nevertheless make clear the need for further research.

Understanding of the problem is enhanced by considering the family under three headings:

1) Individual family members.
2) The family group.
3) The family in its relationship to society.

Reactions of Individual Family Members

These reactions vary through an extremely wide range, from mobilization of "healthy" coping techniques to extremely "pathological" responses. Some of the outstanding factors which help to determine individual responses are: (i) the specific relationship of the individual to the dying person; (ii) areas of conflict mobilization; (iii) the defensive operations employed; (iv) the perception of the situation as a crisis.

THE SPECIFIC RELATIONSHIP WITH THE DYING PERSON

Research in this area has shown the importance of certain "pairings":

1. *Marital Partners.* Increased mortality and morbidity in both widow and widower have been demonstrated in a number of studies, for example, Maddison and Viola (1968), Parkes (1964), Rees and Lutkins (1967), Marris (1958), and Kraus and Lilienfeld (1959). These studies show that death may be pathogenic for the survivors and imply the possibility of contributing factors occurring during the terminal illness, although the duration of illness prior to death shows no correlation with good or bad outcome in widows (Maddison and Viola, 1968).

2. *The Parent and the Dying Child.* The impending death of her child constitutes a massive threat to a mother, who has been shown (Natterson and Knudsen, 1960) to react in three characteristic phases when the terminal illness lasts four months or more. An initial phase of denial is followed by a rational phase, and then by a calm acceptance terminally. It has also been shown that a parent defends against this threat in a way which raises urinary 17-OHCS excretion to levels which are characteristic for that particular parent, and further that these levels are lower for the more effective defenders (Wolff *et al.,* 1964). Chodoff *et al.* (1964) suggested that isolation of affect, denial, and motor activity may be relatively "healthy" defenses in many cases. In an extensive investigation of the parents of children with cystic fibrosis, Meyerowitz and Kaplan (1967) have shown that severe emotional reactions are almost universal, either in response to the diagnosis itself or to the requirements of management. These reactions may include denial, anxiety, and confusion. Important factors in this context would be the degree of identification with the particular child, a conscious or unconscious ambivalence in the parent's attitude to him, the nature and intensity of the fantasies about the child's future which now will not be fulfilled, the dependent needs which have been met by the child, and the degree of libidinization of the relationship.

3. *The Child and the Dying Parent.* The effect of parental death on the child clearly has a close connection with the child's age. Anthony (1940) has outlined the development of the child's concept of death, on which depends his ability to conceptualize the fatal nature of the parent's illness and the irreversibility of the situation which will be created. Before the age of five years, death is equated with sleep and is not considered final. Through the years from five to nine, death is often personified and may be thought of as an event contingent upon the aggressive fantasies or actions of others. It is only after the age of nine that death is seen as a process dependent upon natural laws and characterized by the permanent cessation of vital bodily functions. Fear of death in children is variously seen as a fear of the aggressive retaliation of others, together with a fear of emotional deprivation possibly related to separation anxiety. The effects of the parent's terminal illness on a child are little reported in the literature, although an extrapolation from bereavement studies suggests certain long-term consequences such as the later development of suicidal, delinquent, or frankly criminal behavior, with

less consistent evidence regarding depression and schizophrenia. Clinical descriptions of the child's reactions at the time highlight the guilt which may be produced in him, the effects on him of the mourning behavior of the other parent, and the quality and timing of the explanation he is given. The child, too, will be affected according to his identification with the particular parent, his ambivalence toward him, the extent to which this parent met his dependency needs, and also by the degree of libidinization of the relationship.

4. *Sibling/sibling Relationship.* Important factors here are the extent of present or past sibling rivalry, the age relationship between the siblings, and the degree to which the dying member has filled a parent or child role. Here again we are largely dependent upon the results of research in relation to bereavement (Cain *et al.,* 1964), from which it can be inferred that possible sequelae are disabling guilt, depressive withdrawal, acting-out behavior, and deterioration of school work.

AREAS OF CONFLICT MOBILIZATION

Conflicts may be mobilized in the family member for a variety of reasons. From certain aspects of his own personality development, specific areas of sensitivity touched by the patient or by the illness itself may have resulted; moreover, the stressful situation may promote regression to earlier levels of functioning with revival of the conflicts of that time. Clearly the situation is stressful because of the narcissistic threat implied and because of the concentration of the emotional and other resources of the family on the patient.

Dependency. The dependent needs of the family member are likely to be threatened in several ways. Not only will there be the interruption to the individual's narcissistic gratifications, but there may also be identification with the dying person and with his enforced surrender to a dependent nursing situation. This is particularly threatening to a child, for whom independence is closely tied to ego growth (Anna Freud, 1952). There may also have been a substantial real dependence, emotional and/or financial, on the dying person who is now unable to meet these needs. Reactions may include depression, physical illness, an overprotested pseudo-independence which is extremely fragile, and possibly other more overt psychiatric symptoms.

Aggression. The fact that dependent needs are now ungratified is in itself sufficient to mobilize the family member's aggression. There are also elements of triumph over the dying person, with the presence of magical and omnipotent hostile and revengeful fantasies toward him (Klein, 1945). Hostility may also arise from the management required by the dying person, particularly when the terminal patient is cared for at home and if nursing procedures include repeated cleansing, changing, dressing, or the handling of the patient in particularly unpleasant circumstances. Incontinence, confusion, and the ulceration of advanced malignancy may be repugnant and evoke resentment. Two of our own cases illustrate these problems:

1. A woman was required to nurse her husband through a terminal illness induced by carcinoma which had presumably originated in the parotid gland. He had been ill for twenty-five years, and had endured thirty-two operations. Several years before his death his tongue had been amputated and for eight years he had fed himself by nasal tube. He emitted an extremely bad odor and his face was grossly disfigured.

2. Another woman nursed her husband at home for two years prior to his death, following a major cerebral vascular accident. Toward the end of this period he was doubly incontinent and sometimes needed to have his clothing changed as often as fourteen times in the one day.

The restricted activity of the patient may also evoke hostility, especially if his inability to help himself is used in a passive-aggressive fashion. Child patients are particularly affected by restrictions which lessen instinctual discharge through motor activity, and they may compensate with tantrums or sullen withdrawal which may anger their relatives (Anna Freud). Other ways in which the dying patient may provoke aggression are through certain aspects of his own basic personality, or through the changes therein produced by his illness: for example, depression in severe cardiovascular disease (Dovenmuehle, 1965), fears of desertion and withdrawal in advanced malignancy (Feder, 1965), or the altered mental state in Huntington's chorea (Hans and Gilmore, 1968). Aggression is a particularly likely response where the illness can be interpreted in any way as "self-inflicted": for example, by lack of cooperation, by failure to adhere to a specific diet causing deterioration in the diabetic patient, by injury, neglect, refusal to consult a doctor, or by a past excessive indulgence in smoking when this seems to have been a relevant causal factor. Disappointment over unfulfilled ambitions may also cause resentment, as in the case of a wife who realizes that her husband's terminal illness represents the end of her own hopes.

These aggressive reactions may appear in overt form, they may be displaced to other objects even to the extent of the formation of phobic symptoms, they may be projected to form a paranoid system, internalized resulting in severe depression, or overcompensated by reaction formation to produce excessive concern and "spoiling" of the patient.

Considerable guilt may arise from these aggressive responses and further increase the psychic discomfort. Guilt may also appear if the family member feels in any way responsible for the illness, such as may occur with hereditary fatal diseases (Langsley et al., 1964), or if the family member believes or fears that his own neglect, anger, prejudice, or interference have contributed to the fatal outcome. When nursing procedures cause the patient to suffer, such as may occur in the giving of repeated injections, sadomasochistic problems may arise, with conflicts over "the giving or withholding of comfort" and the relief of pain. We have already mentioned that guilt may be a particular problem in younger children in whom magical thinking is still predominant.

The guilt may be acknowledged in consciousness, or may be reacted against with overcompensatory caring; it may contribute to depression, result in compulsive rituals, or in other physical or psychological symptoms.

Sexuality. Sexual conflicts may be aroused in many ways. Identification with the patient may highlight previous sexual inadequacies or make them conscious, particularly when the terminal illness involves that type of surgery which may activate castration anxiety, or if it arises from carcinoma of the breast or from disease of any other organ which has a sexual connotation. Disease which is mutilating and disfiguring is also important in this connection. Threatened loss of the parent of the same sex may mobilize guilt through Oedipally-based destructive fantasies; on the other hand, impending loss of the opposite sex parent may reactivate incestuous fantasies and their associated guilt. The implications of loss may be even greater for the child, and may contribute to inadequate resolution of the Oedipal situation (Zilboorg, 1937). Anna Freud points out that the feminine castration wish of the male child may be activated in these circumstances and may be damaging to his future masculinity. Pain may also assume sexual connotations in the family member's interaction with the patient and may add further to sadomasochistic satisfactions.

Sublimation or other defenses may need to be mobilized to deal with the family member's instinctual drives when these are no longer able to be gratified for him by the terminally ill person. Sexual acting-out may occur, leading to guilt, or, alternatively, extreme repression may lead to permanent inhibition of sexuality, particularly if at a fantasy level there is a sex-aggression equation.

DEFENSIVE OPERATIONS EMPLOYED

Denial is one of the major defenses mobilized in these circumstances and is often used to an excessive degree. It tends to be exaggerated when parental guilt is marked, or when diagnosis has been delayed, and is maintained longer for those persons at a greater social distance from the dying person—for example, grandparents and distant relatives (Meyerowitz and Kaplan, 1967). Denial may be of the illness itself, or of its fatal nature. It appears in the family members of patients with chronic renal disease (MacNamara, 1967) and is noteworthy in those with fatal hereditary illnesses (Langsley *et al.,* 1964) such as Huntington's chorea (Hans and Gilmore, 1968). It may lead to unreal, magical hopes for recovery. Study of the communications of dying persons (Hinton, 1963; Feder, 1965) shows that many dying patients do have a knowledge of their prognosis despite the lack of real confrontation with it, and the same may well apply to individual family members.

Isolation of affect may appear as a healthy coping device which enables the family member to perform the necessary practical functions for the terminal patient in a rational way. Its excessive use may lead to withdrawal from the patient, as though he were "already dead" (the concept of "social death" mentioned by Kalish, 1968), and thus possibly to his more rapid decline (Weisman and Kastenbaum, 1968). Less isolation of affect may enable the family member to become a confidant to the patient and lessen his speed of deterioration (Lowenthal, 1967).

Sublimation may enable the family member to deal more appropriately with practical problems. Chodoff suggests that it may be the basis of the increased motor activity seen in the parents of leukemic children.

Repression may become excessive, as may *reaction formation,* particularly in the presence of major problems with aggressive wishes and frustration of dependent needs.

Displacement of hostility is especially likely to occur; it may become attached to other family members, or to medical and nursing personnel. Dependent and sexual needs may also be displaced to other family members or outside agents; in the former instance, there may be real danger if intense sexual need causes the generation gap to be bridged in a potentially incestuous way (for example, the dependent and frustrated father whose wife is dying in the hospital and who takes his daughter into his bed in a blind search for some primitive type of gratification).

Projection, particularly of hostile and dependent wishes, may occur on to the patient or another family member. Clinical experience suggests that it is rare for this projection to reach paranoid psychotic proportions.

Introjection of aspects of the patient may occur, with the family member taking on his illness and/or personality characteristics as a defense against the imminent object loss. A possible consequence is an hysterical identification with the dying person's symptoms. In this area, as in so many others, we currently have to rely on clinical impressions rather than on research data.

THE PERCEPTION OF
THE SITUATION AS A CRISIS

The degree to which the terminal illness represents a crisis situation for the family members will depend on the changes in role which are involved or which are seen as likely to ensue, the relative magnitude of the loss for the individual, and the success of previous coping techniques. On theoretical grounds, the fact that terminal illness is inevitably followed by a second crisis precipitated by actual loss is likely to maximize its traumatic potential. In the previously quoted study of the parents of children with cystic fibrosis, it was noted that the reaction to a child's illness was aggravated if there had been a previous death of a child from the same disease.

Reactions of the Family Group

As well as the responses shown by individual family members, there will be a disturbance of the balances and interactions within the small group system of the family itself. The pre-existing family integration will be important in this respect, difficulties being particularly likely if this has been delicately poised, with the now terminal patient in a pivotal position, either because he was its expressive or instrumental leader, or because of his status as family scapegoat. His move into the sick role may call for a substantial reconstitution of family patterns.

Changes in role behavior will occur, and further changes will be anticipated for the future, which will affect work, leisure, interactional and sexual gratifications. Another family member or members may have to assume the position previously held by the patient. Moreover, the tasks involved in caring for him, particularly if he is at home, may require a readjustment of other family functions. A working wife or mother may have to give up her job to care for a sick husband or child. There may be insufficient time and no particular inclination to fill previous leisure roles, and the mother of a dying child may no longer be able to fulfill her sexual role with her husband. There will be an additional work-load if she has to fill the roles of both nurse and breadwinner, as well as the problems of role conflict. Changes in role expectations within the family may occur, and disintegration may result if the consensus necessary for homeostatic balance is not achieved. Meyerowitz and Kaplan have pointed out that younger fathers were significantly more likely to report occupational liabilities resulting from a child's illness, with frequent complaints of inability to accept promotion or transfer because of the illness. Younger families were less likely to have resources in reserve to deal with the problems of physical management; on the other hand, younger mothers were more likely to have close ties with their own families from whom they could derive support. They noted that mothers who had previously been employed outside the home were more likely to hospitalize the child.

Concentration of family resources on the ill member necessitates a readjustment of the established family patterns of gratification. Prolonged illness may leave the family emotionally and financially destitute, particularly in the younger family with less to fall back on and if the terminally ill person has been the breadwinner.

Sick role behavior within the family is important. Other family members may be forced to give up their own "sick role" in the face of the severity and terminal nature of the illness that now confronts them in another member. In certain hereditary diseases the family may carry a considerable burden (Langsley *et al.,* 1964), the disease constituting for them a "guilt-laden family secret," to be spoken of only covertly and with shame, leading them to see themselves as a "doomed" or "infected" family. Certain other illnesses also carry a stigma and this may engender further hostility and guilt within the family.

The family's view of the approaching death as "appropriate" (Weisman and Hackett, 1961), or "on time" (Glaser and Strauss, 1965), will be important, although their opinion may or may not be shared by the patient himself. The reaction to the terminal illness of an elderly member, perhaps an invalid for many years, is certainly different from the response to the impending death of a sick child or a previously healthy young adult.

Communication patterns within the family are frequently modified, decreased, or accentuated in pathological and pathogenic ways. The "conspiracy of silence" about the prognosis is one particular instance of this, by means of which the patient and the family may be denied the opportunity to work through their anxieties, share their remaining pleasures, and plan realistically for the future. One very obvious example arises when death has involved one member of a young or middle-aged couple, where because of this conspiracy there has been no discussion about the possibility or desirability of eventual remarriage for the survivor, a hiatus which may have far-reaching consequences. It has been shown (Kalish, 1968) that there is a tendency to withdraw from the dying person and to direct fewer communications toward him. This withdrawal may result in poorer reality testing, for communication about everyday things is an important means by which this is maintained for the patient and his family (Feder, 1965).

Hospitalization of the patient, or his care at home, is frequently a function of family needs rather than a rational decision based on the demands of the illness; even less does it seem to be a response to the patient's own desires. Wilkes (1965) has reported that the terminal care of cancer patients in the home is seen as satisfactory by at least three-quarters of the relatives involved. Fulton (1965) has pointed out that patients prefer to die at home, but there has been no similar study of family preference. It may be in some instances that hospitalization is a necessity if the family is going to remain an integrated unit. Yet the hospitalization of a child may have the converse effect; the mother may spend the major portion of her time at the hospital with him, leaving the rest of the family deprived of both her physical and emotional presence. Transfer to specific terminal care institutions may present additional difficulties, in that denial can no longer be maintained and the family members may be burdened with further guilt.

Extended family units may provide a wider network of support and additional "role fillers," and their existence may mean that there is less stress on family functioning than in the small nuclear family group. It should be noted that the nuclear family often perceives the extended family as being insufficiently supportive.

The extent to which the terminal illness constitutes a crisis for the family unit is also important. As with individuals, the degree of crisis experienced and the methods of resolution employed will be influenced by previous experience with similar or dissimilar crises, the basic integration of the family, and probably by the presence of concomitant crises. Dysfunction may be shown in psychophysiological symptoms, such as bowel disturbance, or in disturbed psychological and/or behavioral patterns. The effect on parents may be shown by their excessive anxiety over the effects of the situation on the healthy children.

It is worth noting that when the expectation of the death of a patient is reversed for some exceptional reason, and the patient returns to health or to nonterminal invalidity, the family may be involved in a new crisis situation if it has already made an adaptation to the patient's anticipated absence.

Reactions of the Family
in Relationship to Society

The normal two-way interaction between the family and society is modified to some extent when the family contains a terminally ill patient.

Kalish (1966) has demonstrated the tendency for people to maintain a certain social distance from the dying, and has pointed out that the dying actually rate below alien ethnic groups as neighbors. The community has certain expectations of the family's response to the impending death, and such attitudes may create additional stress for the family if consensual validation is lacking. A further issue concerns the presence or absence of practical support, such as the amount and quality of the medical care provided, home nursing facilities, health insurance provisions, and other supportive networks within the community. Meyerowitz and Kaplan have shown, however, that families may perceive the environment as negative and nonsupportive regardless of what is provided. Religious belief and support for this attitude in the community may facilitate the acceptance of terminal illness. Studying the families of patients with chronic and likely to be terminal renal disease, MacNamara found that these families, if mature and controlled in the face of stress, were paradoxically less able to evoke support from the community.

Implications for Practice

The multiple levels of possible dysfunction within the family of the terminally ill patient provide an opportunity for a variety of forms of preventive intervention.

The individual family member. The needs of the individual member, as we have emphasized, can only be understood in the light of knowledge of his own developmental background, the particular roles which may be pathogenic for him, the particular conflicts which are being mobilized, and the defenses which he is using against these. Finally, there is the extent to which the impending death constitutes a crisis situation for him. In the light of this information a plan can be devised for offering him maximum support: This may involve the provision of an opportunity to ventilate his conflicts to an outside person, with or without the mobilization of practical help involving nursing, social, or financial assistance. In more pathological instances, it may require some form of psychotherapeutic intervention to help him look more deeply at his conflicts and work through them, both to manage his present discomfort and to prevent future pathology. In a small percentage of cases definitive treatment of the family member may be essential.

The family group. Understanding of the problems of the family group itself is only possible if there is understanding of the imposed changes in role behavior, the extent to which resources are being concentrated on the ill member, the significance of family concepts of sick role and of death, past and present communication patterns within the family, the extent to which denial is being employed, attitudes toward hospitalization or care at home, the presence or absence of support from the extended family, and finally the extent to which the situation is perceived as a crisis for the family itself. Following such an assessment it may be possible to assist the family members in their adaptation to the new situation, so that they may readjust their interlocking roles and make appropriate decisions about the dying person's care and about their own future. It may also be seen that additional environmental supports are required. Intervention for the family may be introduced when breakdown has occurred, or preferably at an earlier stage when some signs of strain are appearing in the family system, and may take the form of concrete environmental manipulations, counseling, or even psychotherapeutic techniques. Such interventions should be aimed at restoring the stability of the family group to enable it to cope more adequately with the present crisis and with the crisis of the bereavement to come, thus enabling it to return ultimately to a healthy rather than a pathological equilibrium.

The family in relation to society. The important considerations here are the strengthening of the supportive network so that it may better meet the family's needs. It may be important to try to modify community attitudes to the dead and dying, so that people are more accepting and less distancing than they currently appear to be. Experimental evidence (Blackman *et al.,* 1965) makes it clear that people in crisis display psychological symptomatology in inverse relationship to the amount of perceived support in the community network. Our own studies in the particular crisis of bereavement confirm this in very specific ways (Maddison and Walker, 1967). Practical details, such as the provision of adequate health insurance, are also relevant.

The needs of the family which contains a terminally ill patient are likely to be assessed most adequately by a properly trained general practitioner or community doctor, who is possibly the one person whose location and contact with the family are such that he can assess and manage the needs of the individual members and the family as a unit. Members of the clergy and other "caretaking agents" are also strategic persons in any such program of assistance to the family of the dying patient. It is abundantly clear, however, that such persons require a far more detailed and scientific knowledge of the problems and their possible solutions than is currently the case; techniques of mental health consultation (Caplan, 1964) seem uniquely suitable for this purpose.

Recommendations for the Future

Further recommendations must depend upon more thorough research into the factors of greatest significance in determining the eventual outcome of this crisis for the individual, the family group, and the community. Particular types of crisis situations need to be selected and studied by valid research techniques. For example, it should be possible to examine the family crisis caused by the terminal illness of a mother dying with carcinoma, and delineate those influences which differentiate between successful and nonsuccessful coping with it. Subsequently, it will be necessary to devise different techniques of intervention in this situation, and subject them to a controlled study of their effectiveness. It is only then that the persons in care-giving roles to such families can be maximally helped in their tasks of management. Although both theoretically and clinically there are good reasons for assuming that such crises may have pathological sequelae in many instances, firm experimental evidence is still lacking and is essential before any substantial interventive program can be undertaken. From such a baseline of research, more definitive proposals can be evolved which seem certain to make a major contribution to preventive medicine.

BIBLIOGRAPHY

Anthony, S., *The Child's Discovery of Death*, New York: Harcourt Brace, 1940.

Blackman, S., W. Mandell, K. M. Goldstein, and R. M. Silberstein, "An approach to a community mental health theory," in *Proceedings of the 73rd Annual Convention of the American Psychological Association*, Washington: A.P.A., 1965.

Cain, A. C., I. Fast, and M. E. Erikson, "Children's disturbed reactions to the death of a sibling," *American Journal of Orthopsychiatry, 34:*741, 1964.

Caplan, G., *Principles of Preventive Psychiatry*, New York: Basic, 1964.

Chodoff, P., S. B. Friedman, and D. A. Hamburg, "Stress, defenses and coping behavior: observations in parents of children with malignant disease," *American Journal of Psychiatry, 120:*743, 1964.

Dovenmuehle, R. H., "Affective response to life threatening cardiovascular disease," in *Death and Dying: Attitudes of Patient and Doctor*, G.A.P. Symposium No. 11., 1965.

Feder, S. L., "Attitudes of patients with advanced malignancy," in *Death and Dying: Attitudes of Patient and Doctor*, G.A.P. Symposium No. 11., 1965.

Freud, A., "The role of bodily illness in the mental life of children," in *Psychoanalytic Study of the Child, 7:*69, New York: International Universities Press, 1952.

Fulton, R., *Death and Identity*, New York: Wiley, 1965.

Glaser, B. G., and A. L. Strauss, "Dying on time," *Trans-action, 2:*27, 1965.

Hans, M. B., and T. H. Gilmore, "Social aspects of Huntington's chorea," *British Journal of Psychiatry, 114:*93, 1968.

Hinton, J. M., "The physical and mental distress of the dying," *Quarterly Journal of Medicine, 32:*1, 1963.

Kalish, R. A., "Social distance and the dying," *Community Mental Health Journal, 2:*152, 1966.

Kalish, R. A., "Life and death: dividing the indivisible," *Social Science and Medicine, 2:*249, 1968.

Klein, M., "The Oedipus complex in the light of early anxieties," in *Contributions to Psychoanalysis: 1921–1945,* New York: McGraw-Hill, 1945.

Kraus, A. S., and A. M. Lilienfeld, "Some epidemiological aspects of the high mortality of the young widowed group," *Journal of Chronic Diseases, 10:*207, 1959.

Langsley, D. G., R. V. Wolton, and T. A. Goodman, "A family with a hereditary fatal disease," *Archives of General Psychiatry, 10:*647, 1964.

Lowenthal, M. F., P. L. Berkman, and Associates, *Aging and Mental Disorder in San Francisco,* San Francisco: Jassey-Bass, 1967.

MacNamara, M. "Psychosocial problems in a renal unit," *British Journal of Psychiatry, 113:*1231, 1967.

Maddison, D. C., and W. L. Walker, "Factors affecting the outcome of conjugal bereavement," *British Journal of Psychiatry, 113:*1057, 1967.

Maddison, D. C., and A. Viola, "The health of widows in the year following bereavement," *Journal of Psychosomatic Research, 12:*297, 1968.

Marris, P., *Widows and Their Families,* London: Routledge and Kegan Paul, 1958.

Meyerowitz, J. H., and H. B. Kaplan, "Familial responses to stress: the case of cystic fibrosis," *Social Science and Medicine, 1:*249, 1967.

Natterson, J. M., and A. G. Knudsen, "Observations concerning fear of death in fatally ill children and their mothers," *Psychosomatic Medicine, 22:*482, 1960.

Parkes, C. M., "Recent bereavement as a cause of mental illness," *British Journal of Psychiatry, 110:*141, 1964.

Rees, W. D., and S. G. Lutkins, "Mortality of bereavement," *British Medical Journal, 4:*13, 1967.

Weisman, A. D., and T. Hackett, "Predilection to death," *Psychosomatic Medicine, 23:*232, 1961.

Weisman, A. D., and R. Kastenbaum, "The psychological autopsy: a study of the terminal phase of life," *Community Mental Health Journal,* Monograph No. 4, 1968.

Wilkes, E., "Terminal cancer at home," *Lancet, 1:*799, 1965.

Wolff, C. T., S. B. Friedman, M. A. Hofer, and J. W. Mason, "Relationship between psychological defenses and mean urinary 17-hydroxycorticosteroid excretion rates. I: A predictive study in parents of fatally ill children," *Psychosomatic Medicine, 26:*576, 1964.

Zilboorg, G., "Considerations on suicide with particular reference to that of the young," *American Journal of Orthopsychiatry, 7:*15, 1937.

Melvin Krant

IN THE CONTEXT OF DYING

Like all preceding generations, this generation of Americans is undergoing the stresses and tensions that accompany the restructuring of values related to individual human worth on all levels. Our attention is addressed to questions of race and racial problems; to questions of population masses, birth control, and the individual right to abortion; to the meaning of poverty and its "culture"; to questions of the retired, the elderly, the lonely. Changes in patterns of culture and tradition, the growth of democratization on one hand and institutional efficiency on the other, draw our attention also to the problems of the care of the dying. The affluent society is demanded by conscious participants to look at the nonaffluent, and in our field, the affluence of the living now looks at the nonaffluence of the dying. Since medical care is directed almost wholly toward recovery or rehabilitation, the living and recoverable are the affluent. Little direct attention is given to the dying, and in that way they are indeed the nonaffluent.

According to sociologists, the dying individual today is a patient in a hospital or care-giving institution who is to be cared for by a medical system. During the past fifty years, the dying location has shifted from home to the hospital or institution. As traditional geographies have changed, insensitive urban masses have grown and people have been mobilized into nuclear families. With religion seldom subserving him, the dying figure has become a medical-patient problem. Is medicine prepared to accept this shift, this responsibility in existential and functional terms? Probably not, for as long as dying is seen as that of a patient and not that of a man, we have a conceptual problem that medicine is ill-equipped to handle. The dignity of dying, if that term can be used, rests in the dignity of living—a dignity interdependent with the dignity of others, especially us the caretakers, and a dignity to be allowed to all human worth.

As with all social definitions, the problem of function as opposed to concept must be faced. How do we, who now claim an interest in, an affinity for, a responsibility to a group of humans—how do we arrange for the priorities to carry out our mission? Regardless of how we pontificate, if we wish to affect the order of things we need financial aid and certain kinds of power to bring about the change. But first we must ask ourselves what we wish to change.

Do we wish to build special new places to house the dying patient, or shall we devise ways to change things in existing institutions by requesting special wards? Should we think of bringing together new groupings of professionals with special training, or can we rely on the existing professional models, with the hope that educational programs will enlighten and produce better care? Should we consider returning the dying individual to his home and provide support for his family in giving the care there, with ambulant medical care?

Such changes must be paid for. Can we convince the already strained federal budget to pay for the actual building of new institutions, or is this a persuasion for philanthropic foundations? Perhaps we can convince third-party insurance systems to cover home care, as well as in-hospital care. Chronic care is expensive and financially debilitating. Unless we are careful, our newly formed programs for the dying will benefit only the rich and consign the poor to the accustomed indignities even at the end. Medicine is delirious with newly uncovered wonders, all charged with aiding the living to continue in that channel, and at exorbitant costs. New technologies, new medications, new laboratory procedures—how can we compete for the limited dollar-availability when all we are proclaiming is worth and dignity?

Part of the answer rests with power in medical spheres. Who wields it and how are the powerful likely to think and function? The author recently traveled on a World Health Organization Fellowship to look at various systems of physician and psychologic care given for terminal illness. In one country he was invited to participate in a conference at a large university hospital. There was a group of about sixty people in that session, and three hours were spent in discussing various values. In the group were social workers, sociologists, psychiatrists, and psychologists. It was a grand old session except that there wasn't a single clinical physician there. Following the session, the author was advised by the head of social service, "This afternoon you will meet Dr. Y. Dr. Y. runs the cancer service here. We feel we have much to offer to his patients and their families, but he won't let us near those patients. Would you please see what you can do when you meet him?" The author did meet Dr. Y., made rounds with him, talked with him about the various drugs which were being given. He approached each patient in a very paternalistic but loving, kindly "You're doing better, aren't you?" fashion. On returning to Dr. Y's office, the author said to him, "You know, there are several angry people in this hospital—angry in the sense that they think they've got something to offer these patients of yours." Dr. Y's response was, "These are *my* patients—and as long as they are, I'll tell them what to do."

The power here was control over the services offered a large group of patients with advanced cancer. Some of these could certainly have been classified as terminal, but what programs were offered to them was determined solely by the unit's director and not by the available professionals who felt that they also had something important to give.

Care of the dying patient and of his family obviously involves extensive professional performance, and frequently the best care-givers may be nurses, aides, psychologists, social workers, and others who come to know the patient and family. Yet it is the physician who is the ultimate power in any unit, and he can effectively block an open program of care. The physician may view himself as the lonely, solitary figure in decision-making and care-giving. In a way, the educational process he is put through fosters such an exclusiveness.

There appear to be two levels of absence in the physician's education that cause great difficulties in dealing with issues around the dying patient, or perforce, any individual in crisis. The first level is an intellectual one—the medical school and its partner, the teaching hospital, are oriented to medical science and individual patient care and not to major intellectual issues nor to multidisciplined health care and public care thinking. In-depth teaching in psychology, sociology, anthropology, economics, to name a few disciplines, does not occur, so that large-order, interdisciplinary thinking is seldom seen as relevant either in public or private terms. Students go through the medical school unperturbed in general by these large public domains. Geography oftentimes operates to prevent true university participation, for the medical school is near its teaching hospitals and not near the university campus. But geographic proximity does not necessarily result in greater horizons for the medical school. The barriers to this broader and humanistic education reside in conception. The medical school is dominated by medical professionals and the doctor-patient, one-to-one care is really disease-dominated care. This is not wrong; but it does not ensure an understanding of human nature, human worth and values, human perspectives.

Second, the education of the physician, as of the nurse and social science worker, means an education that is almost totally within the framework of that profession. When ultimately the young student-professional finds himself on a ward unit, he enters into ossified role relations with the "other" on the unit, and seldom gets to understand the problems besetting that other professional and the dimensions of that profession's structure. Nurses, for example, are clearly the major care-givers to the in-bed patient, although doctors generate data by examinations and tests to evaluate the disease process. Patients will often communicate differently to a nurse than to a doctor or to a minister, and needs and goals may become confused among the professionals. To be able to deal with staff problems, not to mention patient and family problems, requires respect and honesty among the professionals and an easy world of intercommunication with a sense of sharing authority and responsibility.

These various professional roles are often sex-limited, perhaps in itself the source of intrinsic problems. Physicians in this country are usually males, nurses and social workers usually females. Medicine is the glamorous, hard, cool role, nursing and social work the softer, more emotional role. To promote harmonies on a unit requires tact, patience, and diligence, and the understanding physician may well be aware that leadership usually rests in his hands—leadership, not dominance, arrogance, or aloofness. The separatist education system promotes the feeling of an isolated, lonely role for the physician who stands by himself making important decisions.

As institutions have developed and grown, and more physicians have become full-time in hospitals, especially teaching and university hospitals, the lonely, isolated community practitioner role is no longer applicable, and new ways of dealing with communities with full-time health workers are necessary. In coping with the complex psychosocial problems of people with chronic illness, their terminality and their families, their economic and space-bed needs, and insufficient community resources, people of all disciplines must work together. The physicians' powerful hold on decision-making and program arrangement must be loosened and other workers should be allowed to bring their talents and concerns into appropriate focus.

Another problem that the physician has had to face, especially in the initiating of his professional life, is the defensive depersonalization forced upon him. The young medical student, thrown into a dissecting room with cadavers, has to control his anxieties and perturbations, not by facing and ventilating them, but by denying they exist. He must be cool; professional behavior becomes a closure against his fears. Then on to pathology, where the fact of a man's death is verified in autopsy and organ examination. The patient becomes not a person but a pathology specimen.

The time certainly has come to acknowledge that the quest for educational data requires careful balancing, allowing inquiry and legitimization of feelings and tones. If the student is allowed his humanity in his search for wisdom and imperturbility, he may come to allow the dying man his dignity. This may require the help of a special breed of teacher, or perhaps the members of the Department of Psychiatry. Once discussion and sharing of feelings is permissible, a deeper understanding and interplay with the feelings of others—patients, families, and staff —may emerge.

Medicine's social context is also changing, and this may benefit the dying patient. The notion that the student has come to medical school to become a medical scientist is fading; students now do not run so eagerly to the laboratories as they did in the past. The issues of social and community involvement may be as diverting as was the laboratory from the issues of the dying patient. But the societal sense, made visible and operative in a positive program, may well promote an interest in the worth of caring for the dying and for his family. There is a danger in over-accentuating the societal purposes of medicine, for the student must learn the scientific foundations and modern diagnostic and therapeutic techniques of medicine. But he does not necessarily benefit from behaving like a scientist at a research bench; a societal-oriented alternative may guarantee better and more concerned medical care in the future.

Another issue concerns the phenomena of life in today's large city—loneliness, isolation, street dangers, house dangers, a general level of insanity and uncertainty. The development of these phenomena has accompanied the disintegration of neighborhoods and the community resources available to buffer life's tragedies. The old neighborhoods with their local practitioners, pharmacists, grocers, people-next-door, all concerned, all aware, all knowing, made for gossip, but also for protection and support. The lack of urban practitioners drives people to accident rooms and the big hospital proper. The help of the streets now is replaced by the impersonal extended-care facility. The dying may live a bit longer, but he and his family have lost something essential.

But can the dying be returned to his streets, to his home? As our corporate hospitals have grown and more physicians have become full-time, in-hospital care-givers, and those in practice have moved their offices closer to or within the hospital, less support is available at home. The urban doctor does not even live in the neighborhood of the hospital nor does he often visit in the home. He can now commute to his geographic worksite and depart to his geographic homesite and never even guess what the neighborhood streets are like. This detachment makes the physician, the nurse, often the hospital minister, a foreigner to the ways of the community and completely obliterates the possibility of harnessing community resources to work effectively with him. If the community does work effectively, it does so without his knowledge and participation. Dying at home is made so much harder by these separations —even though technical medicine may prosper.

Re-examination of our institutions, the present-day major resource for care of the dying, clearly shows that the hospital image of doing positive things for the acutely ill patient does not extend to doing positive things for the terminally ill individual. How does one bring change about? Clearly, it cannot be done on moral grounds alone. Doing good for its own sake is seldom an operating force in a cynical, sophisticated society. Care of the dying must become a positive, rewarding, professional experience with an elite corps of care-givers to give it substantial stature in the priority list.

At St. Christopher's Hospice in London, Dr. Saunders allowed the visiting author to wander through the Hospice, free to ask questions of the staff and to sit and talk with patients. The staff meeting that week was formed into a question-search session, with the author as questioner-searcher, and the staff as responder. One young nurse, who insisted that she was not religious-minded, said something striking in response to the question, "How can you work in an institution like this in which so many people die?" She said that she had been a bit jittery when first coming to work there, but that after a while she began to feel that what she was doing was not only important, but that indeed she had become elite. Friends would question and praise her for being able to fill such a desperate need, to do such a remarkable service. This is one key to change. What a remarkable phenomenon, the development of an elitist feeling about one's occupation! What may be necessary is the development of teams of elite personnel who see in their jobs great satisfaction and reward and, in fact, whom society rewards for their services.

The Cancer Unit in Boston (Tufts Medical School—Lemuel Shattuck Hospital) is attempting to embody these principles and to develop new approaches for a teaching institution. The hospital is a chronic disease hospital, mandated for investigation and experimentation into chronic disease states. On the Cancer Unit, attempts are being made to create a truly comfortable interdisciplinary group which sees the medical, social, familial, and psychologic problems of any patient as the living set of problems. The nurses, social workers, aides, medical students, fellows, and residents are all responsible agents for gathering information, and frequent conferences permit sharing of this data and decision-making as to who should attempt to deliver what kind of care. Two sociologists, who make home visits as part of the information-gathering and decision-making process, are also in attendance. There is a "continuing care" nurse who maintains contact with patients at home after discharge. In the planning stages is a program of community at-home care within a given catchment area, and shortly, it is hoped that visits will be made regularly with the visiting nurse association. The lessons of family interaction, crisis resolution, culture, and response are being learned.

The staff has learned that there are people who prefer to come into the hospital to die because they do not wish to be a burden or to inconvenience their families. They have learned to dissipate unfounded fears and concerns, and to train people to manage certain burdens. They have also learned that the guarantee of a hospital bed, if needed, and free and easy communication patterns allow patients to stay at home with their families right through the end.

Now something must be learned about coping mechanisms in grief and bereavement. The attempt is being made to learn how to spot the individual in a family who is a risk for developing serious psychologic and physical disorders in the future, how to intervene therapeutically to prevent grief-loss consequences, and how to bring about better resolution of grief. In effect, grief and bereavement are being studied prospectively, to test the validity of those interventional techniques.

First- and fourth-year medical students are being introduced to these concepts and allowed to share in the labors and profits. They are being taught that to help a man die well is a rewarding and positive experience, not simply that death is the failure of medicine. No secret knowledge is claimed for improving living and dying; but open discussion and shared planning can make it easier for everyone.

The grief process is little known to the hospital, except as a pathologic event leading the individual to the psychiatrist for help. What the role of medicine can be in helping the bereaved through early crisis is something that must be learned by the teacher and taught to the students. In fact, there is no reason why they cannot learn together.

Is there anything special in what is being done? A friend recently asked if taking care of a dying patient did not simply imply giving good medical care to the individual, and demonstrating concern for the family.

This is clearly true, but the key words are good medical care and concern. For in caring for the dying, we are concerned with making living a full and rich experience within the limitations imposed by severe illness. This can be accomplished only by helping a man to resolve the anger, depression, and victimization perceived in fatal illness, and to resolve tensions and conflicts that would rob already diminished and threatened self-esteem and worthiness. This means understanding the anger and effacement in families, the denials and ill-rewarded protectionism that serve to separate families from the patient at the most critical time in his life. Continued care for the family, pre- and post-death, to help them adjust to the mourning period is also needed. All this really is good medical care, but it means psychology, culture, and sociology as well as biology. Dying, death, bereavement, grief, and loss are special things and require special training on the parts of professionals dealing with patients.

Our struggle is to place the human endeavor in proper perspective. From sunrise to sunset and through the dark hours, we participate in the living of a day and night. The beauty of the day culminates in the splendor of a sunset and the peace of the night. And so too with living and dying—our challenge is to bring dignity and peace to the twilight hours and into the night that follows.

W. Dewi Rees

BEREAVEMENT AND ILLNESS

He first deceased; she for a little tried
To live without him; liked it not and died
— SIR HENRY WOOTON

This paper sets out to examine the relationship between bereavement
and the subsequent illness and death of close relatives. The first part re-
views the existing statistical evidence while the second part is a more
conceptual section, illustrated with individual family histories.

That bereavement is associated with an increased risk of mortality
for close relatives is an old concept that has been reported in various
ways in different ages and cultural settings. The epitaph quoted above
discloses the observations of a seventeenth-century poet, although a
modern poet might perhaps more aptly transfer the gender to make the
epitaph read:

> "She first deceased; he for a little tried
> To live without her; liked it not and died"

The main value of present work in this field is that it re-emphasizes the
importance of bereavement as a contributory cause of illness and death,

presents the facts in a manner acceptable to the twentieth-century mind, and provides objective data.

Young Widowed People

A most useful report was published in 1959 by Kraus and Lilienfeld. They examined data based on the 1950 census and all deaths that occurred in the continental United States during the years 1949–1951. They excluded the open-ended age groups of below twenty and over seventy-four, so that their detailed examination is restricted to the age groups twenty to seventy-four. They report that an outstanding feature of the NOVS data is a significant increase in mortality among young widowed people as compared with married people. In the age groups twenty to thirty-four the annual death rate for widowed people is more than twice that recorded for married people of either sex, an increase in mortality which applies to both white and nonwhite people. The highest ratio (average annual widowed person death rate / average annual married person death rate, by age) is for the white male in the twenty-five to thirty-four age group with a ratio of 4.31. In each of the sex groups the ratios decrease steadily with increasing age, although it remains consistently higher than unity for all age groups. The ratios for the widower also remain consistently higher than for the widowed in all age groups.

Details of the causes of death are given only for the age groups twenty to forty-four. A substantial increase in the suicide rate is recorded for young widowers, but not for widows. The suicide ratio for widowers aged twenty to thirty-four is 9.3; for those aged twenty-five to thirty-four it is 6.9, falling to 3.5 by the age of thirty-five to forty-four. The increase in mortality ascribable to all accidents is relatively small, with a highest ratio of 4.4 for widows aged twenty to twenty-four, falling to 2.8 by the age of thirty-five to forty-four. The highest ratio for motor vehicle accidents is also found among widows aged twenty to twenty-four, where the ratio is 5.9, falling to 2.6 by the age of thirty-five to forty-four.

The highest increase in mortality is for tuberculosis, vascular lesions of the central nervous system, arteriosclerotic heart disease, nonrheumatic chronic endocarditis and other myocardial degeneration, hypertension with heart disease, and general arteriosclerosis. The over-all mortality for each of these diseases is at least four times greater for the widowed than the married. The death rate from tuberculosis was particularly high among widowers, where ratios of 8.1, 12.7, and 7.7 were recorded for the age groups twenty to twenty-four, twenty-five to thirty-four, and thirty-five to forty-four. Some of the ratios exceeded 10. The increase in mortality from vascular lesions of the central nervous system among widowers aged twenty to twenty-four was 11.7 times greater than for young married men. Widows aged twenty to twenty-four had a ratio of 14.4 for arteriosclerotic disease, 11.3 for nonrheumatic chronic endocarditis and other myocardial degeneration, and of 10.8 for hypertension with heart disease.

The increase in mortality associated with widowhood ascribable to diseases of the cardiovascular system showed a marked decrease with increasing age in the age groups recorded. It seems, however, that the increase in mortality associated with widowhood among the younger age groups is largely attributable to diseases of the cardiovascular system. Numerically these deaths among young widowed people are far from insignificant. In the United States out of a widowed population of 233,-000 people below the age of thirty-five an average of 1,105 die each year. As the increase in risk for young widowers is twice that of young widows, the annual death rate for young widowers in the United States is about 1 per cent.

Elderly Widowers

The relationship between cardiovascular disease and the increased mortality of elderly widowers compared with married men of the same age groups has been examined by Parkes and his colleagues (1969). Their work was based on a study started by Young and others (1963), who selected a group of 4,486 widowers aged fifty-five and over and compared their mortality rate with that of married men of the same age. They found that for this group of widowers the mortality rate was 1.4 times that of married men and that the increase was restricted to the first six months of bereavement. This increase in mortality for elderly widowers is considerably less than most of the ratios reported by Kraus and Lilienfeld (1959) for younger widowers. Parkes and his colleagues (1969) examined the causes of death recorded for these elderly widowers and found that disease of the heart and circulation accounted for two-thirds of the increase in mortality noted. A significant increase in the mortality rate was found only for the disease group labeled "coronary heart disease and other arteriosclerotic and degenerative heart disease." The comparative ratio for this disease group between the elderly widowers and married men was only 1.7, which again is considerably less than the figures recorded for younger widowers by Kraus and Lilienfeld (1959).

Other Close Relatives

That this increase in mortality associated with bereavement is not restricted to widowed people but also includes other close relatives has been shown by Rees and Lutkins (1967). They examined the pattern of mortality that occurred over a six-year period in a defined population of 5,184 people. They found that during this period 371 people with close relatives died and they compared the subsequent mortality of the 903 close relatives with that of a control group. They found a significant increase in mortality for the bereaved group and that this increase in risk was restricted to the first year of bereavement, which is similar to the findings of Young and his colleagues (1963). Rees and Lutkins (1967) also found that the increased risk for male relatives was 1.8 times greater than for female relatives and that the risk for widowers alone was greater than the over-all rate for all male relatives.

Apart from widowed people there were 747 close relatives in the bereaved group and 712 in the control group. During the first year of bereavement 3.21 per cent of these close relatives died in the survey group, compared with 0.56 per cent in the control group. This increased risk for bereaved relatives was significant, although the risk for widowed people remained considerably higher than for other close relatives. Statistically significant increases in mortality were also recorded separately for bereaved siblings and children, although not for bereaved parents. The absence of a significant increase in mortality for bereaved parents can be attributed to the small number of parents involved or possibly to the reduction in mortality associated with bereavement that accompanies increasing age.

Place of Death

Rees and Lutkins (1967) also noted a relationship between the place at which a person dies and the subsequent mortality of close relatives. The risk of close relatives dying during the first year of bereavement is doubled when the primary death causing bereavement occurs in a hospital compared with at home—and this increase in risk is significant. If the primary death occurs at some site, for example, a road or field, other than at home or in hospital, the risk of a close relative dying during the first year of bereavement is five times the risk carried by the close relatives of people who die at home. This difference in risk is also significant, although the small size of the sample reduces the importance that can be attributed to the result. It was also found that people who die following bereavement are on the average slightly younger than the relatives who predeceased them, and that they die at an earlier age than is usual for the community in which they live. This finding again agrees with that of Kraus and Lilienfeld (1959) that the risk for bereaved people is greater for the younger than for the older age groups.

Morbidity of Bereavement

Few attempts have been made to determine the morbidity in contrast to the mortality associated with bereavement. The findings of Kraus and Lilienfeld (1959) and of Parkes and his colleagues (1969), which have already been mentioned, are relevant in this field, but other data is also available. The medical histories of forty-four London widows as recorded by their general practitioners were examined by Parkes in 1964a. He found that during the first six months of bereavement the consultation rate for nonpsychiatric symptoms increased by half and that this increase in rate was most pronounced for the subgroup diagnosed as osteoarthritis. There was a threefold increase in the consultation rate among widows below the age of sixty-five, and the amount of sedatives prescribed for this group increased sevenfold. There was no increase in the consultation rate for psychiatric symptoms among widows over the age of sixty-five, nor was there any increase in the amount of sedatives prescribed for them. An association between somatic illness and bereavement has also been reported by Wretmark (1959)—peptic ulcer, asthma and eczema; Lindemann (1944)—ulcerative colitis; McDermott and Cobb (1939)—asthma; Green and Miller (1958)—leukemia; and Lidz (1949)—hyperthyroidism.

Stern and his colleagues (1951) found a particularly high incidence of somatic illness among twenty-five elderly people who, following bereavement, attended the old age counseling service of the Department of Psychiatry at McGill University. They found that the most striking feature in this group of twenty-four women and one man was the relative paucity of overt grief and of conscious guilt feelings and the preponderance of somatic illness.

Psychiatric Illnesses

Parkes (1964b) examined the records of 3,245 patients admitted with a mental illness to the Bethlehem Royal and Maudsley Hospitals during the years 1949–1951. He found that ninety-four patients were admitted during the last illness or within six months of the death of a close relative. He found that the number of patients whose mental illness followed the death of a spouse was six times greater than expected but that no discernible relationship existed between the onset of the mental illness and death of other kin. He also found that women had a higher admission rate to a mental hospital following bereavement than men and that the incidence of affective disorders and particularly reactive and neurotic depression was significantly greater among bereaved than among nonbereaved patients. Despite this he found that only 28 per cent of bereaved patients were diagnosed as suffering from neurotic or reactive depression.

A similar relationship between widowhood and mental illness has been made by McMahon and his colleagues (1960), using data recorded during the United States population census of 1950. They report that the point prevalence rate for widowed people admitted to mental hospitals is greater than for married people, but in general is less than for single people or for those who have been separated or divorced. This report differs from that of Parkes (1964b) in showing a higher admission rate for mental illness among widowers than widows.

Parkes (1964b) estimated that of all patients admitted to the Bethlehem Royal and Maudsley Mental Hospitals, 2.9 per cent were admitted within six months of the death of a close relative. He points out, however, that this figure is not an accurate estimate in terms of incidence as the sample contains only a small number over the age of sixty-four and only a small number with psychosomatic illnesses. He found that 28 per cent of bereaved patients were suffering from a "reactive or neurotic depression" compared with only 15 per cent for nonbereaved patients. This group of "reactive or neurotic depression" was the only diagnostic category in which a significant difference (p<.01) was established between the bereaved and nonbereaved patients. He also found that there was a significant difference (p<.02) in the incidence of bereaved women (69 per cent) admitted to hospitals compared with nonbereaved women (57 per cent).

The increased frequency with which women in comparison to men seek psychiatric help following bereavement has been remarked upon by Wretmark (1959). Of twenty-eight patients reported by Wretmark (1959) as being mentally ill following the death of a close relative, twenty-six were women. The duration of symptoms in this series ranged from two days to nineteen years, and the diagnostic categories discerned were reactive depression 57.1 per cent; anxiety state 21.4 per cent; paranoia 3.6 per cent; confusion 3.6 per cent; psychosomatic disease 14.3 per cent. The high incidence of reactive depression (57.1 per cent) reported by Wretmark (1959) is double the incidence (28 per cent) of "reactive or neurotic depression" found by Parkes among bereaved relatives. The discrepancy is even greater with figures reported by Anderson (1949), who reported that 9 per cent of all admissions to the Sutton Mental Hospital were caused by grief. The diagnostic categories given by Anderson were: anxiety states, 59 per cent; hysteria, 19 per cent; obsessional tension states, 7 per cent; manic depressive responses, 15 per cent. This latter group he subdivided into agitated depression, 8 per cent; anergic depression, 4 per cent; and hypomanias, 3 per cent. These figures, however, are based on admissions to a war neurosis unit, where a particularly high incidence of patients with grief reactions would normally have been admitted, and where not all patients suffered from a personal bereavement.

Funerals

Funerals can be dangerous occasions for bereaved relatives. This investigator has never seen anyone collapse at a wedding or christening but has seen people die at funerals. During one funeral service, a sixty-eight-year-old woman, sister of the deceased, collapsed and died before any assistance could be given. Previously, she had been in good health. Autopsy showed death to be due to coronary thrombosis.

On another occasion, an elderly man had collapsed at the open grave of his brother. It was a dull, overcast day, and when the physician arrived at the cemetery he found the man laying on the ground with his friends trying to protect him from the rain by holding a sheet of corrugated zinc over his body. He too was dead. He had a previous history of coronary thrombosis and was currently receiving treatment for auricular fibrillation. His general health was poor and he had been strongly advised not to attend the funeral. His death too was due to coronary thrombosis.

Can We Prevent the Death?

Sometimes death is not so sudden and the physician has an opportunity to help the bereaved. The help given, however, is not always adequate.

A seventy-seven-year-old man lived with a wife who was severely handicapped by Parkinson's disease. She had also suffered from postherpetic neuralgia which at one time was so severe that she became depressed and attempted suicide. She was able to do a little work in the house but most of the chores were done by the husband. He was a remarkably active and youthful septuagenarian, always appearing cheerful and contented. The death of the wife was sudden. It occurred while she was asleep one night, and because of her previous suicide attempt an autopsy was considered necessary. This showed that death was the result of a coronary thrombosis. About two weeks later the man, now living alone, was visited by his physician. He was very dyspnoeic, although he denied the symptoms, and was fibrillating with an elevated blood pressure. Also, he was in left ventricular failure. He improved rapidly with digoxin and diuretics but a few weeks later collapsed in the bathroom. By the time the doctor arrived on the scene he had fully recovered and felt perfectly well. No new pathology could be detected and his heart failure was well controlled, but it was thought best to admit him to a hospital for observation and further investigation. During the night he had an epileptic seizure, and a few hours later a short series of convulsions. Later in the day he had one minor seizure but this time he was connected to an electrocardiogram and it was demonstrated that the seizure was caused by a Stoke-Adams attack. His dose of digoxin was adjusted and the Stoke-Adams attacks ceased. But during the following week, while still in the hospital, he developed pneumonia, failed to respond to treatment, and died.

Separated Relatives

Relatives do not need to live close to one another for bereavement to be fatal. Some years ago, a very self-possessed middle-aged woman and her husband moved into an area and registered with a doctor. During the visit she stated that both felt perfectly well and that she had merely come to make the physician's acquaintance. During the conversation, she reported that she had headaches but that they were not troublesome. Further questioning revealed that three siblings had died from cardiovascular disease during the previous six weeks and that she was now in dread of having a stroke. She was found to have very high blood pressure and the altered sleep pattern and early morning lethargy characteristic of a depressive state. She responded well to treatment with thymoleptic drugs and a diuretic. A few months later two more siblings died. She stopped her treatment, relapsed, and shortly afterward was apprehended for shop-lifting. When charged with the offense, she stated that she did not know why she did it. It is interesting to note that none of the deceased siblings lived close to one another and that they tended to meet one another only occasionally.

Explanatory Hypotheses

Various explanations of the high mortality of widows and widowers, alternative to the "bereavement" effect, have been made, and some of them are valid. The theory of "homogamy" or the "mutual choice of poor risk mates" hypothesis suggests that the unfit marry the unfit. Its influence, however, is likely to be as small as it is improbable that it could produce such a large increase in mortality as quickly as does happen.

The "joint unfavorable environment hypothesis" is an obvious factor in certain instances, such as motor vehicle accidents. Its importance is dependent upon local circumstances and is often greatest at times of disaster, whether this be caused by war or by natural catastrophes.

That a "common infection" may also be an important factor in the increased mortality associated with bereavement is also apparent. Its importance is likely to vary with time and with geographical location. The findings of Ciocco (1940) that during the years 1898 to 1938 there was a significant tendency in Washington County, Maryland, for both spouses to die from tuberculosis, is probably still valid in countries where this disease is endemic, but is unlikely to be as important a factor in Maryland now as in the period covered by the survey.

The remaining important hypothesis alternative to the "bereavement" effect is that the healthy among the widowed tend to remarry and do not appear in the statistics. Kraus and Lilienfeld (1959) have examined this possibility very closely and have shown that if it is a factor at all, then its importance is very small. We are, therefore, left with the conclusion that the large increase in mortality associated with bereavement and, in particular, the large increase in deaths caused by cardiovascular disease is directly associated with the grief reaction of bereavement.

BIBLIOGRAPHY

Anderson, C., "Aspects of Pathological Grief and Mourning," *International Journal of Psychoanalysis, 30:*48, 1949.

Ciocco, C., "On the Mortality in Husbands and Wives," *Human Biology, 12:*508, 1940.

Green, W. A., Jr., and G. Miller, "Psychological Factors and Reticuloendothelial Disease," *Psychosomatic Medicine, 20:*124, 1958.

Kraus, A. S., and A. M. Lilienfeld, "Some Epidemiologic Aspects of the High Mortality in the Young Widowed Group," *Journal of Chronic Diseases, 10:*707, 1959.

Lidz, T., "Emotional Factors in the Etiology of Hyperthyroidism," *Psychosomatic Medicine, 11,* 1949.

Lindemann, E., "Symptomatology and Management of Acute Grief," *American Journal of Psychiatry, 101:*141, 1944.

McDermott, N., and S. Cobb, "A Psychiatric Survey of Fifty Cases of Bronchial Asthma," *Psychosomatic Medicine, 1:*204, 1939.

Parkes, C. M., *et al.,* "Broken Heart: A Statistical Study of Increased Mortality Among Widowers," *British Medical Journal, 1:*740, 1969.

Parkes, C. M., "Effects of Bereavement on Physical and Mental Health," *British Medical Journal, 2:*274, 1964a.

Parkes, C. M., "Recent Bereavement as a Cause of Mental Illness," *British Journal of Psychiatry, 110:*198, 1964b.

Rees, W. D., and S. G. Lutkins, "Mortality of Bereavement," *British Medical Journal, 4:*13, 1967.

Stern, K., *et al.,* "Grief Reactions in Later Life," *American Journal of Psychiatry, 108:*289, 1951.

Wretmark, G., "A Study in Grief Reactions," *Acta Psychiatry et Neurology Scandanavia Supplement, 136:*292, 1959.

Young *et al.,* "The Mortality of Widowers," *Lancet, 2:*454, 1963.

Elisabeth K. Ross

HOPE AND THE
DYING PATIENT

Over the past five years the author and her associates have interviewed hundreds of dying patients. The questions asked were those which always arise when members of the helping professions discuss the patient's needs and care. The many different opinions and suggestions in response were impressive. And yet how seldom, indeed, has the patient been asked to express his opinion as to his needs. This is a summary of what was learned from the patients and what the researchers feel should be taught future members of the helping professions.

The details of this study have been described at length elsewhere. Approximately five-hundred patients have been interviewed, the majority of them hospitalized in a large teaching institution and all of them diagnosed as seriously ill—possibly terminal. The survival of these patients ranged from twelve hours to two years and one month. The ages were from sixteen to ninety-six years. Almost all socioeconomic levels typical of a metropolitan area were represented. Although the majority of them were of Judeo-Christian background, there were also Muslims, Hindus, and atheists. A workshop, held in Honolulu in the summer of 1970, proved that terminally ill patients do not vary in their basic needs despite differences of cultural and/or religious backgrounds. Only the rituals employed differ.

When a patient becomes aware that he has a serious illness, his first reaction is usually shock and denial. This may last from a few seconds to many months, depending largely on his family and the attending physician. Since patients always have a wish to deny cruel reality, one part of them is quite willing to enforce that denial for a while. On the other hand, patients are also aware of the limited time available to handle their affairs and may feel an opposing force. They would like to resolve this denial and handle unfinished business while they still have the capacity for it—physically, mentally, and emotionally. If the force of denial becomes stronger, they may try to search for help. They will turn to those people most important to them, the attending physician and the immediate family. If these people themselves have a need to deny the seriousness of the illness, the patient will soon find himself alone and avoided. The patient's original hope is, "It is not true" or "I hope that my doctor made a mistake." Gradually he will realize that the doctor was right and that he is losing precious time in playing games.

The games people play when confronted with dying are familiar ones. The visitor remarks how well the patient looks when, in reality, he looks terrible. When the patient asks for facts, the subject is changed. The beautiful flowers in the room are admired in the effort to distract him. The patient soon gets the message that he will continue to be visited as long as he does not make undue demands upon the visitor and if he talks about pleasant things rather than "morbid" ones. And so, in essence, he is told how to behave and what to discuss so as not to be shunned and isolated.

The patient's greatest need at all times is hope and reassurance that he will not be deserted. Yet, it is this very need which arouses conflicts in the physician, the staff, and the family, and eventually leads to the devastating isolation that the terminally ill patient experiences. The problem is that all tend to project their own hope onto the patient. In actuality, the patient's hopes change from stage to stage and ultimately are very different from the hopes that the relatively healthy have.

As an example of these changing hopes, the following history is cited. Mrs. C. was a fifty-year-old woman, the mother of two married children, living in a new apartment. She lived near her children and visited them frequently. She worked in a department store and anticipated doing so until her husband's impending retirement. The couple had planned to work as long as possible and enjoy their retirement by traveling extensively, a luxury they could not afford while the children were growing up and being educated. Mrs. C.'s great joy in life had been cooking and caring for her tightly knit family unit.

When Mrs. C. became ill, her family and physician contended that it was all in her mind, that she was nervous and had always been somewhat of a hypochondriac. She tried desperately to continue her work and supplement the family income until her husband's retirement. One day she did as she had seen other employees do. She "took" little things from the shop "for the children." She was apprehended and fired. The shock and shame of this incident was to stay with her for a long time. No one could understand why this reputable lady would behave like a common thief. No one realized that the patient sensed that her days were limited and that soon she would not be able to bring home little things for her loved ones.

Following the loss of her job, Mrs. C.'s pains increased. Another visit to her doctor revealed nothing of significance. Tranquilizers were recommended and the family regarded her increasing somatic complaints as part of her unhappiness and grief stemming from the indignity which she had experienced. A year passed before she visited a consultant; x-rays revealed metastases to the bones.

During the period of uncertainty and physical discomfort, Mrs. C. often ruminated about the death of her parents. Both of them had died of cancer and had suffered long and painful series of hospitalizations. Her only hope was that she did not have cancer. Aware of her concern, the physician and the family decided not to tell her the reason for her discomfort. When she asked her physician, he assured her that she did not have cancer. Mrs. C. was satisfied for a short time. A few weeks later she fainted and fell down the stairs; her appetite became poor and she was barely able to sit in a given position for more than a few minutes. In conversation she assured everyone that she did not have cancer but that her nerves were very bad. This she attributed to her premature retirement. (She had told no one except her immediate family why she had left her job.) She expressed her hope in terms of "recuperating from this," as she had done following previous surgery. She asked for stimulants to regain her strength and appetite.

Often Mrs. C. would hint to her husband that she knew the true state of affairs. He would quickly respond with words of hope and faith and change the subject. He resumed visits to his church and prayed for her complete recovery. He firmly believed that his faith and prayers would bring about this end. For him hope meant recovery. He was unable to conceive of losing his wife "such a short time before retirement." This was to have been the culmination of their life together after the decades of hard work, little leisure, and sacrifice for the children. He spoke of their new apartment, the curtains she wanted, and the trips they planned to take. And all this was not to be fulfilled?

The daughter cried quietly in her bedroom and attempted to hide it from her children and her mother, who was now temporarily residing with her. Her hopes fluctuated between those she shared with her father and the hope that it would be as painless as possible.

Mrs. C.'s son was the most disturbed. He had some medical knowledge and tried desperately to find a cure or some miracle treatment that would prevent the spread of the disease and eliminate the grim prognosis. He spent much of the time making calls all over the country, seeking advice from specialists in cancer care, quacks, parapsychologists, and others. The one thing he was not able to do was to listen to his mother's hopes. He could not share with her *her* needs and concerns.

Each member of the family, in his own desperation, searched for some magical answer and all hope was directed toward the cure, treatment, or prolongation of life.

It was at this time that the author was consulted by the son, who, denying that he had problems, asked for help for his mother and for his sister, who was now nearing a nervous breakdown. When the sister was interviewed, she claimed that she had been nervous all her life and denied needing any help. She asked for assistance for her father and her mother. The father, when seen alone, stated that he could manage quite well but wished to help his suffering wife and children.

It was finally decided to see all members of the family together in an attempt to help them meet this crisis. Although this prevented their projecting their own needs on to other members of the family, the attempt to truly help them failed bitterly. Each member of the family was able to admit that the patient was aware of the seriousness of her illness and wish desperately to share it. They were not able to drop their hope for a cure and to substitute something more realistic for it.

After several weeks, the patient's pain became so overwhelming that she could tolerate it no longer. By then she was on Demerol every four hours and almost totally incapacitated. She continued to express her hope of returning to her apartment "once more," of finding help for her excruciating pain, and—the greatest hope of all—that her family be able to "make it." She no longer hoped for a cure or mentioned retirement. No one of the family was able to listen to her and to share *her* hopes.

A few weeks later, a cordotomy was performed on Mrs. C. When the author visited her, she simply asked her her hopes. The patient smiled for the first time and said, "A little while in my new apartment." The author quietly nodded. The truth was known by both. The family, meanwhile, waited anxiously. They had begged that the truth not be told to the patient since they felt she would lose all faith and confidence in her doctor and her family. All of them had told her that she did not have cancer. The author objected strongly to their explanation that all the pains were simply in her mind and accepted the invitation to visit her as a friend but not as a psychiatrist. To ensure that she knew the true reasons for the visit, the author said, "You know, I presume, that no one performs a cordotomy for psychological pain." She responded, "The two of us knew this all along but it's hard for the others. It's hard for them to face it." The author stayed briefly and assured the patient that she would always be available to her and her family. She quietly pressed the author's hand and said, "My only hope now is that they are strong enough."

The patient knew that she would not be deserted but that her family needed this reassurance even more than she. Hardly a week passed without a telephone call from one of them. They asked for little—just reassurance that they were not alone, that someone, a little less emotional, a little less involved, would be around to listen to them. Their hopes have not changed yet. They will, though, as they witness the strength the patient will demonstrate. She will have someone to talk with about her needs and her hopes. She will not require all available energy to "play the game" and protect her family from "the truth."

What has been learned from many of our patients is the fact that they can and will drop their denial, go through the stages of anger, bargaining, and depression, and then be able to reach the stage of acceptance with its different hopes. They must be assisted in this process and not by the projection of the caregivers' hopes of cure, treatment, or prolongation of life. The patient, once he has faced his finiteness and approaches the stage of acceptance, will alter his hopes to something which will be realistic in the face of his imminent death. Much of his anguish and prolonged suffering can be avoided if his hopes can be supported and reassurance given that care will be continued even though he is beyond medical cure.

Robert Fulton and Julie Fulton

ANTICIPATORY GRIEF:
A PSYCHOSOCIAL ASPECT
OF TERMINAL CARE

Death in contemporary society is increasingly an experience of the aged. Of the two million persons who will die in the United States this year, almost two-thirds of them (62 per cent) will be sixty-five years of age or over, although this age group represents only 9 per cent of the total population. Children under the age of fifteen, on the other hand, account for 29 per cent of the total United States population but only 5.5 per cent of the total deaths (1). This is in sharp contrast to the mortality statistics in 1900, for instance, when proportionally far more children died. At that time, children under the age of fifteen accounted for 34 per cent of the population—approximately the same proportion as today—but this age group accounted for 53 per cent of the total deaths. In the same year, persons aged sixty-five and over accounted for 4 per cent of the total population but 17 per cent of all deaths (2). These changes in mortality statistics are further reflected in life-expectancy figures. A person born in 1900 had a life-expectancy of 47.3 years, whereas a person born in 1967 could expect to live 70.5 years (3).

The context in which dying and death are experienced in the United States has also undergone a significant change. Of the two million deaths that were estimated for 1970, almost two-thirds (64 per cent) will have taken place outside the home in either a hospital or a nursing home (4). The number of persons who will go to such a setting eventually to die can be expected to increase further with Medicare, more sophisticated medical technology, and the progressive segregation of the aged from their families. Medical science, with its associated public health programs, has reduced the mortality rate and prolonged the life-expectancy of millions of our citizens. The extension and bureaucratization of medical health services, therefore, not only have changed the age at which a person can expect to die, but, in addition, have changed the time and place of his death.

The place to which the elderly go to die has recently drawn the attention of medical and social science investigators. Glaser and Strauss have studied the interaction between hospital staffs and chronically ill and dying patients (5). Quint has explored the occupational problems that dying and death present the student nurse (6). Sudnow has focused his research on the manner of treatment accorded dying and dead patients in a public, as opposed to a private, hospital (7), while Kübler-Ross has interviewed the dying patient himself in an attempt to understand more fully the many issues and questions that he must confront with the prospect of his imminent death (8).

These and other investigators have directed their attention to the experience of the dying patient and/or the major problems he presents to the institution and the staff responsible for his care. Little attention, however, has been paid to his survivors. Blauner, giving a possible reason for this, points out that the reversal in mortality statistics over the past few decades has given dying and death a different meaning for the survivors than formerly (9). The change in mortality statistics has directly affected family relations. Blauner observes that the death of an elderly person today need not touch the emotional life of his family nor the social life of a community to the same degree that it once might have. The elderly in contemporary society are increasingly retired from gainful employment and other social activities and are frequently less central to the lives of their families than they were in the past. Greater life-expectancy today, and the sense of having lived out one's life in full, permit the dying person as well as his survivors to accept his death more readily. With the sudden death of a young child, or of a husband or wife in the middle years, there is a sense of the deceased having been cheated out of life and of the survivors having suffered a great loss. In contrast to this reaction, Blauner feels that the quality of a person's death in an institutional setting, particularly the death of an elderly person, does not evoke the same kinds of responses that we have traditionally expected of the bereaved. Medical technology makes possible not only the prolongation of life but also is the basis for repeated and often extended separations of the chronically ill or dying person from his family. Such separations reduce familial and friendship contacts and also serve to weaken social and emotional commitments. The disengagement of the aged from their families, prior to their deaths means, therefore, that their death will little affect the round of life. As Blauner has observed, the death of an important social leader, such as President Kennedy, can seriously disrupt the equilibrium of a modern community. The death of the elderly, on the other hand, less relevant as they are to the life of their families and to the functioning of modern society, does not cause such a rupture (10).

This is not to say that there is no grief felt at the loss of an elderly parent or relative. Rather, it is to point out that the degree or intensity of one's grief at the time of the death is a function of the kind of death experienced. A distinction must be made, in other words, between what can be termed a "high-grief-potential" death and a "low-grief-potential" death. To illustrate: A "high-grief-potential" death can be occasioned by the sudden accidental death of a man or woman upon whom others depend for their physical and/or psychological well-being. Such a death usually will precipitate a series of intense reactions which Erich Lindemann has characterized as "normal grief" (11).

When grief symptoms are seemingly absent, on the other hand, it may mean one of two things: either the survivor is suppressing his feelings of intense grief, which is an important but separate issue in and of itself (12) or, the death did not evoke the emotional reactions Lindemann has described. A death in which these reactions are indeed absent and are not merely suppressed is a "low-grief-potential" death. For many people today the death of an elderly relative occasions only the barest acknowledgment, and such a death might properly be designated as a "low-grief" death. There are many factors which might generate such a response, but one of the most important, we believe, is the phenomenon of "anticipatory grief."

As has been pointed out, the death that a family experiences today is most frequently the death of one of its elderly members. Moreover, prior to death, the elderly member may have been removed from the inner family circle, spending several periods in a hospital or a nursing home prior to admission to a terminal hospital. In any event, the family has experienced periods of separation due to the patient's incapacity or illness. The low-grief response expressed by family members at the time of death may be due to what has been termed by Lindemann as "anticipatory grief" (13). That is, the family members are so concerned with their adjustment in the face of the potential loss that they slowly experience all the phases of normal grief as they cope with the illness or endure the separation prior to the death. Over an extended period of time, therefore, the family members may experience depression, feel a heightened concern for the ill member, rehearse the death, and attempt to adjust to the various consequences of it. By the time the death occurs the family will, to the extent that they have "anticipated" the death or dissipated their grief, display little or no emotion.

"Anticipatory grief" is not a recent psychic phenomenon, nor is it necessarily associated only with death. Both Lindemann and Rosenbaum have found what they would describe as genuine grief reactions in persons who had experienced separation due to the demands of military duty (14). Lindemann cites the case of a soldier recently returned from combat who complained that his wife no longer loved him and that she was seeking a divorce. It was Lindemann's opinion, following a review of the facts in the case, that the soldier's wife had so effectively worked through her grief over the separation and his possible death that, emotionally, she had completely emancipated herself from her husband (15). While this reaction may well form a safeguard against the impact of the actual eventuality of death or a permanent separation, it is apparent that it has important as well as unforeseen consequences for survivors. It has been found, for instance, that a great many of those who are released from military service, jail, or hospitals cannot be reintegrated into their families; in their absence, their families have established new role relationships which no longer include them (16). It may well be that a significant variable in the poor adjustment of men released from prison, as suggested by their high rate of recidivism, is the fact that their significant others are no longer emotionally capable of incorporating them into the family or friendship circle; they are incapable, in other words, of giving them the kind of emotional support they need to make a satisfactory readjustment to the outside world (17).

In each of the above examples of anticipatory grief, family members have worked through their grief without a death actually having occurred.

Appropriate responses and outward expressions of one's emotions in instances of this sort are at best vague and ill-defined. In our society it is considered appropriate either to laugh or to cry—or even to behave casually—when greeting a returning serviceman or someone who has been separated for a long time from the family. The only inappropriate response would be to show a lack of pleasure at the return. At death, however, there is a cultural directive for the bereaved to mourn. Joyful, casual, or business-as-usual behavior is considered both inappropriate and disrespectful.

Culturally, as Volkart has pointed out, we tend to perceive the death of a person as a loss, particularly the death of a close family member. We expect the survivors, moreover, to show grief, because culturally we feel it is natural, proper, and desirable: natural to grieve, proper to show respect, and desirable to get one's grief out of one's system. The question of whether grieving is internally motivated or externally induced is generally not an issue with us. We assume that any observed behavior and the feelings that we impute to that behavior express the relationship between the deceased and his survivors. Regardless of the actual relationship that might have existed prior to the death, we tend to idealize the relationship once death has occurred and to expect expressions of normal grief (18).

This expectation is held not only by the average man, but also by members of the medical profession. They have accepted and internalized these conventional categories of thought long before they became nurses or doctors. There is growing evidence that medical personnel who have attended the deceased patient are highly critical of his family members and friends whose behavior appears, to them, to be inappropriate, incongruous, or callous, and they are responding negatively to family members who display such seeming disregard for their dead relatives (19). To the extent, however, that such behavior is due to anticipatory grief, it is important for medical personnel and other social caretakers to temper their reactions and withhold their judgment of the survivors. To respond angrily or in any other way show disapproval of the behavior of the survivors is to act, in this case, in a lay rather than a professional manner and to aggravate, possibly, an already troubled situation. What must be appreciated here is that the survivors themselves can be just as surprised and disturbed by their lack of response at the death of a close relative or friend as are the medical personnel. The absence of any feeling upon the death can be very disturbing to the bereaved and in the face of the cultural directive to mourn can be conducive to a sense of guilt or a feeling of shame.

Lifton documents a similar guilt reaction in his study of the survivors of the atomic bomb in Hiroshima (20). In recounting life histories of the *hibakusha,* as the Hiroshima survivors are called, a significant aspect of their psychological reaction to the horror and chaos that they experienced was a closing-off of their capacity to feel or to respond to the condition of others. Lifton points out that psychological closure permitted the survivors to function in the situation and to do what they could for themselves as well as for the injured and dying. It was, Lifton believes, an element, nevertheless, in the shame and guilt that swept over these survivors afterward. Their failure to respond to an event as profoundly tragic as Hiroshima was for them a mystifying as well as a demoralizing experience. How could anyone continue to live, eat, and sleep in the face of such a cataclysm? How could anyone go about his daily task of disposing of corpses, comforting the dying, or rendering assistance to the injured without shedding a tear? The psychological closure that Lifton discusses in his essay appears to us to mirror the protective function of anticipatory grief, as well as to reflect its similar consequences. That is, the *hibakusha* were unable to feel any grief at the time it was expected of them, and in reflecting upon this they suffered an extreme sense of guilt. In situations in which grieving is considered appropriate, we not only expect it of others, but also they expect it of themselves. The *hibakusha* responded with guilt and shame at having gone through the death experiences of others with little or no feeling.

One of the unanticipated consequences of anticipatory grief, therefore, is the undeserved critical judgment by others as well as the critical judgment of oneself.

That such psychological factors are at work is illustrated in the research of Natterson and Knudson in which the responses of thirty-three mothers of fatally ill children were studied (21). They reported:

Initially, most mothers (25 of 33) were tense, anxious, withdrawn and readily inclined to weep. They reacted in a disbelieving manner, tending to deny either the diagnosis of the disease or its fatal outcome. They wanted to be with their children as much as possible, often tending to cling to them physically. This staying with the child was sometimes without much regard for the needs of the remainder of the family. Hope for the child was stressed, but in a nonspecific way—"Something will be discovered." They wanted, often in an irrational manner, to try anything in the way of new treatment that might offer hope for a cure (22).

After a period of more than four months, sixteen out of nineteen mothers whose children subsequently died showed calm acceptance of the child's anticipated death. As Natterson and Knudson describe it:

These mothers gradually became less tense and anxious. They stopped denying the diagnosis or its prognosis. Their hope for the child became more specific, often related to particular scientific efforts. A considerable interest in the investigative program often developed at this time. There was a tendency to see the medical problem in its broader aspects, with the beginning of an expressed desire to help all children. Mothers during this period tended to cling less to their own children, encouraging them to participate in school or occupational therapy activities. They often helped in the care of other children on the ward and were generally more social. They spoke more about fulfilling family obligations. In most instances, this reaction gradually gave rise to [a] calm terminal reaction . . . (23).

While Natterson and Knudson chose to describe the change in the mothers' attitude as one of "sublimation," what they observed among the mothers was anticipatory grief.

In sharp contrast to the mothers' behavior was the behavior that was observed among almost all staff members. Initially, the staff members' reactions to a particular child were not marked. As the staff became increasingly involved in the child's problem, they were prone not only to exert themselves more on the child's behalf but also were reluctant to forego any program of medication that might prolong the child's life. Upon the death, it was noted that the staff became depressed, guilty, and self-examining. Such a disparate reaction between the mothers and the staff is potentially fraught with difficulties. Not only were they out of phase, in a manner of speaking, in their responses to the death of the child, but also the emotional response of the medical staff in the terminal stage of the dying could well serve to generate a sense of shame or guilt in the mothers who had worked through their grief. The inability of the medical staff, moreover, to remain dispassionate in the face of what is readily recognized as a tragic death threatened not only to interfere with their medical judgment as to what measures were reasonable in the situation, but also served as a marker of appropriate behavior for the mothers and invited a sense of shame or guilt among those who could not generate comparable feelings.

A retrospective study of twenty families whose children also died of leukemia, by Binger, *et al.,* confirms the anticipatory grief reaction of the parents as reported by Natterson and Knudson (24). The reaction to the child's death by some of the physicians, however, was opposite to the reaction reported by Natterson and Knudson. They write:

The professional has his own problems in coping with the imminent death of a child. He is distressed and often feels guilty about the failure of therapy. Simultaneously he is troubled by his own fears and anxieties about death and feels inadequate to support the dying child and his parents. Faced with these conflicts he often avoids the patient or family or makes himself unapproachable by presenting a facade of business, impatience or formality. Thus at a time when most needed the professional often assumes a neutral or even negative role in contacts with the family of the dying child (25).

It was reported by these researchers that more than a quarter of the families believed that the physician and staff members became more remote as the child's condition worsened. Not only was the child physically more isolated (a precaution taken because of leukopenia and the chance of infection) but he was actively "avoided" by the staff as well.

It should be noted that the origin of the physicians' response in the Natterson and Knudson study, as well as in the Binger study, were in fact the same. Both studies report feelings of inadequacy, guilt, and anxiety among the physicians at not being able to keep the child alive. The differing manner in which physicians chose to respond to these similar feelings points up the lack of appropriate behavioral norms for physicians in this critical area.

Binger, *et al.,* conclude that when professional personnel understand the attitudes of the parents and are prepared to respond to their needs they will become a valuable source of help to the family instead of getting caught up in a situation laden with mutual hostility and recriminations.

Another finding of the Binger study underscores the need for medical personnel to understand the dynamics of grief in order to assist families in such circumstances. The researchers found that in eleven of the twenty families, one or more members had emotional disturbances severe enough to require psychiatric guidance. None, they report, had required such help before. The emotional disturbances included:

several cases of severe depression requiring admission to a psychiatric hospital, a conversion reaction wherein a man was temporarily unable to talk, severe psychoneurotic symptoms and behavioral changes in siblings. In some of the other families, milder disturbances were also reported in both the adults and the children (26).

It is the conclusion of Binger and his colleagues that supportive therapy and counseling for parents and siblings should be considered an essential aspect of total care in order that such untoward reactions to death as these can be both understood and prevented in the future.

But perhaps the most significant implication that anticipatory grief has is for the dying patient himself. While he, along with his survivors, must come to accept his illness and his death, it is a problematical thing for him to know whether his survivors are in fact concerned or grieved to know he is dying. While the answer to this question can be found only within the context of a specific case, there are indications that suggest that this question will loom larger as more and more elderly people, in particular, are removed to nursing homes or terminal-care hospitals. While conclusive evidence is lacking at this time, a number of observers have noted that the visits of family members to chronically ill or dying patients in hospitals or nursing homes diminish in frequency and length soon after their relative is placed in the institution. Riley and Foner report, moreover, on the basis of different studies, that a disproportionate number of deaths occur among elderly patients soon after commitment to an institution (27). While it is, of course, possible that the timing of placements in institutions may be due to the severity of the illness of the patient, nonetheless it is also possible—and deserving of more careful study—that the precipitous rise in patients' deaths immediately following their commitment to the institution may be a response to their removal from their homes. Lieberman, for example, reports that death rates among residents in an old-age home during the first year after admission were more than twice as high as for the same population while it was on the waiting list (28). He concluded, moreover, that early mortality did not appear to be clearly associated either with poor physical health or with age at first admission. Such a finding suggests that still unexplored factors may account for this phenomenon.

We have seen in the case of the leukemia victims that two grief trajectories can operate in the situation of the institutionalized dying patient: As the family comes to accept the death, their emotional involvement diminishes or becomes intellectualized and diffuse, whereas the medical staff may become caught up in the drama of the death and their emotional investment in the patient may increase (29). The turning away of family members at this time, in a psychological as well as a physical sense, can create an insurmountable problem for the patient. At a time when he needs the support, comfort, and reassurance of his family, the phenomenon of anticipatory grief can serve to block such support. The absence of tears or expressions of concern may compel the patient to grieve not only for his own death but also for the seeming loss of his family's love.

In response to the difficult problems inherent in this situation, several different medical centers are sponsoring programs in grief therapy with the hope that paramedical personnel might play a supportive role as surrogate relatives. While this well-intentioned effort is prompted by the highest ideals of medicine and social service, its consequence may be to aggravate an already difficult situation. The professional functionary could play a more valuable role, once he himself understands the dynamics of anticipatory grief, by explaining and interpreting the phenomenon to the patient as well as to his relatives and friends. The patient would be better served if his relatives and friends were to be drawn back into an enlightened relationship with him rather than, as it appears to be proposed, that they be replaced by well-meaning but nevertheless "professional sympathizers."

It should be quite apparent that the task of dying is not simply a polite exchange of confidences or an expression of affection or concern. Dying involves the patient in taking his leave from all of those who have been important to him. The array of questions and issues dealing with such disparate concerns as the education of a grandchild, the marriage of a daughter or niece, the disposition of a ring to a favorite cousin—to say nothing of how old friendships and animosities are to be concluded —can only be the business of the dying patient and those members of his family or friendship group who are immediately and directly involved. To propose a program of professional intervention for more than those patients who are completely without relatives or friends is, in the face of the total number of dying, to assume what would eventually be an impossible task, as well as one which ultimately would defeat its own purpose.

Finally, the effects of anticipatory grief are felt again when the family confronts the funeral. Traditionally, the funeral has served not only as a ceremony to dispose of the dead but also as a supportive and integrative ceremony which aids the bereaved to reorient themselves from the shock of death (30). The funeral, moreover, has had other functions, which, while not readily perceived or understood, are nevertheless important (31). For example, reciprocal social obligations are often reenacted and reinforced in the course of a funeral. In this way, the role of a participant not only reflects his position in the community but the community structure itself is also reaffirmed. Moreover, funerary expectations pertaining to dress, demeanor, and social intercourse both declare and reconfirm family cohesion. The family and the larger kinship system are also acknowledged at the time of a death. Distant family members, moreover, are not only expected to console the immediate survivors but may also share in the expenses of the funeral. Through the participation in a funeral, an individual is presented with and reminded of the various parts and personnel of his social world. The visitation or wake, the funeral service, the interment or disposal service, and finally the concluding family meal all serve to invoke a sense of being part of a larger social whole, just as the observed order of precedence in this rite of passage reminds one that there is structure and order in the social system. The death of a person today, however, is perceived by some as a matter for merely simple disposal. As Blauner has pointed out, the role of the elderly in contemporary society no longer necessitates a funeral such as we have just described (32). The decline in religious beliefs, moreover, and the strong impetus toward "worth" (associated with or identified with one's contribution to society), have merely added to this trend.

It can be argued that the phenomenon of anticipatory grief is also an important variable in this development. A survivor who is emotionally emancipated from a deceased individual will not necessarily feel that the traditional funeral rite is an appropriate response to the death. Rather, he may well believe that the expeditious disposal of the body is most in keeping with the prior reduced status of the deceased, as well as with his own feelings and desires. Anticipatory grief in this context may have positive consequences for the survivor. He has anticipatorily accepted the death and is able to function in his new social environment without the deceased present. To the extent that this is so, he is tempted to dismiss those things associated with the funeral, which historically have served as a religious or social aid to his understanding of the death as well as an aid to his adjustment to it. But, as has been suggested herein, the funeral offers somewhat more than that. It, like other rituals, ceremonies, rites of passage, pageants, and festivals, serves to reinforce a sense of community as it fashions and refashions social bonds. A recent national study concerning contemporary funeral practices shows that in certain areas of the country, particularly on the East and West coasts, there is a tendency for families to modify traditional funeral rites to the point where no one except the immediate family members are present. In addition, there is a tendency with such privatization of the funeral to modify mortuary rites to the barest requirements including, in some instances, the elimination of the public death notice itself (33). While it is probably not true that the traditional funeral will wither away in contemporary America, as Blauner suggests, there is indeed evidence to suggest that for great numbers of people, it will be significantly different from what it has been.

The phenomenon of anticipatory grief serves to play a large part in this transition inasmuch as it allows the survivors to make new and different decisions about the disposal of their dead. Although the phenomenon of anticipatory grief can be functional for the adjustment of the immediately bereaved, it may, as has been pointed out, be dysfunctional for the dying patient as well as for the extended social group. In the case of the privatized funeral, for example, another set of behaviors is attenuated—a set of behaviors which have served historically to maintain and enhance familial, friendship and community relationships. The failure to acknowledge a death publicly not only has humanistic implications for our identity and worth as human beings and political implications for our status as citizens, but also such a failure closes off still another avenue where sympathy, love, and affection may be given and received.

Conclusion

As a psychological phenomenon with social consequences, anticipatory grief confronts us with a two-edged effect. It, like so much else, possesses the capacity to enhance our lives and secure our well-being, while possessing at the same time the power to undermine our fragile existence and rupture our tenuous social bonds.

The intention here has been to point out these several implications of anticipatory grief in order that we may better understand its functioning. In doing so, we may succeed in turning it to our advantage rather than to suffer its consequences through ignorance or misapprehension of its role in our lives.

REFERENCES

1. National Center for Health Statistics, Monthly Vital Statistics Report, Provisional Statistics, Annual Summary for the United States, 1968, Vol. 17, No. 3 (August 15, 1969) Washington, D.C., Table 6, p. 16, and U.S. Department of Commerce, Bureau of the Census, Population Estimates: July 1, 1968, Series, p. 25, No. 400 (August 13, 1968), Table 2, p. 2.

2. U.S. Department of Commerce, U.S. Bureau of the Census, *Special Report: Mortality Statistics 1900—04* (Washington Government Printing Office,

1906), Table 2, p. 22; and the U.S. Bureau of the Census, *Historical Statistics of the United States, Colonial Times to 1957,* a Statistical Abstract Supplement, Washington, D.C., 1960, Table: Series A 71–85, p. 10.

3. U.S. Bureau of the Census, *Historical Statistics of the United States, Colonial Times to 1957,* a Statistical Abstract Supplement, Washington, D.C., 1960, Table: Series B 92–100, p. 25; and U.S. Bureau of the Census, *Statistical Abstracts of the United States: 1970* (91st Edition), Washington, D.C., 1970, Table 65, p. 53.

4. This statement is based upon the fact that the trend is toward greater hospitalization and institutionalization of the chronically ill and dying patient and the data for 1960 which shows that 60% of all deaths occurred in hospital or institution. See *Vital Statistics of the United States,* 1958, Vol. II, Table 57, Public Health Service, Washington, D.C., U.S. Government Printing Office, 1960.

5. Barney Glaser and Anselm Strauss, *Awareness of Dying,* Chicago: Aldine Press, 1965; *see also* their *Time for Dying,* Chicago: Aldine Press, 1968.

6. Jeanne Quint, *The Nurse and the Dying Patient,* New York: Macmillan Co., 1967.

7. David Sudnow, *Passing On,* New Jersey: Prentice-Hall, 1967.

8. Elisabeth Kübler-Ross, *On Death and Dying,* London: Collier-Macmillan Co., 1969.

9. Robert Blauner, "Death and Social Structure," *Psychiatry,* vol. 25, no. 4, November, 1966, p. 379.

10. *Ibid.,* p. 381.

11. Erich Lindemann, "Symptomatology and Management of Acute Grief," *American Journal of Psychiatry,* 101 (1944), p. 187. According to Lindemann, "normal grief" can give rise to such symptoms as sensations of somatic distress, choking with shortness of breath, a need for sighing, an empty feeling in the abdomen, a feeling of tightness in the throat, lack of muscular power and intense distress described as tension or mental pain. In addition to these somatic reactions, Lindemann noted that the bereaved must contend with other grief-related symptoms. That is, the bereaved person will evince a preoccupation with the image of the deceased. He will also feel guilt and will, in certain instances, show extreme hostility. Moreover, he may be unable to execute his normal patterns of conduct. The duration of the grief reaction depends upon the success with which a person does what Lindemann refers to as the "grief work," namely, emancipating himself from his emotional bondage to the deceased and developing new emotional attachments.

12. *Ibid.,* p. 192.   13. *Ibid.,* p. 199.   14. *Ibid.,* p. 199.
15. *Ibid.,* p. 200.   16. *Loc. cit.*

17. For an extensive discussion of the subject of recidivism and the theories of causation associated with it, see Daniel Glaser, *The Effectiveness of a Prison and Parole System,* Indianapolis: Bobbs-Merrill Co., 1964. A rather compelling illustration of anticipatory self-grief is found in John Rosko's book, *Reprieve,* in which he goes to his death calling out words of encouragement and comfort to his guards and the executioner. They, on the other hand, shaken by the prospect of his death, cry as he is strapped into the electric chair.

18. Edmund Volkart, "Bereavement and Mental Health," in Robert Fulton (Ed.) *Death and Identity,* New York: John Wiley and Sons, 1965, p. 279.

19. At a recent symposium on the terminal care of the dying, a hospital staff member expressed strong objections to what she described as the callous behavior of family members upon the death of an elderly relative. She found their behavior so characteristically indifferent to the deceased, particularly at the funeral, that she publicly called for their prohibition from the funeral. Moreover, she proposed that the funeral itself should be conducted from the hospital in order to allow for the attendance of the hospital staff members who, according to her, were usually more concerned over the death of one of their patients than was the bereaved family.

This observation has been increasingly echoed in comments directed to the senior author by nurses and hospital staff members as well as by nursing home attendants and funeral directors over the past few years.

For a discussion of this phenomenon as it affects the funeral see Robert Fulton, "Contemporary Funeral Practices," in Howard C. Raether (Ed.), *Modern Funeral Service,* New York: Prentice-Hall, 1971, pp. 289–320.

20. Robert J. Lifton, "Psychological Effects of the Atomic Bomb in Hiroshima; The Theme of Death," in Robert Fulton (Ed.), *Death and Identity,* New York: John Wiley and Sons, 1965, p. 14.

21. Joseph W. Natterson and Alfred G. Knudson, "Observations Concerning Fear of Death in Fatally Ill Children and Their Mothers," *Psychosomatic Medicine,* Vol. XXII, no. 6, (November-December, 1960), pp. 456–63.

22. *Ibid.,* p. 459.   23. *Ibid.,* p. 460.

24. C. D. Binger *et al.,* "Childhood Leukemia: Emotional Impact on Patient and Family," *New England Journal of Medicine,* 280 (February 20, 1969), pp. 414–18.

25. *Ibid.,* p. 415.   26. *Ibid.,* p. 417.

27. Matilda Riley and Ann Foner, *Aging and Society,* New York: Russell Sage Foundation, 1968, p. 591.

28. Morton A. Lieberman, "The Relationship of Mortality Rates to Entrance to a Home for the Aged," *Geriatrics,* Vol. 16, no. 10, 1961, pp. 515–19.

29. Natterson and Knudson, "Observations Concerning Fear of Death . . . ," p. 462.

30. See, for instance, David G. Mandelbaum, "Social Uses of Funeral Rites," in Robert Fulton (Ed.), *Death and Identity,* New York: John Wiley and Sons, 1965, pp. 338–60; *see also,* Emile Durkheim, *Elementary Forms of Religious Life,* New York: Macmillan Co., 1926; Bronislaw Malinowski, *Magic, Science and Religion and Other Essays,* Boston: Beacon Press, 1938, p. 33 ff; Robert Hebenstein and William Lamers, *Funeral Customs the World Over,* Milwaukee: Bulfin, 1963.

31. Robert Fulton, "Contemporary Funeral Practices," in Howard C. Raether (Ed.) *Modern Funeral Practice,* New York: Prentice-Hall, 1971, pp. 289–320.

32. Robert Blauner, "Death and Social Structure," passim.

33. *Ibid.*

*Edward H. Futterman, Irwin Hoffman,
and Melvin Sabshin*

PARENTAL ANTICIPATORY MOURNING

Anticipatory mourning constitutes a major task in the adaptation of parents to the expected loss of a child. A fatal illness, such as leukemia, which combines an inevitable outcome with an often prolonged period of expectation, illuminates the various aspects of anticipatory mourning as they unfold and interact. In this study, formal interviewing of twenty-three sets of parents with leukemic children as well as informal contact with over one hundred additional families with children suffering from a variety of malignancies formed the empirical base for generating hypotheses regarding adaptation. Despite the wishes of parents to thwart the inevitable course of the disease and to maintain their investment in the cherished child, mourning invariably begins before death. Our observations have led to conceptualization of anticipatory mourning as a series of functionally related aspects or "part processes" (18). Our goal is to define these part processes and to suggest hypotheses concerning their evolution, integration, and adaptive implications.

Anticipation, Anxiety and Mourning

While the phenomenology and theory of mourning *after* death have been subjects of considerable attention, theoretical considerations of anticipatory mourning have been sparse (4, 26, 31, 37). Recent investigations of families coping with fatal illness have revealed a range of adaptational responses by family members, including a variety of behaviors which might be considered as expressions of anticipatory mourning. We have not, however, encountered systematic attempts in this literature to examine the evidence for anticipatory mourning or to explore the particular theoretical ramifications of this phenomenon. This paper represents a preliminary effort in this direction, serving as a basis for more rigorous analysis of data (22).

In discussing the concept of anticipation, Fenichel states, "The prerequisite of an action is, besides mastery of the bodily apparatus, the development of the function of judgment. This means the ability to anticipate the future in the imagination by testing reality, by trying in an active manner and in a small dosage what might happen to one passively in an unknown dosage" (8). Much psychoanalytic literature bears on the anxiety which often accompanies anticipation. Freud, for example, noted, "Anxiety has an unmistakable relation to expectation; it is anxiety about something" (10); and further, "Anxiety comes to be a reaction to the danger of a loss of an object." (10). Subsequent literature exploring the functions and consequences of anxiety in anticipation of physical or psychological harm has been voluminous. Notable among recent discussions of the subject from an adaptational framework are those of Janis (24) and Lazarus (25). The former describes the effects of warnings in terms of response sequences, whereby the individual, in response to objective or "reflective" fear, ideally adopts an attitude combining both vigilance and self-reassurance in "compromise formations" leading to realistic and adaptive behavior. In this model, maladaptation is associated either with "blanket reassurance" (denial) which results in failure to take necessary precautionary steps or with "indiscriminate vigilance" which leads to irrational overreactions (24). Lazarus, in his theoretical integration of the stress literature, defines threat as "the anticipation by the individual of a harmful occurrence" (25). He views anxiety as one among a number of possible responses to threat which occurs, specifically "when a clear coping impulse has not replaced the primary reaction to threat" (25).

In contrast to the work on anxiety and anticipation, studies and discussions of mourning as an adaptive response to expected future loss have been relatively rare. While Freud dealt with mourning almost exclusively in terms of actual object loss, he did note that awareness of the transience of existing objects could lead to a "foretaste of mourning" (12). The phenomenon was first described as a clinical entity by Lindemann, who wrote:

A common picture heretofore not appreciated is a syndrome we have designated *anticipatory grief*. The patient is so concerned with her adjustment after the potential death of father or son that she goes through all the phases of grief-depression, heightened preoccupation with the departed, and review of all the forms of death which might befall him, and anticipation of the modes of readjustment which might be necessitated by it (26).

Pollock also notes,

In instances where death is anticipated as a result of long-standing debilitation, acute mourning reactions may occur prior to the actual death. In several patients, whose parents were dying of malignant conditions, the shock response came when the patients first heard of the hopeless malignant diagnosis, and only very slightly when the actual death occurred. In these persons, the ego was able to react to the upset in the present reality more gradually so that when death supervened much preparation had already been done. . . . Grief responses may antedate the actual death . . . the reaction here is that the lost person is already lost in the internal milieu even though the death has not occurred in reality (31).

Rosner discusses a special case of anticipatory mourning in which an individual's preoccupation with a potential future loss served to defend him against grief over an actual loss he had suffered (33).

Reports of anticipatory mourning reactions are prevalent in the literature pertaining to adaptation of parents to fatal illness in children. Richmond and Waisman discovered that parents tended to become increasingly involved with other children on the ward of the hospital as the hope for the survival of their own child waned (32). Natterson and Knudson noted that mothers of leukemic children reached a stage of disengagement from the sick child and acceptance of his fate as the time of death grew near (27). In most instances, when the stage of acceptance was not reached, they found that duration of illness was less than four months and that acute grief reactions at the point of the child's death were more common. Friedman *et al.* actually employed the terms "anticipatory grief" and "anticipatory mourning" (9). Under these headings, which they used interchangeably, the authors subsumed a variety of behaviors, including the waning of hope, emotional turmoil, depressive symptoms, and progressive detachment from the dying child. In connection with the prevalence and course of anticipatory grief these authors wrote:

The amount of grieving in anticipation of the forthcoming loss varied greatly in the individual parents, and in a few, never was obvious at any time during the child's clinical course. However, in most, as noted by others (27), the grief process was usually quite apparent by the fourth month of the child's illness, frequently being precipitated by the first acute critical episode in the child's disease. Grieving then gradually evolved as the disease progressed and any death on the ward had a potentiating effect (9).

Hamovitch found that following initial expressions of apparent disbelief, which were more "holding actions" than "basic denial," parents "seemed to move almost immediately into a mourning pattern" (21). Most recently, Binger reported that "From the initial diagnosis through the illness of a child and his subsequent death parents manifested all aspects of 'anticipatory' as well as subsequent grief reactions" (3). Drawing precise conclusions from these observations as to the course of anticipatory mourning is made difficult by the lack of clarity and consensus in the definition of terms describing the various aspects of the process.

Adaptive Dilemmas in Anticipating
The Loss of a Child

The work of mourning involves gradually relinquishing emotional investment in the dead or dying person (11, 31). With regard to postbereavement mourning Freud wrote: "Mourning occurs under the influence of reality testing; for the latter function demands categorically from the bereaved person that he should separate himself from the object, since it no longer exists" (10). Pollock has observed that "this absence is not only perceived but is confirmed by the repeated confrontations of the external world and is finally noted and remembered" (31). In anticipatory mourning, the consequences of reality testing are more complicated. Not only is the person present and alive, but also evidence that he will die is often obscure or hidden and must be taken at the word of the physician. Moreover, unlike post-bereavement mourning, anticipatory mourning must be balanced against the realistic task of continuing emotional investment in the dying person with, perhaps, even increased energy devoted to his care.

Nevertheless, we have found that, even while maintaining hope and mastery activities throughout the course of the child's illness, the parents in our study usually began disengaging from the child before his death. Such disengagement is emotionally hazardous since it runs counter to the tasks of caring for the child's needs and promoting his development. Parents are, therefore, particularly vulnerable to guilt which may result from the emotional detachment that accompanies anticipatory mourning. Compensatory restitutive efforts, on the other hand, may lead to symbiotic clinging and stifling overinvolvement with the sick child, neglect of one's own needs as well as those of other family members, general family disruption, and inability to deal with the demands of reality.

Most of our work has been with families in which a child has been diagnosed as having leukemia. The characteristics of this disease intensify and prolong the caring versus mourning dilemma confronting the parents. Modern chemotherapeutic agents have extended the average life expectancy of the leukemic child to more than two years, and there is a growing number of children who have survived five years or longer. Medical advances have also reduced the morbidity of these children so that long symptom-free periods of remission are quite common. The apparent health of the child over long periods of time along with reports of ongoing research encourage parents to hope for life. On the other hand, death is still considered the inevitable outcome of leukemia within a few years of onset, and the predictable unfolding of the illness, with its increasingly frequent relapses and ever shorter periods of remission, serves to confirm the diagnosis and fatal prognosis. Throughout, successful adaptation requires that parents maintain a dynamic balance between those tasks involving continued investment in the physical and emotional well-being of the child on the one hand, and the task of anticipatory mourning on the other.

Sample and Method

Most of the parents of the twenty-three families who were formally interviewed, as well as many of the other families seen informally, were middle-class or lower middle-class, Catholic, suburban residents of Illinois. The parents ranged in age from their early twenties to their late fifties. The sick child was an only child in just one of the families interviewed, and in fourteen of twenty-three families there were two or more healthy siblings at the time of the diagnosis. Descriptive data on the interviewed families are summarized in Table I. On the whole, in line with Hamovitch's findings, most socioeconomic variables in our sample did not seem to systematically affect the course of adaptation (21). On the other hand, although formal religious affiliation did not appear to be a major factor, qualitative idiosyncrasies of religious beliefs did sometimes influence the expression of some aspects of anticipatory mourning.

The interviews, which were recorded and transcribed whenever possible, were conducted at various points during the course of the child's illness and after the child's death. There were a total of forty-five interviews involving twenty-three families. Table II summarizes the distribution of the interviews over time and over families. As the table shows, interviews were distributed over the course of the illness from the time of diagnosis through the terminal phase and beyond the child's death, thereby generating data on the course of adaptation. Five families, who were the first to participate in the study, had one or two post-death interviews only. However, even in these instances, rich retrospective data were obtained on reactions and coping during the course of the child's illness. A total of eighteen families were interviewed one to three times while the child was living, of which five had one post-death follow-up

TABLE I

Descriptive Data On the Interviewed Families At the Time of Diagnosis

A: THE PARENTS

N	Intact Couples	Divorced Mothers	Average Age		Age Range	
			M	F	M	F
23	21*	2	33	37	20–51	22–58

Religion		
Catholic	Protestant	Mixed
14	8	1

Occupation		
Blue collar	White collar non-professional	White collar professional
7	13	3

* One father died during the child's illness.

B: THE CHILDREN

N	Males	Females	Age Intervals			Average Age	Number of Siblings				Average Number of Siblings
			2–5	6–9	13–14		0	1	2–4	5–7	
23	11	12	11	10	2	6	1	8	8	6	2.7

TABLE II

Interview Distribution

		During Illness * (Months since Dx)				Post-death (Months since death)	
		0–2	2–12	12–24	24–48	0–6	6–20
Number of families	Interview span						
13	1–3 during illness	7	5	3	6		
5	1–3 during illness and 1 post-death	2	5	4		5	
5	1–2 post-death					2	6
Total 23							
	Interview subtotals	9	10	7	6	7	6
	Family subtotals	9	8	6	4	7	4

NOTE: Total interviews = 45 (40 tape-recorded and transcribed)
Range of interviews per family = 1–4
Average interviews per family = 2.0

* Eight of 32 interviews conducted during the course of the child's illness were obtained during periods of medical relapse. Two of these eight were obtained during the terminal hospitalization of the child.

interview. During the course of the illness, nineteen interviews were obtained in the first year following diagnosis, while thirteen were obtained after more than one year had elapsed. In six instances interviews were conducted more than two years after the diagnosis was made.

In order to permit as much spontaneous generating of issues by the parents as possible, interviews were loosely structured and not rigorously standardized as to content. We felt that the circumstances dictated that "standardization of conditions of rapport," in Guttman's terms, take priority over standardization of questions asked or specific areas covered (19). For similar reasons, the timing of the interviews was also less regular and standardized than might have been possible under other circumstances. While the effects of these and other methodological factors will be fully determined in systematic content-analysis of the data (22), the interviews clearly show much similarity with respect to the adaptational issues that they raise, thereby allowing us to draw preliminary conclusions regarding the nature and course of parental anticipatory mourning and its relationship to other aspects of adaptation.

Definition of Anticipatory Mourning

Anticipatory mourning is defined as a set of processes that are directly related to the awareness of the impending loss, to its emotional impact, and to the adaptive mechanisms whereby emotional attachment to the dying child is relinquished over time. We have found it useful to consider other related adaptive tasks of equal importance in the total adaptation of families as outside the core of anticipatory mourning. Some of these are discussed in more detail elsewhere (23,13, 36). They include, for example, the task of maintaining family life-style and integrity, the task of maintaining a sense of mastery and confidence (including dealing with helplessness, anger and guilt), and the task of caring for the child's needs and promoting his development. In some instances, these tasks overlap or are mutually reinforcing, while in others they appear to conflict, forming what we have called adaptive dilemmas. Successful adaptation seems to involve a dynamic, ongoing synthesis of coping processes related to a variety of adaptive tasks posed by the child's fatal illness.

Empirically, we have observed a series of interwoven and interdependent part processes which, taken as a whole, form the task of anticipatory mourning. These processes emerge and reach prominence at different points in time. Their evolution during the course of the child's illness is marked by complex interaction with each other and with other coping processes. Inspection of our clinical data suggests the sequential emergence of the following part processes of anticipatory mourning.

1. *Acknowledgment:* Becoming progressively convinced that the child's death is inevitable.

2. *Grieving:* Experiencing and expressing the emotional impact of the anticipated loss and the physical, psychological, and interpersonal turmoil associated with it.

3. *Reconciliation:* Developing perspectives on the child's expected death which preserve a sense of confidence in the worth of the child's life and in the worth of life in general.

4. *Detachment:* Withdrawing emotional investment from the child as a growing being with a real future.

5. *Memorialization:* Developing a relatively fixed conscious mental representation of the dying child which will endure beyond his death.

Acknowledgment

Lazarus has emphasized the importance of cognitive activity in the coping process, stating that, "for threat to occur an evaluation must be made of the situation to the effect that harm is signified" (25). Acknowledgment, which is largely an outcome of such cognitive activity, refers to the process by which parents become progressively convinced of the fatality of their child's illness. This process involves a continual struggle between hope and despair. Ideally, appraisal of reality mediates between the degree of active preparation for death and the amount of hope maintained. Our findings are consistent with the observation by Bozeman *et al.* that "intellectual acceptance did not constitute a static belief but was just one aspect of the mother's adaptation to threatened loss, which shifted with the extent of the perceived threat" (5).

Like Binger *et al.* (3), we found that most parents suspected that their child had leukemia or at least that he was very seriously ill before the diagnosis was officially presented by the physician or the hospital staff. Persistence of the child's symptoms despite customary therapeutic efforts, accompanied by active searching, reading, and questioning by the parents, led to suspicions and dread in the pre-diagnostic period. These suspicions tended to mitigate the emotional impact when the diagnosis was finally confirmed and presented in the hospital. In some instances parents reported feelings of relief that at last they knew what was wrong and could do something about it.

Once told of the diagnosis and prognosis, all parents indicated recognition of the child's fatal condition. This acknowledgment marked the beginning of anticipatory mourning. Feelings of disbelief were generally quite ephemeral. Friedman *et al.* (9), describing early reactions, also noted that "the majority of parents appeared to intellectually accept the diagnosis and its implication, rather than to manifest the degree of disbelief (27) and marked denial (5) described by others." In fact, although hope was universal, there were no instances of absolute denial in all of our data. As stated by Friedman *et al.*, "Unlike massive denial, hope did not appear to interfere with effective behavior and was entirely compatible with an intellectual acceptance of reality. That the persistence of hope for a more favorable outcome does not require the need to intellectually deny the child's prognosis is of clinical significance, as it differentiates hope from defense patterns that potentially may greatly distort reality" (9).

Improvement in the child's condition and the achievement of remission as a result of treatment heighten the parents' dilemma by validating the diagnosis on the one hand and discrediting it on the other. The "mixed message" of reality perception is illustrated in this statement by a mother whose daughter was on the verge of her first remission:

When your kid looks terrible it makes you feel terrible. You don't know what it is and it is the unknown that will scare you. . . . And then when I saw her I realized that, well, she looked a little better. And like right now she looks great. I mean she's pudgy and these signs have disappeared. But still I know that inside she still has all this. I think she's fooling a lot of people because you can't see it from the outside.

Typically, families exhibited determination to hold on to acknowledgment of the fatal prognosis even when the course of the illness was long and relatively benign. One mother, whose daughter was in her fourth year of virtually symptom-free survival since the time of diagnosis, remarked, "Part of me believes that there is nothing wrong with her. But there is a little part deep in my heart that knows there's got to be something. I'm sure you're not lying to me." Another mother offered a retrospective account of the course of her acknowledgment and the cognitive efforts that it demanded in the following comments to her child's physician after the death:

Each time he was better you kept reminding us "Now, remember, this is only a stage he is in: it can turn anytime." And I kept reminding myself, "Well, this is borrowed time. Anything can happen." Sure, we knew what was going to happen! We still had him around. It wasn't something that was dragged away from you in a split second.

Sometimes, insistence upon facing the truth had a fierce quality, and false reassurance from relatives and friends was unequivocally rejected. One father reported, "I almost chewed my wife's head off one night when she had the gall to say to me that one of her friends said that our son was well." Parents often felt more comfortable with people, such as other parents with fatally ill children, who shared their level of awareness of the fatal prognosis.

In spite of the persistence of acknowledgment on some level, periods of remission did tend to raise the parents' hope that there might have been some mistake or that their child might be the exception to the rule. The same mother quoted above, whose child was in her fourth year of remission, remarked, "This is four years and I don't believe it. I really think I am going to wake up some day and it's all going to be a dream." Relapse, therefore, particularly if it was manifested clinically, came as a blow and reawakened feelings of despair. Typically, over the long course of the illness a series of such remissions and relapses had a cumulative impact upon the parents so that their acknowledgment progressively deepened to the point of resignation. By the terminal period, during the final vigil at the child's bedside, only faint residuals of hope remained.

We view acknowledgment as an evolving process in complex interaction with reality events and with other processes. There are continual alternations among levels of awareness which are integrated into a total adaptive pattern. Hopeful statements are often tinged with resignation, while pessimistic remarks are laden with hope. One mother asserted, "Each day we accept it more, because each day that he lives we've got a better chance that there's gonna be a cure found." A father, in a simple statement, epitomized the whole dilemma and the complex integrative coping that it requires by advising, "Plan for the future, but not with your heart and soul." Despite the many day-to-day and even moment-to-moment fluctuations in the dynamic synthesis of acknowledgment and hope, the progressive deepening of parental awareness of the fatal prognosis served to facilitate the emergence and unfolding of the other part processes of anticipatory mourning.

Grieving

Grieving refers to the process in which parents experience and express the emotional impact of the anticipated loss. We view grief as a combination of affective responses such as shock, numbness, confusion, diffuse anxiety, pain, and psychosomatic responses, as well as more differentiated and focused sadness or depression over the impending or actual loss. The overt signs of emotional turmoil may vary greatly in intensity, form, and timing. In our own previous work (23) and in the writings of other authors (26, 31, 9) the terms *anticipatory mourning* and *anticipatory grief* have been used interchangeably. In this discussion, however, we are distinguishing anticipatory mourning as the over-all generic process from grieving as one of its component part processes.

In early reactions to the diagnosis, less differentiated and more diffuse forms of grieving seem to predominate. Along with other investigators (5, 9, 21) we have found that shock and numbness were common as immediate reactions. As one mother said, "I listened, but I don't know what he (the doctor) said." Numbness quickly gave way to pain, sadness, and crying. Hyperactivity, psychosomatic manifestations, and insomnia were also most often present in the first month or two following diagnosis. In general, during this early period of turmoil, work routines and family life were often disrupted. Parents frequently felt overwhelmed and the grieving seemed to be primarily reactive and passive.

As one mother put it, "When the doctor hit me with the diagnosis, it was like being hit with a brick."

As the initial turmoil subsided, more stable and controlled patterns of overt grieving emerged. We have been impressed by the extent to which parents succeed in actively inhibiting, channeling, and timing their grieving behavior in coordination with other adaptive tasks with which they are confronted. One expression of the parents' control over their grieving is in their choice of confidantes. In line with other authors (5, 9, 3), we found that parents make highly selective use of a variety of social resources as they reach out for emotional support. In general, parents weigh the vulnerability of others as well as their potential value as sources of support in deciding how much to confide in them or to shield them. A typical pattern was one which attempted to maintain family equilibrium by shielding the sick child and, to a lesser extent, his siblings from awareness (14, 3, 9). Some parents resolved to do much of their grieving alone, "I have my times when I'm low but nobody sees me. I go and have my good cry and I'm okay." But most found some person or persons, either spouse or others, with whom they shared their deepest feelings. A common attitude was verbalized by one mother who said, "I think that you have to have somebody to talk to, no matter who it is. Someone that you can confide to and who will just let you talk. . . . I think that helps an awful lot."

Another aspect of active regulation of grieving involved parents' deliberate timing of their expressions of grief. Frequently, apparent absence of grief actually reflected intentional postponement or delay of overt grieving in the interest of other coping processes such as activities designed to prolong the life of the sick child or to maintain the normal equilibrium of the family. "I save my crying until after the children are asleep," one mother said, illustrating a common coping strategy. A longer-term perspective is reflected in one divorced mother's remarks when her child seemed to be doing well:

It's still in there. I know this. And I imagine that if she ever gets to a bad point again I will probably be more sad about it. But I hope to get out of it. I mean that's the only thing I can do because I still have another child. I don't know if that's right or wrong but I figure I've got two children not just the one, and I can't just sit around and mope that Brenda's got leukemia.

The integrative adaptive functioning which such delay of grieving represents is overlooked in the literature when it is described solely in terms of denial or suppression. The latter terms emphasize the person's need to reduce or avoid emotional pain as an end in itself. They neglect the long range adaptive plan and the sheer courage that may be involved in such behavior. In fact, prolonged delay of catharsis may be chosen as a coping strategy even when a parent perceives that immediate overt grieving could bring relief. Delay of grieving, as a response to very real adaptive dilemmas facing the parents, illustrates vividly the effective operation of the synthetic function of the ego under severe stress.

Over the course of time we have also observed that the quality of grief tends to be modified so that it becomes more differentiated and focused. In place of the acute emotional pain characteristic of the early reaction, a more tempered sense of melancholy emerges, accompanied by active articulation and evaluation of the loss that is impending. This mellowing of grief occurs in conjunction with increasing reconciliation, detachment, and memorialization.

As the grief experience becomes increasingly differentiated and articulated, it also becomes less intense and overwhelming. The over-all pattern, however, is marked by many transitory fluctuations in the intensity and quality of grieving throughout the course of the illness. Along with acknowledgment, the intensity of grief tends to peak at times of diagnosis and relapse and in the terminal period. However, unlike acknowledgment, the successive peaks of grief decrease in strength. Relapses, and particularly the first relapse, may also bring a temporary recurrence of the early, less differentiated, more passive-reactive type of grief (5, 9, 3).

Overt grieving may also be triggered by a variety of contingencies, including temporary separations from the sick child, the deaths or relapses of other children, and a host of chance events, such as statements made by the sick child himself or by others, or any number of things that the parents may read, see, or hear. In another paper (23) we described several manifestations of grieving (not distinguished in that paper from mourning) that we observed in the outpatient clinic waiting room, including "proxy mechanisms" (17), whereby parents facilitate their own grieving as they become involved in the loss and grief of other families. Two examples of such proxy mechanisms are the development of "anticipatory mourning alliances," in which parents involve other families in their own emotional distress, and the process of "psychological adoption," in which parents become attached to other children and grieve over those losses in rehearsal for the loss of their own child.

Grieving, as an essential aspect of parental anticipatory mourning, is a complex coping process whereby parents accept, articulate, and express the emotional impact associated with their acknowledgment of the anticipated loss. While antecedent to reconciliation and to the other part processes of anticipatory mourning, grieving is, in turn, continuously modified in quality and intensity by their development over time.

Reconciliation

The extent to which a person feels good about himself, about others, and about life, that is, his characteristic level of "confidence," as defined and elaborated by Benedek, is jeopardized when he suffers unexpected misfortune. While acknowledging the similarity between "confidence" and Erikson's concept of "basic trust" (7), Benedek uses the former term to emphasize "the ongoing reciprocity of the interpersonal and intrapsychic processes which bring about structural changes not only in the child, but also in the mother" (1). The discovery of a fatal condition in a child threatens the confidence level of parents and can lead potentially to guilt, blame, and bitterness. Reconciliation refers to the parents' development of a perspective which preserves their sense of confidence in the worth of the child's life and in the worth of life in general in spite of acknowledgment of the child's fatal condition. From the viewpoint of Lazarus's theoretical system, reconciliation may be seen as a form of "cognitive reappraisal" in which the stress is reinterpreted in a manner which neutralizes some of its potentially damaging psychological force (25). Reconciliation is preparatory to detachment and a necessary part of the work of mourning. Before the parents can let go of a child, they strive to make it all right to let go by assuring themselves that the integrity and worth of self, others, and life will not be destroyed by the child's death. In this sense, reconciliation, which may continue in post-bereavement mourning, is a necessary dimension of the work of anticipatory mourning as well.

A number of authors have touched upon aspects of reconciliation in their discussions of parental adaptation to childhood fatal illness. Friedman *et al.* discussed the "search for meaning" as it affected resolution of feelings of responsibility for the child's disease (9). Along with other investigators (3, 5) they have also reported on the role of religion in providing parents with a consoling metaphysical or philosophical framework for understanding the child's death. However, we have not discovered empirical or theoretical writing which has considered explicitly the integral relation of these coping mechanisms to the processes of anticipatory and post-bereavement mourning.

Redefining the child's death in a way that reduces its feared or awesome implications constitutes one form of reconciliation. For example, a father stated, "A child is more fit to die than an adult because he hasn't lived long enough to do anything wrong"; and a widowed mother remarked, "You know that if this child is going to die at least she is not alone. She's in heaven with her father." Redefining the child's death may take on an even more pronounced positive coloring, as exemplified by a father's declaration, "If the good Lord is willing enough to do so much for me, I certainly can contribute something to him. I should be willing to give back some of his gifts to me. Life is so joyous. If you look at it from this respect, death itself should be happy." On the other hand, redefinition can also be expressed in negative terms whereby life is seen as so dismal that death comes to be regarded as a relief. Such may be the case in the later stages of the child's illness, when there is often a wish for an end to the child's suffering.

Another form of reconciliation, which usually has less of a religious flavor, involves seeking consolation from the past and present life of the child. This aspect includes appreciation of the quality of the child's life, of the care that the child received, or of the duration of his survival from the time of diagnosis. For instance, one mother was consoled that her child had good parents and a good life as long as it lasted: "I'm glad we did take that trip. . . . I don't think we cheated him out of anything." Another mother stated, "I'm thankful he's been around this long. The guy told me nine months and here it is four years."

Another type of reconciliation involves surveying one's life from a broad perspective and concluding that, however painful the prospect of losing a child might be, there is still much to live for. This kind of activity can be described as "counting blessings" and is usually a realistic affirmation of the conviction that all is not lost. Many parents focus upon the fact that at least they still have other children to care for or a good marital relationship, or good friends or rewarding work. This aspect of reconciliation is particularly important as an attitude adjustment which wards off feelings of bitterness, restores confidence, and sets the stage for active redirection of energy away from the dying or deceased child and toward other valued objects and interests.

The following is an example of a particularly poignant and integrative expression of reconciliation, reported by a mother in a retrospective account, seven months after her child's death:

The baby came three months before Harold died. . . . I wish I had spent more time with him alone and not have had the distraction of the baby. But on the other hand, when he was ill at home I used to go into the bedroom and sit with him and with her, and talk to them both. I used to feed her sitting there next to him so I could be with him and talk to him. And then I did tell him about his own birth. I remember telling him about the ride to the hospital, which I thought was particularly beautiful. Sentimental, perhaps, but it made me happy to tell him and I think he was happy to hear about it. And I told him how much we wanted him and how proud Daddy was that he had sons. . . . I felt I had to cram in a lot of things in a short time. And it's tragic, but perhaps, we live in a family, and many times children don't know these little things. You just never get around to telling them. But this was a time when I planned: 'What do I want this child to know about us, about himself, about our family, about our philosophy, about our relationship?' And even if nothing else matters. Even if all our philosophy and religion or anything is rather irrelevant, at least I felt that we did the best job that I knew that I could do at that time. I don't mean to say there were no failures. There were times that I felt that, perhaps, I should have done differently. But I feel satisfied before God and man and for myself. And I don't say this proudly. I just say it as a fact.

Reconciliation in some form or forms has been apparent in all the families we have interviewed. While it may begin as early as the period of diagnosis, reconciliation becomes more fully articulated over the course of time. It facilitates the mellowing of grief on the one hand and the progress of detachment on the other. Reconciliation is an active coping process. While it has restorative and healing effects, it may also foster a new articulation or critical review of values, goals and philosophy of life.

Detachment

The work of mourning includes the difficult task of gradually relinquishing emotional investment in the dying child. Bowlby describes the urge to recover the lost object in the early phases of post-bereavement mourning (4). Similarly, in anticipatory mourning we see many examples of the urge to retain the object that is being lost. On the other hand, signs of detachment are also observable before death. Lindemann called attention to the problems that could be caused by "psychological emancipation" from the object prior to its actual loss (26). Chodoff *et al*. pointed to the same phenomenon in parents of fatally ill children, noting "gradual detachment of investment from the child who became less a real object than, in a sense, already a memory while still alive" (6). A number of other investigators have observed parental detachment from the dying child, particularly in the latter stages of his illness (32, 27, 9). In fact these authors generally restrict their documentation of anticipatory mourning to evidence of detachment combined with evidence of grief.

Indications of detachment from the fatally ill child include direct and overt signs, such as physical withdrawal from the child or visible redirection of energies toward other family members and other areas of interest, as well as more covert mental processes, such as wishing to get away from the child, wishing it were over, or diminished fantasy about the child and his future. Even clinging to and indulgence of the sick child, as we will explain, can be viewed as indirect evidence that the process of detachment is taking place. Nearly all the parents we have observed have demonstrated some signs of detachment from the dying child.

Parents exercise a degree of control over the process of emotional detachment just as they do over the other part-processes of anticipatory mourning. In particular, the timing of detachment seems to be related to more or less firmly held parental expectations about when the child will die. If the child dies "on time" (16) detachment is balanced against other adaptive tasks so that care of the child is maintained to the end, even while adequate preparation for the loss is achieved. In these instances, the signs of detachment during the course tend to be primarily covert or indirect, with direct expressions emerging only in the terminal period. The psychological hazards of detachment for both parent and child become more pronounced when the child survives longer than expected. In such instances, premature detachment can lead potentially to neglect of the child's emotional and/or physical needs, with concomitant parental guilt during the course of the illness and following the child's death. In one case, a mother expected her child to live eighteen months based upon the average life-expectancy of children with leukemia at the time of diagnosis. When that time and more had passed, this mother expressed an eagerness to move on and become reinvolved with other aspects of her life as a parent and as a member of the community. She seemed increasingly impatient with the burden of caring for her daughter as compared with the positive attitude with which she had earlier taken up this challenge. However, as was characteristic of almost all parents in her predicament, this mother continued to manage her detachment sufficiently well so that no significant neglect of the child's needs was apparent up to the time of this writing, four years since the diagnosis was made. Contrasting with the adaptive problems arising when the child's survival exceeds expectations are those occurring when the child dies sooner than expected. One father, who underwent a stormy reaction following the death of his son felt cheated because he had anticipated a three-year period of survival and his child had not lived that long.

As they struggle with the dilemma of simultaneously retaining and relinquishing investment in the dying child, most parents, at one time or another, cling to the sick child or indulge his needs at the expense of other family members. Clinging is a complex phenomenon which has multiple meanings and functions. It may be a manifestation of intensified anxiety about temporary separations, subjectively associated with the impending permanent loss. In this connection, clinging may also defend against the parent's wishes to withdraw from the sick child and to be relieved of the burden of his care. In one family, for example, transient school phobic episodes developed as expression of intense separation anxiety and mutual ambivalence of mother and daughter whenever there was an apparent increase in the threat of death (15). In general, clinging behavior tends to increase at points of relapse or other evidence of deterioration in the child's condition (23). As an expression of the urge to hold on to the object soon to be lost, clinging resembles the savoring of cherished transient objects (12) or the familiar experience of embracing loved ones prior to separating from them. In this sense, clinging can be viewed as an integral normative aspect of the process of detachment. In our experience clinging has been a temporary coping response, limited by reality testing and rarely causing significant premature arrest of the child's developmental progress.

Detachment usually accelerates in the terminal period. At times, hospital personnel have complained about a family's seeming lack of concern, callous behavior, and disinterest in a child who has been ill for a prolonged period of time or who has had a prolonged terminal phase. In one instance, after hospital staff expressed concern about her failure to visit, a mother admitted to one of the investigators on the phone that she "could not bear it" any longer and that she had made a conscious decision to devote more time to other family members, relegating care of the sick child to relatives and to the hospital. A lesser degree of detachment was illustrated by a mother who became attached to a number of other children on the ward, describing one of them as her "flower child." When her dying daughter became jealous and sought more attention, the mother became irritated and lost her temper. On the whole, however, even when overt signs of detachment were present, parents maintained care of the child's physical and emotional needs through the terminal period and to the point of death. In fact, most parents were very active at this time making sure everything possible was done even while preparing themselves for the end.

Detachment and continuation of the provision of adequate care and love to the sick child are not mutually exclusive. Despite the dilemma involved, parents were usually capable of integrating both coping processes. In some instances, preventive therapeutic efforts may be useful in helping families to accept their feelings of detachment from the sick child. This type of support tends to reduce guilt feelings and latent resentment and actually frees energy that can be devoted to improved emotional and physical care of the child (23).

In this discussion of detachment we have been referring to a process of emotional disengagement from the sick child as a real, growing individual with a normal future. Detachment prepares parents for the actual loss of the child and permits them to have energy available to deal with other life problems and to reconstitute their relationships with other family members when the child dies.

Memorialization

Memorialization refers to the process by which the conscious mental representation of the dying child is molded into a relatively permanent form which will endure beyond the child's death. The fixed image of the child, the product of memorialization, expresses the way his parents want to remember him. Through this process the memory of the child and certain of his attributes become stabilized for parents and fixed in their minds. The practices of establishing memorials and of composing eulogies are familiar as ritualized aspects of post-bereavement mourning. In a less formal sense, Orbach observed idealization in the case of a mother whose child died of leukemia: "Soon after his death she was aware of her idealization of him and of utilizing this ideal as a standard for comparing him with her other children to their disadvantage" (29). However, the possibility that such processes may begin on a psychological level before the actual death has received scant attention in the literature.

Operationally, we are defining memorialization in terms of two relatively distinct tendencies: progressive abstraction and progressive idealization. *Progressive abstraction* is the process by which parents begin to think of their child in terms of global characteristics or traits rather than in terms of specific behaviors in specific circumstances. To the extent that a portrait of a child is primarily developed on the basis of such generalizations or abstractions it is subject to less modification through repeated observations of the child's behavior and development.

In other words, the child's image becomes more frozen or fixed and less available to reality testing. *Progressive idealization,* or eulogization, of the child refers to the gradually increasing preponderance of positive characteristics in the parents' image of the sick child. Perception becomes increasingly selective and biased so that negative attributes are de-emphasized, ignored, or forgotten. An extreme form of idealization is *enshrinement,* which denotes the tendency to conceive of the child as having other-worldly characteristics. When a child is enshrined, he is usually viewed as saintly, with wisdom, insight, understanding, goodness, or sufferance far beyond what is normally ascribed to children. While it is conceivable for parents to memorialize a child in derogatory terms, we have encountered only positive memorialization and suspect that in our culture negative forms would be associated with psychopathology.

An illustration of how the quality of portrayal of the child can vary along the dimensions of abstraction and idealization is offered by the following pair of statements made by a father describing his fatally-ill daughter:

1. One of the high points in her life—about three weeks ago she won the citizenship award for the eighth grade in junior high school. . . . After that she told her mother she had been working on that ever since fifth grade.
2. She was good in almost everything she tried.

The first statement is concrete and observational rather than abstract. It clearly praises but does not enshrine the dying child. The second statement is much more generalized and idealizes her more. To the extent that memorialization is occurring, we would expect to find increasing presence of abstraction and idealization in statements parents make about the dying child over the course of the illness. We are currently testing and refining a system for content analysis of interview material which will enable us to test some of these hypotheses more systematically and provide a picture of the course of memorialization during the illness and after the child's death.

Enshrinement, as a special form of idealization which characterizes the child in other-worldly terms, often has a religious quality, and its presence, especially when explicit or strong, seems related to antecedent religious beliefs in the family. The following is a dramatic example of the phenomenon of enshrinement involving a report by a mother of her interaction with her son in the hospital a few days before his death:

Marshall asked me how Jesus made people. And I started to explain like you would normally to a four-year-old. And he said, "No mommy, I know now!" And that helped more than anything anyone could have said or done. I think he was shown a way through God to answer the question I could not answer.

Full enshrinement is relatively rare as compared with the other expressions of memorialization we have described. Also, unlike progressive abstraction and idealization, which are observable as gradually increasing phenomena, enshrinement is often manifested in single dramatic events or extraordinary moments of experience.

With the subsequent death of the child, the fixed images, ascribed meanings, and symbolic interpretations of the child's behavior combine to form the basis of myths about the child which become a part of the family's self-image. What begins as memorialization also evolves into part of the family's philosophy of life and its ways of integrating death into its value systems. The interaction of memorialization and reconciliation is particularly evident in these instances. For example, one mother, in an interview conducted seven months following the death of her ten-year-old son stated:

In our faith we believe that we can pray to the dead and ask for their intercession. I remember the moment he died. It was my first feeling; and I kissed him and sat by his bed and held his hand for a while and just felt: "Well, now the child has become more the man." In other words, I felt the passing on to a better life. He knows more than we do and can perhaps now influence and help us.

Benedek has noted the importance of the image of the child in the mental life and development of the parents. She states, for example, "Parents meet in their children not only the projections of their own conflicts incorporated in the child, but also the promise of their hopes and ambitions. The parents, each in his own way, have to deal with the positive as well as the negative revelations of himself in the child" (2). Parental projections are particularly evident and important in determining the specific content of memorialization. One mother, for example, interpreting the regressive behavior of her seven-year-old daughter, stated:

And I often wondered if there was a reason for her going backwards. Just goofy things. . . . but sometimes I think maybe she is doing this for my benefit—something to remember her by—like a gift.

Through memorialization the task of detachment is made less painful in that some of the original investment in the child can be transferred to the mental representation of him which endures beyond his death. However, significant investment in the real child is retained until the end, leaving important aspects of the work of mourning to be accomplished in the post-bereavement period.

Adaptation and Maladaptation
In Anticipatory and
Post-Bereavement Mourning

After the death of the child, there was usually a deepened sense of acknowledgment of the loss and a brief upsurge of acute grief, soon followed by further reconciliation. Presence of grieving at this time testified to the significant emotional investment in the child that had been maintained through the entire illness, while the limited intensity and duration of post-bereavement turmoil testified to the work accomplished in anticipatory mourning. Natterson and Knudson described the most common reaction immediately following the death as one of "mixed expression of calm sorrow and relief" (27). Their observation that more acute distress in this period was related to short duration of illness is consistent with our view of anticipatory mourning as a multidimensional process which requires time to unfold and develop. Friedman *et al.* reported that the few parents in their study who did not display anticipatory mourning "experienced a more prolonged and distressing reaction after the death" (9).

Unlike Binger *et al.* (3), we have observed few instances of severe psychopathology, severe maladaptive behavior, prolonged turmoil, or permanent family disruption in our sample of parents. The discrepancy in these findings may be due to differences in the nature of the samples, in the medical and psychosocial care provided, or in definitions of disturbance. In those few families in our study showing evidence of severe impairment of functioning, signs of disturbance were apparent during the course of the illness as well as following the death. Furthermore, maladaptation was associated with aborted, extreme, or distorted manifestations of anticipatory mourning. One father, who began blaming his wife for his daughter's illness soon after the diagnosis, never showed signs of mellowing of grief or of reconciliation while the child was alive, and had to be hospitalized after the child's death when he threatened his wife with physical harm. Another father failed to progress in his anticipatory mourning beyond tenuous acknowledgment mixed with poorly controlled reactive grieving, even though the child survived more than eighteen months from the time of diagnosis. After the death, he became severely distraught and paranoid, and was, for a time, unable to function. He continued to resist genuine acknowledgment, claiming that his son was "healthy except for his leukemia," and blaming the death upon medical mismanagement rather than upon the disease itself. One month after his son died, he remained agitated and bitter, although the struggle toward reconciliation had begun:

What the devil! Billions of people have died since Adam and Eve and the world goes on. I'm sure it'll go on regardless of what happened to us or not. There's people that are in worse shape than we are. What the hell would we do if an atomic bomb hit and everybody was, uh, infected with radiation— is that how you say it? Then what do you do? Like the Japanese. You see everybody dying. That's something. This was fast. It's over with. But I'm still bitter regardless. It's my son. And this—this is what bothers me. The thing that makes me so mad or embittered is the fact that—all this negligence. This lack of—lackadaisical: "Oh the hell with it." "I'll have a cigarette." "I'll be there in a minute." I don't say that we weren't let off easy as far as cost goes . . . A lot of people don't know what love is. I explained that to you; the different kinds of love. And this is why I say. We love our kids. I don't give a damn if somebody else doesn't. And this is everyday— people murder their children. They put them in a basket and leave them on steps. Well, we don't feel this way about it.

In a third instance of serious disturbance, a mother who had a history of psychosis and of fanatic religiosity refused to acknowledge the fatal prognosis, stating, "As far as I'm concerned Lila's not sick. . . . I've asked Him not to take her and I believe that He's not going to take her. And I prayed with my minister, and that meant two of us had agreed and so she's all right!" Less than two months following diagnosis, the mother, in an example of extreme premature detachment, withdrew the child from medical care, saying that she was placing the girl "in the hands of God." The child died at home a few months later.

After the death, an aberrant form of reconciliation was developed by tying the child's life to a rigid delusional system, and memorialization was expressed by an exaggerated enshrinement of the deceased four-year-old daughter:

That child having leukemia has helped many people in Christ. I feel that Lila was a born missionary. I think a book should be written about her life. In just that little time people learned to love her, learned to trust, learned to respect and learned to think more about the Supreme Being. Lila was beautiful; she lived a beautiful life and was a darling child. She was adored. She was loved by those who met her. Almost three hundred people viewed her body. People came from out of town, Chicago, everywhere. She reached out into the world. She touched a lot of people. People from overseas sent condolences. . . .

This mother's ego resources were not sufficient to deal with the sustained tension associated with the adaptive dilemmas of anticipating the child's death over a long period of time. Instead of caring for the child while at the same time proceeding through the various phases of anticipatory mourning, she had to let the child die prematurely and then compensate for her guilt through grandiose forms of reconciliation and memorialization.

These few cases of maladaptation contrast with the *adaptive* anticipatory and post-bereavement mourning that was characteristic of the overwhelming majority of parents in our study. In general, the evolving part processes of anticipatory mourning were integrated with each other and with other adaptive tasks. The course of the over-all process was marked by balanced responsiveness to the multiple demands of reality and by progressive change over time. The death of the child, however painful for the parents, could be adaptively integrated by the continuing mourning process in the post-bereavement period.

Conclusion

Post-bereavement mourning has been conceptualized as a normative adaptation to the loss of an object (31). Similarly, anticipatory mourning is a normative adaptation to impending loss, and illustrates coping processes occurring in response to a prolonged "accidental crisis" (7). A process view of normality (35) including the concept of phasic interweaving of a series of variables (20, 34), seems most appropriate for describing adaptation to this kind of stress. We have described parental anticipatory mourning in such process terms, deriving hypotheses and propositions about adaptation from the data, in keeping with the particular need for empiricism in this area (28). More work remains to be done in order to assess how valid the suggested processes and part processes are, and whether they can be reliably measured.

In our culture, the death of a child is, perhaps, the most poignant of conceivable losses (30). Nevertheless, despite the many adaptive tasks and dilemmas posed by the fatal prognosis of leukemia in a child, the overwhelming majority of parents in our study demonstrated remarkable resources in coping with this stress. Anticipatory mourning, a major aspect of the parents' adaptation, involved a cumulative series of interdependent and continually interacting part processes. These were: acknowledgment, grieving, reconciliation, detachment, and memorialization. The task of mourning was well-advanced but rarely completed by the progression of these part processes before the death, and significant work remained to be accomplished in the continuing mourning process after bereavement.

REFERENCES

1. T. Benedek, "On the Psychic Economy of Developmental Processes," *Archives of General Psychiatry*, *17:*271–76, 1967.

2. T. Benedek, "Parenthood as a Developmental Phase." *Journal of American Psychoanalytic Association*, *7:*389–417, 1959.

3. C. M. Binger, A. R. Albin, R. C. Feuerstein, J. H. Kushner, S. Zoger, and C. Mikkelsen, "Childhood Leukemia: Emotional Impact on Patient and Family," *New England Journal of Medicine*, *280:*414–18, 1969.

4. J. Bowlby, "Process of Mourning," *International Journal of Psychoanalysis*, *42:*317–40, 1961.

5. M. F. Bozeman, C. E. Orbach, A. M. Sutherland, "Psychological Impact

of Cancer and its Treatment—Adaptation of Mothers to Threatened Loss of Their Children Through Leukemia I," *Cancer 8:1–19*, 1955.

6. P. Chodoff, S. B. Friedman, and D. A. Hamburg, "Stress, Defenses and Coping Behavior: Observations in Parents of Children with Malignant Disease," *American Journal of Psychiatry, 120:*743–49, 1964.

7. E. Erikson, *Identity and the Life Cycle,* New York: International Universities Press, 1959.

8. O. Fenichel, *The Psychoanalytic Theory of Neurosis,* New York: W. W. Norton, 1945, p. 42.

9. S. B. Friedman, P. Chodoff, J. W. Mason, and D. A. Hamburg, "Behavioral Observations on Parents Anticipating the Death of a Child," *Pediatrics 32:*610–25, 1963.

10. S. Freud, (1926) "Inhibitions, Symptoms and Anxiety," *Standard Edition,* Vol. 20, London: Hogarth Press, 1959, pp. 185, 169, 172.

11. S. Freud, (1917) "Mourning and Melancholia," *Standard Edition,* Vol. 14, London: Hogarth Press, 1957.

12. S. Freud, (1916) "On Transience," *Standard Edition,* Vol. 14, London: Hogarth Press, 1957.

13. E. H. Futterman, and I. Hoffman, "Crisis and Adaptation in Families Anticipating the Death of a Child" in E. J. Anthony and C. Koupernik, *Death in Childhood* (in press).

14. E. H. Futterman, and I. Hoffman, "Shielding from Awareness: an Aspect of Family Adaptation to Fatal Illness in Children," *Archives of the Foundation of Thanatology, 2:*23–24, 1970.

15. E. H. Futterman, and I. Hoffman, "Transient School Phobia in a Fatally Ill Child," *Journal of the American Academy of Child Psychiatry, 9:*477–94, 1970.

16. B. Glaser, and A. L. Strauss, *Time for Dying,* Chicago: Aldine, 1968.

17. W. A. Greene, "Role of a Vicarious Object in the Adaptation to Object Loss," *Psychosomatic Medicine, 20:*344–50, 1958.

18. R. R. Grinker, Sr., *Psychosomatic Research,* New York: W. W. Norton, 1953.

19. D. Guttman, "Psychological Naturalism in Cross-Cultural Studies" in E. P. Willems and H. L. Rausch, *Naturalistic Viewpoints in Psychological Research,* Chicago: Holt, Rhinehart and Winston, 1969.

20. D. A. Hamburg, and J. E. Adams, "A Perspective on Coping Behavior: Seeking and Utilizing Information in Major Transitions," *Archives of General Psychiatry, 17:*277–84, 1967.

21. M. B. Hamovitch, *The Parent and the Fatally Ill Child,* Los Angeles: Delmar Publishing Co., 1964, p. 116.

22. I. Hoffman, "Parental Adaptation to Fatal Illness in a Child" (Doctoral dissertation, University of Chicago, in preparation).

23. I. Hoffman, and E. H. Futterman, "Coping with Waiting: Psychiatric Intervention and Study in the Waiting Room of a Pediatric Oncology Clinic," *Comprehensive Psychiatry, 12:*67–81, 1971.

24. I. L. Janis, "Psychological Effects of Warnings," in G. W. Baker and D. W. Chapman (Eds.) *Man and Society in Disaster,* New York: Basic Books, 1962.

25. R. S. Lazarus, *Psychological Stress and the Coping Process,* New York: McGraw-Hill, 1966, p. 33, 310, 44.

26. E. Lindemann, "Symptomatology and Management of Acute Grief," *American Journal of Psychiatry, 101:*141–48, 1944.

27. J. M. Natterson, and A. G. Knudson, "Observations Concerning Fear of Death in Fatally Ill Children and Their Mothers," *Psychosomatic Medicine, 22:*456–65, 1960.

28. D. Offer, and M. Sabshin, *Normality,* New York: Basic Books, 1966.

29. C. E. Orbach, "The Multiple Meanings of the Loss of a Child," *American Journal of Psychotherapy, 13:*906–15, 1959.

30. E. S. Paykel, Life Events and Acute Depression (Paper presented at Annual Meeting of the American Association for the Advancement of Science, Chicago, December, 1970).

31. G. Pollock, "Mourning and Adaptation," *International Journal of Psychoanalysis, 42:*341–61, 1961.

32. J. B. Richmond, and H. A. Waisman, "Psychologic Aspects of Management of Children with Malignant Diseases," *American Journal of Diseases of Children, 89:*42–47, 1955.

33. A. A. Rosner, "Mourning Before the Fact," *Journal of the American Psychoanalytic Association, 10:*564–70, 1962.

34. E. Ross, *On Death and Dying,* New York: Macmillan, 1969.

35. M. Sabshin, "Psychiatric Perspectives on Normality," *Archives of General Psychiatry, 17:*258–64, 1967.

36. M. Sabshin, E. H. Futterman, and I. Hoffman, "Empirical Studies of Healthy Adaptations" (in preparation).

37. L. D. Siggins, "Mourning: A Critical Survey of the Literature," *International Journal of Psychoanalysis, 47:*14–25, 1966.

Institutional Care

Cicely Saunders

A THERAPEUTIC COMMUNITY: ST. CHRISTOPHER'S HOSPICE

Among all our professions, there is something which we have in common and which is relevant in both different cultures and settings. Whatever our role, we are concerned *with persons* and we are concerned *as persons*. It is for this reason that I am including photographs of some individuals and families I have known—pictures which will bring the images of other persons in front of you.

Who are the dying? Is it the patient who, near the end of her illness, appears not to recognize the fact, or the one who does recognize it at a much earlier stage and lives on with that knowledge? Is it the patient who so completely accepts a long-term disability that she forgets it while she carries on with the business of meeting those around or the elderly, frail or well and active? Or is it after all a member of the staff? We need to remind ourselves that we are not thinking about "the dying" but about all of us—the whole family of man.

Elisabeth Kübler-Ross (1) has expressed clearly many of the things

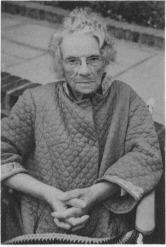

Photo 1

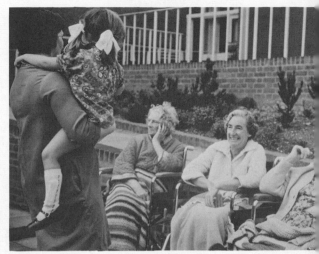

Photo 2

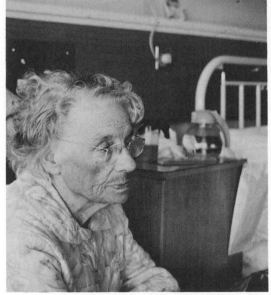

Photo 3

Photo 4

we had already recognized as well as some that we had not seen before. How do dying people feel? What stages of thought may they go through (or perhaps telescope together) as they approach and advance through the process of dying?

Photo 1 shows the mixture of defiance, denial, and demand that we must surely recognize. For us it was coupled with the constant complaint "It's your pills that are making me feel ill." Such a person is hard to meet and help. *Photo 2* shows how she turns away into isolation as an orderly picks up her child in the Hospice garden and meets a group of patients nearby. *Photo 3,* taken a few weeks later, shows the overwhelming feeling of depression, weariness, and longing. But on that same day, *Photo 4,* she is beginning to meet us, perhaps even to accept what is happening. Some two weeks later she was still taking her medication when she chose and was maintaining this much control of the situation.

The Hungarian refugee in *Photo 5* suffers from the added isolation of a language barrier. He could be reached by the symbols and sacraments of his own Catholic faith and also by sharing with us the pictures of his family in the folder in his hand, but the person who really comforted him was the patient in the next bed. Cheerful, untidy, and a rather heavy drinker, this man took life as it came, and in *Photo 6* he also takes death very much as it comes. (He died some two weeks later.) He was allowed to spend much of his time out in the local public house until three days before he died. In *Photo 7* he comes in saying, "Let me be in the picture with my friend." The Hungarian shows the wistful longing that is so typical of the bereavement of the dying. Some people have hands that we can take and some have fists that say, "Stay away." I think one has to remember that however important touch is at most times, it can also be an intrusion. But my Irish friend just goes ahead in simplicity and can get away with it, as shown in *Photo 8*.

Can we, as professional helpers like the nurse in *Photo 9,* have the spontaneity and capacity for meeting the lonely patient? This man had few friends or family. All these pictures are taken with the patients' permission for them to be used in talks and teaching, and each patient is given up to six copies as "royalties." This man did not have enough people to give his six away to, but he showed them, one by one and identical to everyone who came into the ward. How does one manage to care, as the girl does in the photo, and be prepared constantly to come in and give this kind of friendship? It can be done if you have the support of a concerned group, preferably a mixed group. Not only do we share in frequent discussions, but patients and their families also meet outside the Hospice with staff and their children. The nurse in *Photo 10* giving tea to patients and relatives, with her small son "helping" her, and the noisy water game of some of the playgroup for the children of married staff in the background, are part of a therapeutic community which includes many volunteers and a small group of elderly residents in their own wing. The time a few of them so willingly give has helped us with problems of communication.

Language may not be the only barrier. *Photo 11* shows a girl with motor neurone disease who, having lost her speech, could communicate with us by blinking in Morse code. With the help of one of these elderly residents she could communicate—not merely in the "Yes" or "No" or single words to which these patients are often limited but, instead, in a series of letters. I recall some of these written soon after her admission —"In my heart I feel I can't give up fighting"—and the change when she wrote a few months later:

I am awfully concerned about K. and wonder if you think there is any way I can help her. I long to be able to go over and comfort her, particularly at those times when she is so distressed and frightened. I know she gets tired easily so hesitate to suggest spending too long a time with her. On the other hand I have all the time in the world if you think it would help her if I sat with her, and although I cannot reach out and hold her hand, she can hold mine. Mother or the nurses could always come and let me know, I am writing to you in the first instance because you know what would be wise. If you think I could help in this way I should like to write to K. myself.

And finally,

Last year I used to weep because I wanted to go home. I seemed to have lost everything which means so much to me—and now I have so much—in fact, all that matters. My attitude towards death has utterly changed. I know now I shall be completely healed and am going Home. If I weep when patients die, they are tears of joy for them.

I cannot exaggerate the importance for that girl of being able to express her thoughts and to share her journey into acceptance, nor for her elderly friend to know her and to be the channel of communication.

But more than lack of speech can cut off our meeting with others. The man in *Photo 12*, with his sons eagerly listening to him, was seen first at home by the nurse in charge of our visiting service. His bed was in one room, and the rest of the family was in another with a shut door between them and an atmosphere of anger and fear creating a further

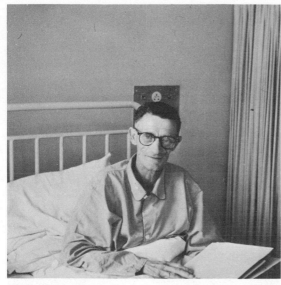

Photo 5

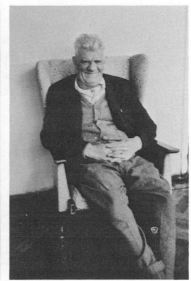

Photo 6

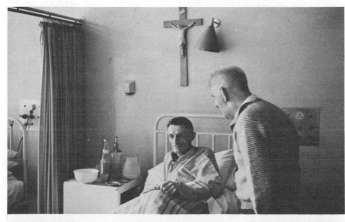

Photo 7

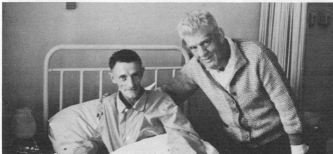

Photo 8

barrier. As he came into the Hospice and his pain was relieved, they met again the father they had been shutting out of their consciousness and they continued to do so until he died.

We have many instances which show the importance to a dying person of welcoming the whole family, including the children and grand-

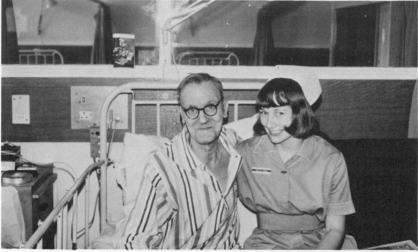

Photo 9
Photo 10

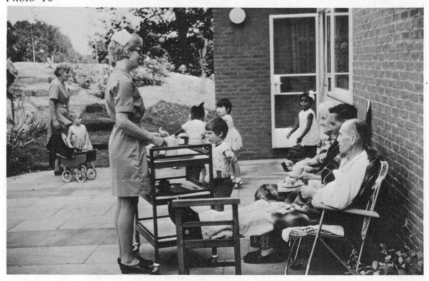

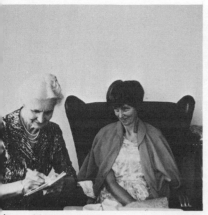

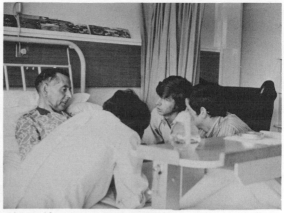

Photo 11

Photo 12

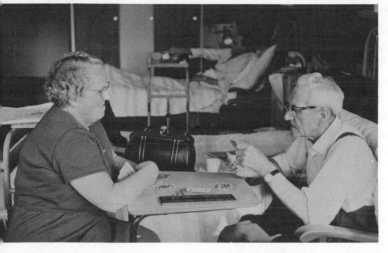

Photo 13

children. Visits which are full of unspoken farewells may have a strong element of joy if there is a baby to take the central place—often sitting on the patient's bed. We allow children of all ages to visit, and we find that they do not seem to be frightened. They are encouraged to run around or to help when they wish. It appears that if young children visit a grandparent or parent, they notice a smile and a few words rather than how sick they are. To remember illness and death in such a context is far less traumatic than an apparently meaningless disappearance by ambulance and then no more contact.

We feel that it is our responsibility to give relief of physical distress

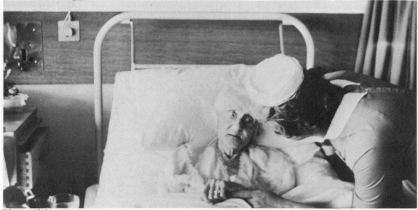

Photo 14

in a concerned, supportive atmosphere so that all this can happen spontaneously. Sometimes there are remissions and a person who has felt engulfed by pain and distress finds that time for living is given back to him. Depth in time is more important than length, but borrowed time is very precious. If it seems suddenly that you have more time than you expected, there may be a new awareness. Over and over again, I believe, we have seen the best part of a life at its ending, made fuller by the sense that it has been given back for a while.

Relief of pain can take away tension from a patient and despair and guilt from his spouse (2, 3). Physical and mental distress are closely interwoven, and we cannot always distinguish between their treatments. The regular dose of analgesic averts the threat as well as the fact of pain and relieves anxiety as well as physical distress. Distress and suffering are so often self-perpetuating as tension grows, but relief also leads to further relief. Our aim is the constant control of pain so that a patient can take part in any suitable activity and enjoy the open visiting hours which so many families fill faithfully. The man in *Photo 13* was admitted directly from the outpatient department of another hospital in unrelieved pain. We did not need to change the drugs prescribed but only to give them on a regular schedule rather than on demand. Once this was done, he could enjoy himself much as he had done at home.

We try to support patients at home if it is possible. Some have been helped to remain there, actively caring for their children till near their death. Two families met constantly over a period of several months in their visits to the Department and came to know each other well. When the first patient, a mother of two-year-old twins, went downhill and died after a brief admission, this was a great blow to the others. Their discovery in the next two weeks that the grandmother had moved into her house to take over, and that life was beginning again with continuity for the twins, was a great comfort and strength. The second mother, who was facing her own death, could begin to believe that life would start again for her children also.

The breathing space given by the control of physical pain may enable people to come through mental distress. One elderly lady settled down to write her life story and in doing so sorted out a great deal of resentment and bitterness from the past. Parting may be filled with bitterness as well as with sorrow, and we may not know why so often it fades away as it does. We cannot change what has happened to us but we may change its meaning. She achieved this, and the consequent release led to such an improvement in her physical condition that she was able to return home and deal with some unfinished business. She returned to die peacefully two months later.

I am reminded also of a patient, now dead, who had been in and out of the Hospice for nearly two years, all this time putting up such a facade that we felt we were never meeting him. When he came back for the last admission, things fell into place and he seemed suddenly to achieve reality and self-acceptance. Two days before he died he said to me, "You know, I was thinking last night, I *am* a silly fellow. Why do I make such a fuss?" A confession, a preparation, and letting go at last.

There is certainly a place here for the more traditional approaches of religion. We see this, but for our part we want to define religion more widely and see it as the field of the relationships of one person to another, commitment in the context of a common life (4, 5). We are only going to meet these people and understand something of what is taking place if we are on their level, moving at their speed. Our Matron (Director of Nursing) shows this as she goes round the wards, *Photo 14*. If we pay true attention, we find often that those who are considered retarded or confused are not so but are still very much themselves.

We do not move our patients out of the ward when they come to the moment of death. Families may stay around for many hours and often speak of the support of the whole group, of staff in particular but also other patients and their families. We fill the gap ourselves if there is no

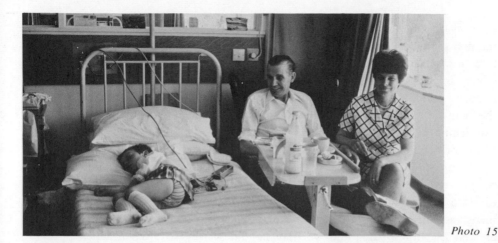

Photo 15

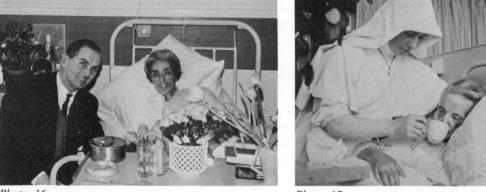

Photo 16

Photo 17

family member to sit with a dying patient during the last hours. A visiting student, a volunteer, or perhaps a staff member may remain with the patient until death comes.

As we face these demands, we find a great deal of strength comes from the patients themselves. We have recorded many of the ways in which people have found their own way through. We have seen the importance of pleasure, brought perhaps by a young student or volunteer. We have seen two people finding a union in adversity which they failed to find before. Among the very small number who have ever spoken to us of a wish for voluntary euthanasia was a young man. He talked of it as a way out of increasing dependence and yet went on making of that very dependence a constantly deeper relationship with his wife. His

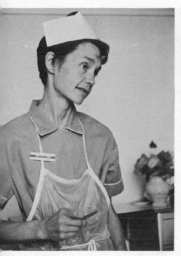

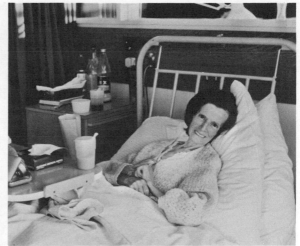

Photo 18   Photo 19

views would change from day to day as his relationship with us also deepened, and we could discuss it freely. We did not always agree, but we continued to talk and shared what we could. The last picture I have of this couple showed a warmth and happiness together which was a vindication as well as a challenge. He died peacefully in his sleep a few weeks later.

Part of the care of dying patients is the recognition of the moment when active treatments such as chemotherapy, blood transfusions, and other procedures are no longer relevant to a patient's real need. Too determined a perseverance with such measures can only detract from the peace and dignity of death and limit the possibilities of relationship. Such a recognition and the concentration on treatment for relief of pain enabled the family in *Photo 15* to go on meeting like this until a few days before the young man's death. *Photo 16* was taken three days before the next patient's death. She was helped to say her goodbye with all her courage and dignity, without the confusion of tubes or of yet more hopeless surgery for an obstructive bowel lesion. Both these patients demanded considerable skill on our part to enable them to go on living together with those they loved until they died. Even if we were alone, most of us would choose to have two cups of tea on our last afternoon rather than the distress of yet another infusion, as shown in *Photo 17*.*

The nurse in *Photo 18* has just carried out "last offices" ** for a pa-

* Photograph from St. Joseph's Hospice, London.
** Laying out a body.

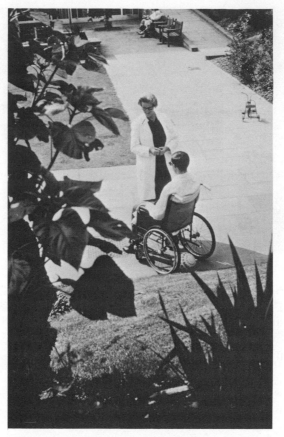

Photo 20

tient whom she loved. It was not an intrusion on her privacy or on the patient's to take this photograph—we knew them well enough. How does one do this, for this kind of caring is costly.

Our help comes foremost from some of our patients. Several of us use *Photo 19* often. This patient sums up many of our thoughts about a "good death." She knew she was dying and was as ready to go as she was to stay until the time came. After her death we found a paper in her locker with "I am in His hands" written over and over again all down the page.

Many have inspired us by the courage that may develop during a long illness. Others have been with us for only a short time and yet have left vivid memories. There is much satisfaction and challenge to be found as one constantly meets people at their moment of maximum individuation and maturity, at the moment when they sum up all that they are as they come to die.

A few of our patients are with us for two to three years with slowly progressive neurological diseases. I was discussing this meeting with one of them, a policeman now about forty-five years old and in the third year of his illness, (*Photo 20*). He referred to what he saw in our wards as a "bringing together illness." He meant not only the bringing together of skills, but even more the bringing together of families, of the lonely person with the staff, of patient with patient. His best friend in the ward had been a man from Brixton Jail. One of the stories he told me was of the day when he was out to the bathroom and Jock from Brixton came to say, "There's one of your lot inside. I'm not sure which one of us he's looking for!" He also spoke about the staff, how they would sit on the patient's bed or locker for a few minutes. "It's what you do with your odd moments that counts." He said, "They let you be yourself," and, "It's easier, you know, when you accept the facts, for then some of the complexities fall away." It is still a battle to reach and keep this calm, but his final remark was, "I don't know what is around the next bend, but I do know it's all right."

We have a modern, vivid picture of the Resurrection in the Hospice, and we send a reproduction of it to the families on the first anniversary of a patient's death. You can interpret this as you wish. It may be in the

Photo 21

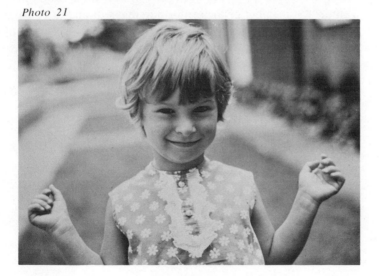

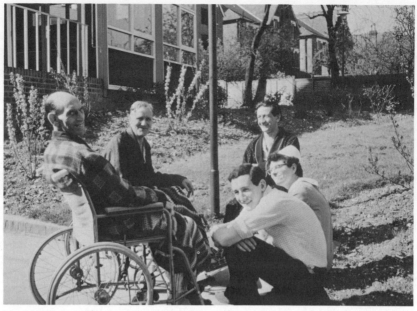

Photo 22

traditional way, it may just be in a feeling of light out of darkness. Light and darkness? I do not think you can have one without the other. Death is part of life and there is something about death that gives life its quality—and helps it to new beginnings. So I end with the joy of a child from our Playgroup, *Photo 21,* and a group, *Photo 22,* which includes a student, a member of the senior nursing staff and three patients, two of whom died within a fortnight of that picture. These are some of the psychosocial aspects of terminal care. But perhaps our most important question is—"How do we find this community wholeness and fit the dying patient and his family, and ourselves, into the whole of life to which we all belong?"

REFERENCES

1. E. K. Ross, *On Death and Dying,* London: Tavistock Publications, 1969.

2. C. M. Saunders, "The treatment of intractable pain in terminal cancer," *Proceedings of the Royal Society of Medicine, 56:*195, 1963.

3. C. M. Saunders, "The symptomatic treatment of incurable malignant disease," *Prescribers' Journal, 4:*68, 1964.

4. J. Macmurray, *Persons in Relation,* London: Faber, 1961.

5. Ibid., *Religion, Art and Science,* Liverpool: Liverpool University Press, 1961.

PHOTOGRAPHS

Nos. 1, 2, 10, 12, 18, 20, 21 by Grace Goldin *
Nos. 3–9, 11, 13–17, 19, 22 by Dr. Cicely Saunders

* Mrs. Goldin's efforts were supported by United States Public Service Grant #5R01-HS-10063-04.

Rose Dobrof

COMMUNITY RESOURCES AND THE CARE OF THE TERMINALLY ILL AND THEIR FAMILIES

The Stories

ITEM I

Many homes for the aged reserve their infirmary or hospital beds for their own infirm residents and admit only the healthy aged from the community. In the home where I was a staff member, the first step in the process of screening out unacceptable applicants was an assessment by our medical staff of the applicant's health status as reflected in doctor's and hospital reports. If, on the basis of these reports, it was determined that the applicant was unacceptable, the task of telephoning the family to inform them of the decision was delegated to the social service staff.

In the jargon of the institution, these were "medical rejects" and for obvious reasons all of us dreaded making those calls. Recently, one of such calls assigned to me was to the sixty-seven-year-old sister of an eighty-five-year-old maiden lady who, according to the report from her own doctor, was a severely impaired brain syndrome patient. As I dialed the number, I looked over the identifying information. The younger sister was a widow; her only son lived in California; the two sisters shared a one-bedroom, third-floor apartment in a once proud, now rundown, neighborhood. Both received Social Security benefits, and they supplemented this income by drawing on their meager and fast-disappearing savings.

The sixty-seven-year-old sister answered the phone, and I identified myself, and told her of our decision and the reasons for it, as gently as I could. We explain our requirements at the beginning of the intake procedure, and at that point, some families, recognizing that their aged member cannot meet the requirements, withdraw the application. Others hope against hope that the applicant will be more like herself again, and continue with the application. At the point of formal rejection some are usually not surprised and often have begun a search for an alternative arrangement. Still others can see no alternative, and they may deny the accuracy of the medical evaluation. If they do grant its accuracy, they may respond with an angry attack on an institution which presents itself as a haven and refuge for the old, but refuses to take the ill or impaired old person whose need is clearly great and most urgent.

The sixty-seven-year-old sister did none of these things. Her voice was pleasant, her tone well-modulated, as she asked me some intelligent, thoughtful questions about the level of care we provide in our Domiciliary section and the reasons for our admissions policy. Then, "Excuse me, just a minute, Mrs. Dobrof." I heard her voice change to a shriek. "See, sister, now what am I going to do? You're not crazy enough for the mental hospital, but you're too crazy for the Home. See what you've done to me! There's nobody who will help me." Then a few seconds of silence, and I heard again the pleasant voice, "Thank you so much for calling me, Mrs. Dobrof. It was kind of you to take the time." And a click, informing me that she had hung up.

ITEM II

Eighteen months ago a fourth child was born to a lower-middle class family in New York City. The infant was a genetic anomaly, so grossly impaired, and with so serious a cardiac condition, that her life expectancy is now reckoned in months. The baby remained in the hospital for several months, partly because its hold on life was a tenuous one, partly in order to complete exhaustive diagnostic and evaluatory procedures, and partly because the hospital staff feared the impact of its presence on the family, whose financial resources were meager, whose apartment was already crowded, and whose psychic strength was already strained by the birth of such a child.

The tests were completed, the bleak message conveyed to the parents, and the baby's health status was stabilized. The infant no longer required the resources of the acute treatment hospital. A regimen of medication and care was prescribed, and the bed in the pediatric section of the acute treatment hospital was urgently needed for another baby. There was no place to send her except home to the family. The state facility for retarded children would accept her but not until—and if—she reached the age of two years and six months. Voluntary child-care institutions have long waiting lists, and in addition the grossness of the impairments and the brevity of this child's life expectancy made her unacceptable to them.

So the baby went home. Ten months later, pushed beyond her physical and psychological strength, tortured by her feelings that the baby was a punishment for her sins, and bedeviled by her deeply-felt wish to prove herself sufficient to her tasks, the mother made a feeble and unsuccessful attempt to kill her baby. And so the baby was returned to the pediatrics unit in the acute treatment hospital, where it remains—a case, labeled "disposition pending."

ITEM III

A young family, mother and father in their thirties, children in elementary school and junior high, all struggling with the normal problems of family life, is suddenly confronted with problems of quite a different order.

The wife's sister, (also in her thirties), to whom the young family is very close, a career woman who lives in an apartment nearby, did not feel well. After weeks of assuring her family that she must be just tired and maybe nursing a cold, she finally went to the doctor. He had her admitted to the hospital, where his diagnosis of cancer was confirmed and a mastectomy performed.

Six months later, the thirteen-year-old son became ill with leukemia. For more than three years the family alternated between hope and despair: a second operation, followed by cobalt treatments for the sister; several hospitalizations, numerous blood transfusions, periods of remission (the good times) for the son.

The family was fortunate in some respects. They were upper-middle-class and prudent people, so both sister and parents had major medical and hospitalization insurance, and both had savings accounts. Moreover, they were surrounded by friends and neighbors who helped with the day-to-day tasks of living.

But three years later both sister and son were dead—first, the sister; three months later, the son.

In the three years, marked by frequent hospitalizations of both patients, the family connected with no professionals except the two attending physicians and the nurses on the floor. At no point did the Social Services Departments of the hospitals enter the case. When the patients were at home, their families cared for them and did not know about or seek out the services of Cancer Care, the Visiting Nurse Association, or a family service agency.

A month after the death of her son, four months after her sister's death, the mother collapsed in a neighbor's living room. Following this, she was hospitalized for several weeks in the psychiatric unit of the hospital where her son had died.

ITEM IV

Recently, a serious young social work student visited me in my office. Her field work placement is in the Social Services Department of one of the most prestigious teaching hospitals in New York. This morning she had been sent to make a home visit at the apartment of a post-stroke patient who had been discharged from the hospital last week.

The patient is seventy-nine; her husband is eighty-one. The patient, the student learned, had been "going down hill" for at least two years before this hospitalization. She was frequently incontinent, increasingly forgetful, and recently was preoccupied with fears that her husband had fallen in love with the fifty-seven-year-old widow down the hall. The husband, a diabetic with a severely ulcerated leg, had called the hospital because, even with the help of a Visiting Nurse Association nurse once a week and a home-health case worker three times a week, he couldn't manage the care of his now bed-ridden wife.

Our student had made her visit, heard the husband's story, seen the wife, and called her supervisor. Now arrangements were being made for the patient's admission to a nearby proprietory nursing home with which the hospital has a transfer agreement and which has an occupancy rate of under 80 per cent. The paper work—certification of the patient, and so on—would take several days.

Why hadn't the patient been sent directly to the nursing home from the hospital? Our student wasn't sure. "When I asked, all I got was some interdepartmental buck-passing. To tell you the truth, I don't think anyone really thought about any possibility except that the patient would go back home."

ITEM V

There is a social worker in New York State who serves as a member of the staff of a community-health center for thirty-five hours a week; for a certain number of hours per week he is an independent entrepreneur—a broker who, for a fee, guarantees to the families of the old, impaired, or infirm a service called Home-finding. In the seller's market of 1970, he represents the buyer, finding for him a nursing home, home for the aged, state mental hospital, or private psychiatric facility which will accept the aged parent, and hopefully at a price the family can afford to pay.

The Point of the Stories

I am reasonably certain that none of these stories is shocking in the sense of revealing information that is not already known to social workers. Each one can, from experience, undoubtedly top my stories. Certainly their choice of a vocation testifies to their concern.

My intent in beginning with this litany of personal suffering and institutional failure is to use these stories to help identify the precise nature of our failure and then make suggestions for action. Thereby, I hope we will avoid the trap of concluding that our problem is one solely of not enough community resources, and that our only hope is more.

This is not to say that I think we have enough, but only that the addition of institutions, health centers, and personnel will not in itself guarantee effective, accessible, appropriate services. A more critical look must be taken at the organization of services, the mechanisms used to guarantee integration of services, the patterns we developed to insure accountability—that is, continuity of work with an individual or family until the task is completed.

Returning to our cases for a moment to see if we can make more specific the reasons for our failures, we note that with the exception of the cancer-ridden sister and son and the possible exception of the genetic anomaly, the patients whose stories I've told may not, at first glance, fit the conventional picture of the terminally ill. And for certain purposes, they might better be classified as "the chronically ill." But the process of dying, like so many other events in the life cycle, has changed significantly in this century. Acute illness is no longer the major cause of death. Instead, death occurs more often now as the final event in an insidious, long-term process (1). In increasing numbers the patient dies not at home but in a hospital or long-term care facility (2).

Several years ago in our Home, a beautiful, devoutly religious eighty-six-year-old man was maintaining the death watch at the bedside of his aged wife. Her cancer took its pain-wracked time, and during one of those days I sat with him and he talked of his faith in God. It had not been shaken in this ordeal; he still did not question God's ultimate goodness or purpose. "But oh, Rose, it hurts so bad and it lasts so long."

Thus did he summarize the dying process of today, and thus are the patients in my stories dying in typical fashion for this period of time, their cause of death, a chronic illness; the duration of the terminal period not known with certainty, and perhaps very long; and death likely to occur in an institutional setting, not at home.

Now to the specification of our failure to provide the kind and quantity of community resources which these patients and their families needed.

The eighty-seven-year-old brain syndrome patient and her sister are the victims, of course, of a shortage in institutional provisions for the increasing numbers of severely impaired aged in our population. But the short supply of such facilities is not the only cause of our failure here. More facilities, as presently organized, would not solve their problem. The problem is the lack of integration among the agencies and institutions in the network of services for the aged.

Specialization among institutions, and careful specification of the societal task assignment of each institution and the nature of the services it is prepared to offer, have been altogether understandable and largely functional concomitants in the development of our health and welfare institution. Specialization has encouraged the development of truly expert professions and professionals; it has aided in the accumulation and dissemination of new knowledge about the etiology and treatment of many of the ills that beset us; it has been important in the mobilization of public support for efforts on behalf of selected patient groups. But specialization among agencies and institutions has led also to gaps and broken connections in the service network, so that individuals fall, unserved, into these gaps. Or services become fragmented and individuals, regardless of the multiplicity and diversity of their ills, remain whole and forced to travel from specialist to specialist, agency to agency, in search of the services and resources they need (3).

The brain syndrome patient, described above, went unserved. She was too impaired for the voluntary home for the aged; not psychotic enough for the state mental hospital, which no longer admits "the simple senile" patient whose condition is organic, and therefore, irremedial; not sick enough physically, and likely to live too long for the proprietory nursing home, which limits its intake to the short-term rehabilitation patient or the equally short-term terminally ill. More of the same, therefore, carries no guarantee of help for this patient and her sister unless it is accompanied by community coordination of agencies and institutions with respect to their programs, policies and objectives, in order to close the gaps among these agencies; and unless it is accompanied by integration of services to the individual client to insure accessibility, delivery, and continuity of the services she requires (4).

The picture for the tragic little baby and her family is a better one now than it is for the two old sisters—or than it was before the baby's mother's desperate act forced the hospital to respond. The use of an acute hospital pediatric bed for the baby is at this point the only possible alternative, albeit a poor one in social planning terms. The removal of the baby from the home and the sustained casework help provided by the hospital social worker hopefully will shore up the reserve strength in this family and permit it to continue as a nurturing, stable unit in the months and years after the death of the baby.

In addition, the hospital social worker, with the knowledge and permission of the family, has assumed the crucially important role of service coordinator. In view of the fragmentations and gaps in service, some organizational pattern must be developed which assigns to one worker in one agency or institution this responsibility for coordination of services. In this instance, the hospital social worker is doing what the family could never do on its own. Among other things, she is pushing aggressively to cut organizational red tape to effect placement of the baby in a State institution at the earliest possible date. The hospital worker has also referred the family to the Retarded Infant Service, which, among other activities, provides home-makers to families like this one. The retarded child may no longer be in the home, but the mother still needs help with her home-making tasks in order to regain her emotional health and build new reserves for the difficult months ahead.

As a general comment about home-maker services, it should be stated that this service is urgently needed by most families with a chronically or terminally ill member. It is also a service which is in critically short supply in most communities. Most home-maker agencies or departments have long waiting lists and often must make painful priority decisions among families whose need for the service is equally desperate.

For several years the National Council for Homemaker Services has recommended to the Congress that a broadened definition of eligibility for in-home-care be incorporated into Titles XVIII and XIX of the Social Security Act and that the range of homecare services which are reimbursable under these Titles be similarly broadened. These recommendations are based on the belief that a home-maker service is indispensable in our industrialized, urban society and, therefore, must be among our first-line services, with sanction and funding a governmental responsibility.

The tragedy of the doomed baby and her family obviously was not aggravated by the absence of resources alone. The lack of institutional facilities for such babies must be labeled as a moral and programmatic failure of monstrous proportions. However, there are other failures. Among these are the gap between service institutions which, in this case, has been created by the voluntary institution's limitation of its service to the less impaired, educable child and the State institution's minimum-age requirement.

Use of an acute hospital for what is essentially custodial care is clearly a misuse of a scarce resource. But if provision of custodial care is an inappropriate task for this type of hospital, it is just as clearly a task beyond the abilities and resources of most families. In theory, most of the doctors, nurses, or social workers staffing our hospitals and working with the families of the grossly impaired and retarded would agree that a baby like this one should probably not be cared for at home. In practice, however, the dearth of institutional facilities and the inadequacy of those which do exist make placement of these children a long, tortuous process. Facing this misery with the family, hospital staff members often find it too painful to say, "Yes, your child should be in an institution. It will profit him little from being in a home environment, and the small gain will be at a tremendous cost to the family." Instead, the worker, implicitly or explicitly, conveys the message to the family that the child belongs at home, and that the care of the child, although fraught with difficulty, should not be beyond the capabilities of the family.

Or often this second message need not even be delivered. The family itself—molded by a twentieth-century version of the Puritan Ethic with its emphasis on individual and family responsibility and on the salutory nature of pain and despair—believes that care of the child is a God-given task. Therefore, failure to shoulder this burden is a sin against God and a sign of human inadequacy.

Think for a moment of the 1930s, when thirteen-million men, one quarter of the nation's labor force, were unemployed and walked the streets in a desperate search for work—a search made all the more corrosive to their sense of self by the gnawing feeling that they themselves were somehow to blame for their plight, that their families were hungry and scared and cold because they were not competent enough to find and hold a job. They did not see themselves as one of thirteen-million men in the same boat; rather, they saw the thirty-nine million who were working, and they were ashamed that they were not among the so favored.

Similarly, many among the parents of the retarded and the impaired are bedeviled by feelings that they should care for their child and that their inability to do so reflects their own inadequacy—not society's. The family's own sense of inadequacy is confirmed by the professional's inability to deal honestly and openly with the societal failure to provide sufficient resources. The burden of guilt they already carry is thereby compounded.

Our failure to deliver needed community resources to the young mother (and her family) in time to prevent her collapse after the deaths of her sister and her son can be accounted for by reasons different from those already described. In retrospect, it is obvious that two terminal illnesses, occurring almost simultaneously, and removing from the family group two key members, represented a mortal threat to the integrity of the family unit and the mental health of the surviving members. Both attending physicians knew the whole story, as did a number of the nurses who cared for the patients during their hospitalizations. Why then was there no offer of nonmedical services made to the family during the harrowing months of illness, or after the two deaths?

One cannot attribute this failure solely to the lack of community resources; both hospitals had well-staffed social service departments; the family was eligible for the services of Cancer Care, a relatively new and very effective and innovative private agency; in the community, an excellent Family Service agency operated, well organized and staffed, and able to provide casework treatment, a home-maker service, and referral, if necessary, to other community resources.

In this case, their failure may be attributed to a defect in the organization of services, a defect which in turn reflects the failure of our professions and institutions to move beyond "conventional wisdom" and values. With respect to organization of services, in most hospitals the attending physician for the private patient is the undisputed captain of the treatment team, and referral to or orders for any hospital service are his responsibility. Thus, the social worker in the hospital has no official knowledge of the private patient and no entry into the case, except at the request of the attending physician.

Our nation's system of values and beliefs holds the explanation for this organizational pattern and the physicians' failures to make the referral to the Social Services Department.

I spoke before of the mother's feelings of guilt because her inability to care for the retarded child was a sign of weakness; of the unemployed man's belief that his joblessness was his own fault. These feelings of self-depreciation, deeply imbedded as they are in our value system, carry with them the logical corollary that financial security and family stability reflect individual competence and the adequacy of family members. The assumption is that the individual's and the family's ability to manage for themselves without help from community social welfare agencies should be taken for granted.

Thornton Wilder, in *The Eighth Day,* captures these ideas and beliefs in a particularly apposite way. He tells of Goshen, the poorhouse in Coaltown, a midwestern town:

To go to Goshen meant that your life, your one life, had been a failure. The Christian religion as delivered in Coaltown, established a bracing relation between God's favor and money. Poverty was not only a social misfortune; it was a visible sign of a fall from grace. God had promised that the just would never suffer want. The indigent were in an unhappy relation to both the earthly and heavenly orders (5).

The family struck by the double tragedy of the illnesses and deaths of the sister and the son was a financially secure and stable family. Hence, the assumption in this case that even facing such crushing losses its members needed no outside help, except that of the technical services of the doctors and the nurses. If this had been a poor family, their need for such concrete services as home-health-care would have been obvious; and, further, their need for counseling, supportive casework services would have been assumed, since society accepts the condition of poverty as prima facie evidence of inadequacy and dependence.

More community resources, therefore, could not have removed the obstacle between this family and the help its members needed. What is required instead is, first, a reassessment by the professions involved of the rarely explicit, usually hidden assumptions made concerning their clients' and patients' need for help; and second, reexamination and restructuring of the organization of professional services within the hospital, including the way in which tasks are assigned to various professional departments.

The failure in the case of the aged, post-stroke patient, who was sent home to be cared for by her even older husband, reflects professional and institutional defects of the same order. "Buck-passing" among departments is frequently symptomatic of ambiguity in task assignments within the hospital and of the lack or malfunction of organizational mechanisms designed to insure development of individual treatment plans and delivery of the services required to implement these plans. Just as the family of the retarded child needed a social worker to act as a traffic manager to coordinate the activities of the various community agencies providing services to the family, so also, within the hospital or institution, the task of service coordination must be assigned to one staff person or professional department.

But coordination of services, while necessary, is not in itself sufficient, if failures such as this are to be avoided in the future. Here, too, we must examine professional staff attitudes and assumptions. Remember, the social service student had the impression that everyone simply assumed that the wife would return to her own apartment, to be cared for by her husband. It was only after his frantic call to the hospital, and the student's home visit and firsthand assessment of the situation, that the staff assumption was proved to be in error and a different plan for the patient's care was worked out.

In making the initial decision, the staff had clearly made the most elementary kinds of errors. The husband had not been consulted, nor had his ability to care for his wife been evaluated. How can we account in a teaching hospital for a disposition decision being made in so cavalier a fashion, based on such fragmentary and incomplete information? The staff response to lack of resources both in the hospital and in the community account, at least in part, for our failure in this case.

Hospital staffs are characteristically undermanned and overworked, harassed by the problems and needs of the patients, harassed by the demands of their staff colleagues for information, decisions, plans. In this day of acute shortage of hospital beds, disposition planning is a high priority item, and the slowness of the process causes a struggle between the medical staff, who need a bed for the critically ill patient, and the social work staff, unable, in the face of the lack of resources in the community, to find an appropriate institution or nursing home placement.

It is altogether understandable, therefore, that the social worker and the doctor, noting that the post-stroke patient has a loyal husband and an apartment to return to, breathe a sigh of relief, give the order for discharge, and notify the husband of the time his wife will be ready to be taken home—without asking if this is really a viable plan. How able is the husband to care for his wife? Are there children who can help? Is the apartment big enough for the rented hospital bed? Where are the laundry facilities for the frequently soiled linens and nightgowns?

In sending the wife home to her husband's care, the staff is supported by our value system, as reflected in the marriage vow "in sickness and in health." But in New York City in the twentieth century, these words cannot be interpreted to mean that the obligation of the eighty-one-year-old man to his senile and bed-ridden wife can be fulfilled only by his caring for her in his apartment, and that his placement of her in an extended care facility is a dereliction of his duty to her. Nor does the marriage vow require one to sacrifice his own health in order to care for the other. In a very real sense, this old man was trapped—just as was the mother of the retarded baby—by his own and the professional's implicit assumptions about the responsibilities of husband to wife and family to child, and by their limited and distorted view of the way in which the responsibility was to be discharged (6). The old man was able to call for help almost immediately upon his realization of his entrapment; the mother of the retarded baby was slower to recognize her captivity. The societal failure lies in the fact that neither was given help until it was almost too late and then only when they asked for it.

And finally, our broker in institutional care for the aged. Surely there would be no need for or profit from such an enterprise if this were not a seller's market, one in which the demand far outstrips the supply. An adequate supply of community resources—including but not limited to institutional beds—would seem in itself to obviate the necessity for a broker. Yet, the reality in many of our communities is not one just of the absence of resources. Our picture of reality must include the inaccessibility of the resources which do exist; the narrowness with which many agencies and institutions define their services and the clients they will accept; the rigidity and complexity of their organization, which seems to the client like a Kafka novel, a maze of red tape, a forest of rules and regulations, so that the client is unable to travel the road to service without a guide, unable to negotiate the system without the broker.

Conclusions

This is a bleak picture of community resources and professional practices, and all of us know that it is not the complete picture. Many hospitals in New York City have, over the years, developed innovative, effective programs of comprehensive care and have tested a variety of patterns of service delivery which go far toward guaranteeing accessibility and continuity of care. Community mental health centers, funded with a mix of philanthropic and government monies, are located in many neighborhoods and provide important direct services, and in addition are the crucial link from neighborhood to large medical centers. At Jacobi Hospital, the Genetic Counseling Service in the pediatrics service is an exciting, largely Foundation-funded program of comprehensive and continuing service to these children and their families, with continuity of service guaranteed to the family even after the placement or the death of the affected child. Montefiore Hospital, founded originally as a home for the chronically invalid, has become a major medical and teaching center. But in the process it has continued to fulfill its original obligation to the chronically ill, and its program includes as well a multitude of services to the chronically and terminally ill in their homes, and to the families of the patients.

The one characteristic which all of these innovative programs have in common is that all of them developed because of the failure of available resources to respond to the unmet needs and the unsolved problems. None of them, however, represents a simple addition of more of what we had. All of them have involved a new kind of service or a new pattern of organization or vehicle for delivery of the service.

Home-health care developed largely because of the shortage and the high cost of inpatient hospital care. Group therapy emerged from the crucible of World War II, when the shortage of trained personnel and the pressure to return emotionally incapacitated soldiers to active duty led the professionals to try the short-cut of therapy in a group, instead of in the one-to-one relationship. Extended care facilities are a partial answer to the shortage of personnel and beds in acute treatment hospitals. The training and employment of paraprofessionals is a response to the chronic and increasingly short supply of the traditional health-care professionals.

I emphasize now that although all of these programs and services were created by shortages, their effectiveness lies not in addition to what *is,* but rather in the development of new, less expensive resources, or in the more effective organization and staffing of existing facilities and programs. Similarly, in each of the examples used for the purposes of our discussion, the lack of resources was not the only reason for the lack of effective service to the terminally ill and their families. Rather, in each case, the failure to help reflected poor use of what we do have: fragmented services; the absence of integration at the case level; the absence of coordination at the community level; internal organizational pathology, resulting in buck-passing among the staff; the lack of an effective system of accountability; and the presence of a maze of red tape for the patient. Our failures reflect also our unawareness of the implicit beliefs we have about the nature of the responsibility of family to member. We are unable either to re-examine the appropriateness of these beliefs in twentieth-century America, or to monitor their sometimes untoward impact on our work with the families who need our help.

If we focus our attention only on the lack of resources and the need for more, we are blinded to the possibility of creating new and better services and programs. We are foreclosing the possibility that necessity may mother new and better inventions. And if we focus only on the shortage, we are doomed always to failure, for there never will be enough, we will always need more. Even in the richest and most socially responsible of societies, there is an inevitable lag between the discovery of individual needs, the development of ways to meet those needs, and the public sanction and support for these ways. So, if our only hope is more, if even as we work for more there is nothing we can do with what is, then success in helping can never be until tomorrow, and failure to help is always our daily companion. To hope and work for tomorrow, while still hoping and working today, is not an easy task. But it is not one which we may escape, and in the end I believe with F. Scott Fitzerald that

The test of a first-rate intelligence is the ability to hold two opposed ideas in the mind at the same time, and still retain the ability to function. One should, for example, be able to see that things are hopeless and yet be determined to make them otherwise (7).

Surely this is the test we who work with the terminally ill and their families must face, and surely our goal must be to make our work something other than hopeless.

REFERENCES

1. M. Cherkasky, "The Hospital as a Social Instrument: Recent Experiences at Montefiore Hospital" in Knowles, J., *Hospitals, Doctors and the Public Interest,* Cambridge, Mass.: Harvard University Press, 1965, pp. 93–110.

2. E. W. Burgess, "Family Structure and Relationships," in *Aging in Western Societies: A Comparative Study,* Chicago: The University of Chicago Press, 1960, pp. 271–99.

3, 4. A. J. Kahn, *Theory and Practice of Social Planning,* New York: Russell Sage Foundation, 1969, pp. 267–304.

5. T. Wilder, *The Eighth Day,* New York: Popular Library Edition, 1969, pp. 46–47.

6. A. I. Goldfarb, "Clinical Perspectives," in *Psychiatric Research Report 23,* American Psychiatric Association, February, 1968, pp. 176–77.

7. F. S. Fitzgerald, *The Crack-Up,* New York: A New Directions Paperbook, 1956, p. 69.

Ethical Issues

Fred Rosner

EUTHANASIA

"To be or not to be, that is the question," a dramatic pronouncement by Shakespeare's Hamlet, has taken on new meaning in the age of cardiac transplantation, artificial hearts and kidneys, pacemakers, defibrillators, respirators, and the like. Medical progress has made possible significant extention in years of human life over that of a half century ago. However, not always is man's period of usefulness to himself or to society lengthened commensurate with his increased life span. How far should today's physician go, with a host of devices at his disposal, in keeping a patient alive who is no longer useful to himself or to society?

Few physicians would deny that extraordinary efforts with the use of mechanical devices need not be maintained when one is dealing with a deeply comatosed, aged patient who has had a cerebrovascular accident and for whom there is no hope of restoring useful or happy existence. The same holds true regarding a patient dying of an incurable malignant brain tumor. On the other hand, most physicians will agree that sudden death in a young person due to shock from infection, drowning, or asphyxia should be treated very vigorously. All resuscitative attempts at restoring respiratory and cardiac function must be made in this potentially reversible situation.

The moral courage required to make the decision as to when to use extraordinary measures to prolong life or when to stop them is considerable. The minimum medical or nursing care, such as nutrition, warmth, and change of body position, must be given to all patients. Beyond that, the decision usually rests with the physician. It is certainly medical opinion and judgment which form the basis for deciding whether there is any reasonable or even remote hope for recovery. It is said that "if the doctor is sincerely and selflessly trying to do the best for his patient, he is more likely to take the right course than if we try to draw up hard-and-fast rules to guide him in all cases" (1). However, much more than the physician is involved in a critically ill or incurably ill patient. The patient, the family, and society need also be considered.

The patient may be the type of individual who values his life and independence above all else; or he may be one who does not wish to become a burden on his family and requests to be put out of his misery, not objecting if the *coup de grace* were administered prior to physiological death. The family may be obsessed with the fear of not being able to cope with the situation and even if they decide to do the best they can, the physical burden may become too much to bear. Not infrequently does a terminal cancer patient involuntarily drain his relatives physically, emotionally, and financially. Society in general is very much concerned about the problem of terminal care and questions such as where do people die, under what conditions do they die, and to what extent society has made adequate provision to deal with the medical and social aspects of the dying patient. Voluntary organizations, religious orders, philanthropic bodies, service organizations, nursing groups, and individuals, as well as local and national governmental agencies, should all be involved in society's attack on the problem.

Definition of Death

Before embarking on a discussion of euthanasia, including classification, terminology, exemplification of the problem, and legal and religious attitudes and arguments for and against this procedure, it seems useful to briefly discuss death and the definition of death. The need for such a definition has been re-emphasized by the recent heart transplants. In addition, the increasing use of life support systems has rechanneled attention to the time and technique of the diagnosis of death. Public attitudes toward this problem in historical and current times have been reviewed (2). Death is the final diagnosis and, traditionally and by common law, the authority to make it has been vested in the physician. But the swift pace of today's medical developments, particularly organ transplantation, brings with it issues that are clouding the traditional definition of death.

A philosophical view of death was pronounced by Biorck (3) when he stated:

Is death a force in itself? I think not. We often project that word upon what is in fact the last phase of life. A cancer sucking out our last ounce of energy, a suffocation depriving us of our breath, a delirium of the heart throwing us into recurrent convulsions may all be experienced as an enemy force, internal, yet alien to us, the herald of Death. It may be that some of us succumb to an enemy within us. But this enemy is Disease, not Death. A human being may be dying. He is never dead. If he is dead, he is no more a human being. Death is in itself nothing. But it leaves a dead body behind, perceptible to our senses, and, in addition, among those nearby a feeling that something imperceptible has gone.

Medical and legal definitions of death are similar in certain respects but differ in other respects (4). Even among various physicians or medical groups, there is no unanimity of opinion nor uniformity of criteria. Further compounding the problem is the fact that there are different types of death, each with a different definition. There is physiologic death, intellectual death, spiritual death, and social death (5). Religious criteria to define death may be at variance with either those of the medical or legal professions.

The criteria for defining death acceptable to many physicians include complete bilateral, pupillary dilatation with no reaction to local constricting stimuli, complete abolition of reflexes, complete cessation of spontaneous respiration, absence of measurable blood pressure, and a flat electroencephalogram (6).

At the 1968 national meeting of the American Medical Association, guidelines for organ transplants were approved by the House of Delegates. One of the major guidelines states (7):

When a vital single organ is to be transplanted, the death of the donor shall have been determined by at least one physician other than the recipient's physician. Death shall be determined by the clinical judgment of the physician. In making this determination, the ethical physician will use all available, currently accepted scientific tests.

How does one ascertain the irreversibility of the process of life? The Ad Hoc Committee of the Harvard Medical School to Examine the Definition of Brain Death has arrived at a definition of irreversible coma (8). The Canadian Medical Association named its own committee of experts to come up with a legal and ethical definition of death.

At what point need a physician no longer attempt resuscitation? The 22nd World Medical Association meeting in Australia in 1968, adopted a statement, to be known as the Declaration of Sydney, which states in part that a physician's determination of death "should be based on clinical judgment, supplemented if necessary by diagnostic aids, of which the electroencephalograph is the current most helpful single one." Drafters of the statement admitted its indefiniteness and stressed that there are no precise scientific criteria nor a definition for what is the moment of death.

When is the dying patient beyond help? When is the physician guilty of a grave moral and religious sin by not doing everything possible to "maintain" his patient? Just as one cannot properly define health as the absence of disease, it seems totally inappropriate to define death as the absence of life. Society in general and the medical and legal professions in particular are currently struggling to arrive at an acceptable definition of death.

The Catholic Church is on record as not requiring a physician to use "extraordinary" means to prolong life of a hopelessly ill patient (9). The term "extraordinary" is not defined, however. The Church is also opposed to the removal of hearts from persons certainly not dead (10). The Church requires "clear and reasonable" evidence for death before a heart can be removed for transplantation. However, "clear and reasonable" remain to be defined. For Christians, unlike Jews, there are sacramental rites to be accorded to the dying person prior to the departure of the soul from the body and, therefore, it seems imperative that a proper definition of death be available.

Jewish law defines death as the absence of spontaneous respiration and the cessation of cardiac action. This classic definition of death in the Talmud and Codes would be set aside if prospects for resuscitation of the patient, however remote, are deemed feasible.

Euthanasia: Terminology and Classification

The word "euthanasia" is derived from the Greek "eu," meaning well, good, or pleasant and "thanatos," meaning death. Webster's dictionary defines euthanasia as the mode or act of inducing death painlessly or as a relief from pain. Euthanasia is popularly spoken of as "mercy killing." A less painful term used by euthanasia societies is "merciful release" or "liberating euthanasia." Some people classify euthanasia into three types: Eugenic, medical, and preventive. A more meaningful classification speaks of eugenic, active medical, and passive medical euthanasia. Eugenic euthanasia would encompass the "merciful release" of birth monsters and socially undesirable individuals such as the mentally retarded and psychiatrically disturbed. Perhaps an extreme example of this method of extermination was the Nazi killing of all the socially unacceptable or socially unfit. To many, this Nazi practice as well as all eugenic euthanasia is considered nothing less than murder, and thus there are very few proponents of this type of euthanasia.

Active medical euthanasia is exemplified by the case where a drug or other treatment is administered, and death is thereby hastened. This type of euthanasia may be voluntary or involuntary, that is, with or without the patient's consent.

Exemplification of the Problem of Euthanasia

Many physicians have had to wrestle with the problem of an incurably ill, suffering patient. For example, on December 4, 1969, a general practitioner in Manchester, New Hampshire, ended a cancer patient's suffering by injecting a substantial quantity of air into the patient, intravenously. He was acquitted. On March 9, 1950, a woman in Stamford, Connecticut, shot and killed her father who was dying of incurable cancer. She was acquitted.

The problem is far from localized to the United States. In December, 1961, Giuseppe F., having settled in France, was struck with an incurable disease. He summoned his brother Luigi and convinced the latter to kill him, which Luigi did. The jury acquitted Luigi.

One of the most famous instances exemplifying many of the problems surrounding euthanasia is the case of Maurice Millard, M.D., son of the founder of the British Euthanasia Society. Dr. Millard told a Rotary meeting: "To keep her from pain . . . I gave her an injection to make her sleep." His objective as specifically stated was to relieve pain, not to put an end to the patient's life. An outcry in the British press followed, labeling the incident a "mercy killing." Although the British Euthanasia Society admitted that from a strictly legal sense mercy killing is murder, it backed Dr. Millard by insisting that "every doctor must be guided by his own conscience." Many physicians disagreed, saying euthanasia is only legalized murder. Others cited the Hippocratic oath which states: "I will give no deadly medicine to anyone if asked, nor suggest any such counsel." Still others were of the opinion that the Hippocratic oath refers only to premeditated murder. The medical council refused to act against Dr. Millard unless the family of the deceased lodged a formal complaint. However, the family consented to Dr. Millard's actions. Thus, all the ingredients to emphasize the problem of euthanasia are present in this case: the incurable patient in great pain, the request for euthanasia by patient and family, and the physician's acquiescence and participation.

The list of examples one could cite is endless. The aforementioned illustrative cases serve as background for the ensuing discussion.

Legal Attitude Toward Euthanasia

Although suicide is not legally a crime in most American jurisdictions, aiding and abetting suicide is murder. Euthanasia in the United States, even at the patient's request, is legally murder. In England the Suicide Act enacted into law in 1961 states that it is no longer a criminal offense for a person, whether in sickness or in health, to take his own life or to attempt to do so. However, any individual who helps him to do so becomes liable to a charge of manslaughter. Euthanasia *per se* does not exist in the law books of France and Belgium, and in both countries it is considered premeditated homicide. However, a bill to legalize euthanasia for some "damaged" children came before the Belgian government on November 26, 1962, following the famous Liege trial involving parents, relatives, and a physician charged with murdering a thalidomide-damaged child.

In Italy euthanasia is only a crime if the victim is under eighteen years of age, mentally retarded, or menaced or under the effect of fear. More tolerant attitudes also exist in Denmark, Holland, Yugoslavia, and even Catholic Spain. In Russia, euthanasia is considered "murder under extenuating circumstances" and punishable with three to eight years in prison. Switzerland seems to have the most lenient legislation. The Swiss penal code was revamped in 1951 and distinguishes between killing with bad intentions, that is, murder, and killing with good intentions, that is, euthanasia. In addition, in 1964, passive euthanasia was legalized in Sweden.

Even in the countries where euthanasia is legally murder, "the sympathies of juries toward mercy killings often cause the law to be circumvented by various methods, making for great inequities of the legal system."

In 1935 the first Euthanasia Society was founded in England by C. Killick Millard, M.D., for the purpose of promoting legislation which would seek to "make the act of dying more gentle" (11). In 1936, one year after the founding of the Society, a bill was introduced into the House of Lords which sought to permit voluntary euthanasia in certain circumstances and with certain safeguards. Following a rather heated debate, it was decided that "in view of the emergence of so many controversial issues, it would be best to leave the matter for the time being to the discretion of individual medical men—the bill was rejected by 35 votes to 14."

Another Voluntary Euthanasia Bill was debated before the House of Lords on March 25, 1969. The Bill, which was moved by Lord Raglan, makes it lawful for physicians to give euthanasia, provided that the patient has signed a declaration (in the first place for three years, and then has re-executed it for his lifetime), and that this has not been revoked. It entitles a patient to whatever drugs may be required to keep him free from pain and it clarifies the law in circumstances when a patient is in such stress that he cannot be relieved by ordinary drugs. Lord Raglan maintained that everyone should be allowed to die when and how they chose and not in a way chosen by someone else. After considerable debate, the bill was rejected. The Euthanasia Society of England is active today and its goal is to see implemented a "plan for Voluntary Euthanasia which would permit an adult person of sound mind, whose life is ending with much suffering to choose between an easy death and a hard one; and to obtain medical aid in implementing that choice" (11).

In 1938, three years after the inception of the British group, the Euthanasia Society of America, Inc., was founded by Charles Francis Potter. This nonsectarian, voluntary organization, rather than seeking to have legislation enacted to legalize euthanasia, is attempting to achieve a more enlightened public understanding of euthanasia through dissemination of information. This goal is being strived for through discussions of euthanasia in medical societies and other professional groups, research studies and opinion polls, dissemination of literature, a speaker's bureau, and other responsible media of communication.

Other euthanasia societies have arisen in Sweden and Japan. Support for these societies and their work comes from various other groups, such as the American Humanist Association and the Ethical Culture Society. Opposition to euthanasia is also strong, however. Thus, the Academy of Moral and Political Sciences of Paris voted on a motion completely outlawing, forbidding, and rejecting euthanasia in all its forms. In addition, the Council of the World Medical Association, meeting in Copenhagen in April of 1950, recommended that the practice of euthanasia be condemned (12). The debate continues and some of the arguments presented by proponents and opponents of euthanasia will be presented here.

The problem has been well stated by Filbey (13). "When a tortured man asks: 'For God's sake, doctor, let me die, just put me to sleep,' we have yet to find the answer as to whether to comply is for God's sake, the patient's sake, our own or possibly all three." Even if the moral issue of euthanasia could be circumvented, other questions of logistics would immediately arise: Who is to initiate euthanasia proceedings? The patient? The family? The physician? Who is to make the final decision? The physician? A group of physicians? The courts? Who is to carry out the decision if it is affirmative? The physician? Others?

Euthanasia: Pros and Cons

Arguments for and against euthanasia are numerous, have been and continue to be heatedly debated in many circles, and will be only briefly summarized here.

Opponents of euthanasia say that, if voluntary, it is suicide. Although by British law, suicide is no longer a crime, Christian and Jewish religious teachings certainly outlaw suicide. The answer offered to this argument is that martyrdom, a form of suicide, is condoned under certain conditions. However, the martyr seeks not to end his life primarily but to accomplish a goal, death being an undesired side product. Thus, martyrdom and suicide do not seem comparable.

It is also said that euthanasia, if voluntary, is murder. As one writer aptly put it: "Euthanasia must be defined within the knife's edge area between suicide and murder." Murder, however, usually connotes premeditated evil. The motives of the person administering euthanasia are far from evil. On the contrary, such motives are commendable and praiseworthy, although the methods may be unacceptable.

A closely related objection to euthanasia says that it transgresses the

Biblical injunction "Thou shalt not kill." To overcome this argument, some modern Biblical translators substitute "Thou shalt not commit murder" and, as just mentioned, murder usually represents "violent killing for purposes of gain, or treachery or vendetta" and is totally dissimilar to the "merciful release" of euthanasia.

That God alone gives and takes life as it is written in Deuteronomy 32:39: "I kill and I make alive" and Ezekiel 18:4: "Behold, all souls are Mine," and that one's life span is divinely predetermined, is not denied by the proponents of euthanasia. The difficulty with this point, however, seems to be the question of whether euthanasia represents shortening of life or shortening of the act of dying.

To complete the religious argumentation, it is said that suffering is part of the divine plan with which man has no right to tamper. This phase of faith remains a mystery and is best exemplified by the story of Job.

It is further argued by opponents of euthanasia that since physicians are only human beings they are liable to error. There is no infallibility in a physician's diagnosis of an incurably ill patient, and mistakes have been made. Dr. I. M. Rabinowitch, in an address on the subject of euthanasia delivered before the Medical Undergraduates Society of McGill University on March 21, 1950, quoted his own case. Eighteen years earlier a diagnosis of carcinoma of the esophagus had been made, yet Dr. Rabinowitch was very much alive when he spoke at McGill University eighteen years later. Such mistaken diagnoses are exceedingly rare, but they do occur. The same is true of spontaneous remission of cancer, which has been reported, however, only in very rare instances.

The need for euthanasia today is minimized by some because of the availability of hypnotics, narcotics, anesthetics, and other analgesic means sufficient to keep any patient's pain and distress at a tolerable level. This fact, in general, may be true, but occasional patients develop severe pain which is refractory to all drugs and which requires surgical interruption of the nerve pathways for relief.

The Hippocratic oath or a similar vow taken by all physicians is conflicting. On the one hand, it states that a physician's duty is to relieve suffering, yet, on the other hand, it also states that the physician must preserve and protect life. This oath is used as an argument by both proponents and opponents of euthanasia.

A very valid point of debate is the suggestion that if euthanasia were legalized for incurably ill, suffering cancer patients, then extension of such legislation to the grossly deformed, psychotic, or senile patients might follow. A recent editorial stated: "If euthanasia is granted to the first class, can it long be denied to the second? . . . Each step is so short; the slope so slippery; our values in this age, so uncertain and unstable . . ." (14).

Further debatable questions are the sincerity of patient and/or family in requesting euthanasia. A patient racked with pain may make an impulsive but ill-considered request for merciful release which he will not be able to retract or regret after the *fait accompli*. The patient's family may not be completely sincere in its desire to relieve the patient's suffering. The family also wishes to relieve its own suffering. Enemies or heirs of the patient may request hastening of the patient's death for ulterior motives. These and further arguments both for and against euthanasia are discussed at greater length by Fletcher (12), Sperry (15), and others.

CATHOLIC ATTITUDE TOWARD EUTHANASIA

In at least five places (Matthew 5:21, Matthew 19:18, Mark 10:19, Luke 18:20, Romans 13:9) the New Testament contains the Biblical admonition "Thou shalt not kill." Based on this, the attitude of the Catholic Church in this matter is cited as follows

. . . The teaching of the Church is unequivocal that God is the supreme master of life and death and that no human being is allowed to usurp His dominion so as deliberately to put an end to life, either his own or anyone else's without authorization . . . and the only authorizations the Church recognizes are a nation engaged in war, execution of criminals by a Government, killing in self defense . . . The Church has never allowed and never will allow the killing of individuals on grounds of expediency; for instance . . . putting an end to prolonged suffering or hopeless sickness . . . (16).

Thus we see a blanket condemnation of active euthanasia as murder by the Catholic Church, and therefore a mortal sin. The reasons behind this teaching include the inviolability of human life or the supreme dominion of God over His creatures and the purposefulness of human suffering. Man suffers as penance for his sins, perhaps for the spiritual good of his fellow man. Suffering teaches humility and helps the Catholic identify with his crucified Lord.

Passive medical euthanasia is treated quite differently. The Church distinguishes between "ordinary" and "extraordinary" measures employed by physicians when certain death and suffering lie ahead. In this day of auxiliary hearts, artificial kidneys, respirators, pacemakers, defibrillators and similar instruments, the definition of "extraordinary" is unclear and nebulous. Pope Pius XII, in the last year of his life, issued an encyclical not requiring physicians to use heroic measures in such circumstances. Thus, passive euthanasia is sanctioned by the Catholic Church. In an address to the congress of Italian anesthetists on February 24, 1957, the Pope further stated: "Even if narcotics may shorten life while they relieve pain, it is permissible."

PROTESTANT ATTITUDE TOWARD EUTHANASIA

In the Protestant Church there are "all possible colors in the spectrum of attitudes toward euthanasia." Some condemn it, some favor it, and many are in between, advocating judgment of each case individually. Perhaps the greatest Protestant advocate of legalized euthanasia is the Anglican minister Joseph Fletcher. His three main reasons are the following: (1) Suffering is purposeless, demoralizing, and degrading; (2) Human personality is of greater worth than life per se; and (3) The phrase "Blessed are the merciful, for they shall obtain mercy" is as important as "Thou shalt not kill."

JEWISH ATTITUDE TOWARD EUTHANASIA

The Jewish attitude relating to our subject has been described in detail (17) and summarized by Jacobovits (18) as follows:

. . . any form of active euthanasia is strictly prohibited and condemned as plain murder . . . anyone who kills a dying person is liable to the death penalty as a common murderer. At the same time, Jewish law sanctions the withdrawal of any factor—whether extraneous to the patient himself or not —which may artificially delay his demise in the final phase.

However, the discontinuation of instrumentation and machinery which is specifically designed and utilized in the treatment of incurably ill patients might only be permissible if one is certain that in doing so one is shortening the act of dying and not interrupting life. Yet who can make the fine distinction between prolonging life and prolonging the act of dying? The former comes within the physician's reference, the latter does not.

It might be of interest to mention that probably the first recorded instance of euthanasia concerns the death of King Saul in the year 1013 B.C. At the end of the first book of Samuel (Chapter 31:1–6) we find the following:

Now the Philistines fought against Israel, and the men of Israel fled from before the Philistines and fell down slain on Mount Gilboa. And the Philistines pursued hard upon Saul and upon his sons; and the Philistines slew Jonathan and Abinadab and Malchishua, the sons of Saul. And the battle went sore against Saul and the archers overtook him and he was greatly afraid by reason of the archers. There said Saul to his armor-bearer: "Draw thy sword, and thrust me through therewith, lest these uncircumcized come and thrust me through and make a mock of me. But his armor-bearer would not; for he was sore afraid. Therefore, Saul took his sword and fell upon it. And when the armor-bearer saw that Saul was dead, he likewise fell upon his sword and died with him. So Saul died and his three sons, and his armor-bearer, and all his sons, that same day together.

From this passage it would appear as if Saul committed suicide. However, at the beginning of the second book of Samuel, when David is informed of Saul's death, we find the following: (Chapter 1:5–10)

And David said unto the young man that told him: "How knowest thou that Saul and Jonathan his son are dead?" And the young man that told him said: "As I happened by chance upon Mount Gilboa, behold Saul leaned upon his spear; and lo, the chariots and the horsemen pressed hard upon him. And when he looked behind him, he saw me, and called unto me. And I answered: Here am I. And he said unto me: Who art Thou? And I answered him: I am an Amalekite. And he said unto me: Stand, I pray thee, beside me, and slay me, for the agony hath taken hold of me; because my life is just yet in me. So I stood beside him and slew him, because I was sure that he would live after that he was fallen. . . ."

Many commentators consider this a case of euthanasia. Radak (Rabbi David Kimchi, A.D. 1160 to 1235) specifically states that Saul did not die immediately on falling on his sword but was mortally wounded and in his death throes asked the Amalekite to hasten his death. Ralbag (Rabbi Levi ben Gerson, A.D. 1288 to 1344) and Rashi (Rabbi Solomon ben Isaac, A.D. 1040 to 1105) also support this viewpoint, as does Metzudath David (Rabbi David Altschul, seventeenth century). Some modern scholars think that the story of the Amalekite was a complete fabrication.

Conclusion

One recent writer asked a series of provocative questions (19):

When confronted with a dying or apparently dead patient, a physician is challenged. What should he do? Should he acknowledge defeat and make life's final moments as peaceful and as comfortable as possible, or should he use all the resources at his command to postpone clinical death? After clinical death, that is, when spontaneous respiration has ceased and the heart has stopped beating, should a physician delay biological death or the permanent extinction of life by keeping tissues alive with stimulators, respirators and other resuscitative devices? If he does, for how long should he do it? For only as long as necessary to win time for restorative measures to take effect, or, if these fail, indefinitely, to have a living bank of organs for later transplantation? When a patient with a cardiac pacemaker, artificial heart or respirator has irreversible brain damage and is moribund, is he murdered by the physician who turns off the current?

This writer's opinion is that "a person dying is still a person living, and he keeps his elementary human rights up to the moment when life becomes extinct"(19). But precisely when is life extinct? When is death irreversible? When should extraordinary resuscitative measures be employed, and for how long? When may they be withheld? The attitude of physicians and others toward euthanasia from a purely moral standpoint is enunciated by Karnofsky (20) as follows:

It is ethically wrong for a doctor to make an arbitrary judgment, at a certain point in his patient's illness, to stop supportive measures. The patient entrusts his life to his doctor, and it is the doctor's duty to sustain it as long as possible.

REFERENCES

1. B. Whitlow, "Extreme Measures to Prolong Life," *Journal of the American Medical Association, 202:*374–75, October 23, 1967.

2. J. D. Arnold, T. F. Zimmerman, and D. C. Martin, "Public Attitudes and the Diagnosis of Death," *Journal of the American Medical Association, 206:*1949–54, November 25, 1968.

3. G. Biorck, "Thoughts on Life and Death," *Perspectives in Biological Medicine, 11:*527–43, Summer, 1968.

4. M. M. Halley and W. F. Harvey, "Medical vs. Legal Definitions of Death," *Journal of the American Medical Association, 204:*423–25, May 6, 1968.

5. H. K. Beecher, "Ethical Problems Created by the Hopelessly Unconscious Patient," *New England Journal of Medicine, 278:*1425–1430, June 27, 1968.

6. J. Z. Appel, "Ethical and Legal Questions Posed by Recent Advances in Medicine," *Journal of the American Medical Association, 205:*513–16, August 12, 1968.

7. "Ethical Guidelines for Organ Transplantation," *Journal of the American Medical Association, 205:*341–42, August 5, 1968.

8. "A Definition of Irreversible Coma. Report of the Ad Hoc Committee of the Harvard Medical School to Examine the Definition of Brain Death," *Journal of the American Medical Association, 205:*337–40, August 5, 1968.

9. "The Pope Speaks Prolongation of Life," *Osservatore Romano, 4:*393–98, 1957.

10. Msgr. F. Lambruschini, quoted in the *New York Times,* January 25, 1968.

11. "A Plan for Voluntary Euthanasia," London, The Euthanasia Society, 1962, p. 28.

12. J. Fletcher, "Euthanasia: Our Right to Die," in *Morals and Medicine,* Princeton, New Jersey: Princeton University Press, 1954, Chapter 6.

13. E. E. Filbey, "Some Overtones of Euthanasia," *Hospital Topics, 43:*55–61, September, 1965.

14. "Euthanasia," editorial, *Lancet, 2:*351–52, August 12, 1961.

15. W. L. Sperry, "The Prolongation of Life. Euthanasia-pro and Euthanasia-con," in *The Ethical Basis of Medical Practice,* New York: Paul B. Hoeber, Inc., 1950. Chapters 10–12.

16. I. M. Rabinowitch, "Euthanasia," *McGill Medical Journal, 19:*160–75, 1950.

17. F. Rosner, "Jewish Attitude Toward Euthanasia," *New York State Journal of Medicine, 67:*2501–06, September 15, 1967.

18. I. Jacobovits, "The Dying and Their Treatment. Preparation for Death and Euthanasia," in *Jewish Medical Ethics,* New York: Bloch, 1959, Chapter 11.

19. F. J. Ayd, "What is Death?," *Medical Counter Point, 1:*7–14, March, 1969.

20. D. A. Karnofsky, "Why Prolong the Life of a Patient with Advanced Cancer?," *CA, Bulletin of Cancer Progress, 10:*9–11, 1960.

Thomas A. Gonda

ORGAN TRANSPLANTATION AND THE PSYCHOSOCIAL ASPECTS OF TERMINAL CARE

Introductory Comments

Recent dramatic developments in human tissue transplantation have raised a number of personal and social issues with respect to the care of the terminally ill that are novel as well as inordinately complex. As has often been the case in other areas, the technical and scientific advances in tissue transplantation have far outstripped our ability to deal with and resolve the problems and questions that they have created on levels of personal and social interaction. There is evidence, however, of a rising concern in this area whose intensity can be gauged by the small but burgeoning literature that deals with psychological, ethical, moral, legal, and social issues in the artificial maintenance of life and in the therapeutic uses of human tissue. This is reflected in the annotated bibliographies compiled in each of the past two years by Hall and Swenson (5) of the National Clearing House for Mental Health Information.

The technical feasibility of organ transplantation was demonstrated in experimental animals by Carrell and Guthrie (1) at the turn of the century. Many years were to pass before Lower and Shumway (6) succeeded in supporting circulation with a transplanted heart and before immuno-suppressive and tissue-typing techniques were developed that could *begin* to handle the awesome problems of the rejection phenomenon. At the present time, the transplantation of kidneys and hearts from donor to recipient is essentially a problem of medical treatment with difficulties that may lead some to conclude that the practical and reliable transplanting of major organs is a vision of the distant future. More often than not, however, we have been surprised at the swiftness and ingenuity of achieving solutions to seemingly insuperable scientific and technical problems. So, we must prepare ourselves on the humane, ethical, and moral levels before the reality of mass transplanatation is upon us. Moreover, it is a fact that regardless of overall frequency or long-term failure, each instance of organ transplantation *now* used in terminal care involves to one degree or another all of the psychosocial issues presented herein as well as many others.

At the risk of being obvious, it is important to emphasize the fact that the kidney is a paired organ, whereas the heart is single. This means that living donors as well as cadaver donors may be used in kidney transplantation, while the heart transplanatation procedure is limited to cadaver donors. One further biotechnical fact differentiating kidney and heart transplantations is the existence of an artificial kidney that allows first a prolonged period of preparation of the recipient and donor, and also permits maintenance of life of the recipient in the event of rejection of the donated organ. The currently available artificial hearts, on the other hand, allow recipients only very brief moments of survival.

Although the relationship between donor and recipient is exceedingly intricate, for purposes of exposition it will be helpful to delineate those personal and societal issues that are primarily donor-related issues from those that are primarily recipient-related.

Donor-Related Issues

THE LIVING DONOR

In considering the donor-related problems of heart and kidney transplantation, we immediately encounter the question of whether or not a vital organ, even if paired, should ever be taken from a living donor. Although the law clearly permits this procedure provided the donor is an adult who is fully informed of the consequences and risks, a look at actual practices suggests that the choice to become a living donor is made under a number of pressures which would exist even if it were true that donors always survive and that one kidney was actuarially as good as two. Data establishing the certainty of long-term donor survival is not available.

The responsibility to procure the live donor is most commonly assigned to the recipient or to members of his family. In most instances the donor candidate is a genetically-related member of the recipient's immediate family. The numerous potential psychological stresses and intrafamily conflicts introduced by the need for organ donation make a choice that is free of coercion virtually impossible. Examples of the kinds of stressful and coercive situations that have been described include: a) family interpersonal dynamics that subtly pressure one member into unwanted donorship status; b) disruption of families in instances in which one of the siblings refuses to be considered as an organ donor; c) guilt of a family member who refuses to donate an organ, leading to psychopathologic reactions including suicide; d) persistent feelings of omnipotence and control over the recipient; e) transgression of cultural beliefs that call for a special need to maintain body integrity, with eternal damnation the consequence if one is unwhole or if all of one's body parts are not buried together. Even when the donor is consciously motivated primarily by humanitarian considerations, and even when he is viewed as a hero by friends and relatives, residual ambiguities and conflicts at deeper levels can be incapacitating in the long run. Whereas often in renal transplantation the related donor's grief reaction ends suddenly as the recipient's condition improves, extreme donor reactions of anger and/or grief are not uncommon when a kidney is rejected by the recipient.

Live donors who are unrelated to the recipient are nearly always motivated by reasons of self-benefit; all the more so when no prior social relationship has existed between donor and the recipient. More often than not, such "volunteers" are severely disturbed individuals for whom the act of being a donor has serious self-destructive implications. It may be suggested that obtaining special privilege (early parole for a prisoner) or substantial earthly goods (significant cash payment) in return for the sale of an organ are both healthy and ethically acceptable motivations. Notwithstanding, the social wisdom of such transactions is highly questionable. At the very least, the subordinate issues of tax consequences and warrantees would soon arise were organs ever declared salable property having a fair market value.

The high cost of organ transplantation forces emphasis on the question of who pays for the surgical procedure undergone by the donor, including for the care of unforeseen complications. Since the recipient must find his own donor, the issue of whether or not the recipient should be responsible for payment of the costs incurred by the donor is very real. Some insurance companies have recognized such charges as appropriate.

Even if the issues entailed in the practice of organ donation by adults are fully resolved, the problem remains as to whether or not a vital organ should ever be taken from a live donor who is a minor.

THE CADAVER DONOR

The primary issues relating to organ transplantation from cadaver donors involve the problems of defining death, the procurement of cadaver donors, and the effects of transplantation upon the donor's family.

The most difficult problem involved in the definition of death is to specify the precise moment that death occurs. The exact time of death often has critical legal importance, but the criteria for diagnosing death are purely matters of medical judgment. Advances in resuscitation and heart bypass techniques have necessitated revisions in the diagnosis of death to include central nervous system ("brain") death. Silverman and coworkers (8), in their analysis of a questionnaire sent to members of the

American Electroencephalographic Society, disclosed that of 1,665 patients reported to have isoelectric electroencephalograms, there were only three with truly linear records who recovered some cerebral function, and all three had drug-induced coma. Other changes in the diagnosis of death can be foreseen. However, what seems of continuing importance is that there be no distinction between "medical" and "legal" death. Is there a better definition at this stage of our knowledge than to state that the time of death is when the attending physician says it is? In view of this and until there is a better answer, is it not imperative that the determination and pronouncement of death be made by physicians who have no connection with the transplant team?

Sanders and Dukeminier (7) have defined the fundamental issue in the procurement of cadaver donors as "what claims to cadavers by what persons should be recognized and protected by society." They suggest that the most important policy question is the protection of the bodily integrity of the living. How might advocates of euthanasia respond to this question? Other central principles they outline which are involved in the procurement of cadaver organs are: a) the ethic to use cadaver organs to save the life of some other person; b) the ethic to respect the wishes of the decedent in the disposition of his body; c) the ethic to salvage cadaver organs in such a way as to minimize the traumatic effect of the procedure upon the bereaved relatives; and d) the ethic to take into account any religious objections to cadaver transplants. Within the past two years several states have adopted as law versions of the Uniform Anatomical Gift Act that address many of the issues related to these central principles.

Based on their experiences with families of cadaver donors at Stanford University Hospital, Christopherson and Lunde (2) concluded that donation of vital organs can be a meaningful part of the normal grief process if pathological motivations are absent and if the transplant team recognizes the special needs of donor families at this time and is willing to provide them with assistance. They point out that anonymity, or at least not meeting the recipient, is a very important donor family "need." An issue stemming from these observations is whether or not homotransplantation requiring cadaver organs should be performed at institutions that are not in a position to deal effectively with the psychosocial aspects of the procedure, that is, to evaluate the psychological status and motivations of prospective donors and to deal carefully and immediately with emotional problems in the donor families as well as those of the recipient.

Recipient-Related Issues

With the recipient we once more, in somewhat different form, meet the issues associated with informed consent and family involvement. Informed consent as it relates to the recipient presents essentially the same problems as informed consent in any serious major surgical procedure. Explaining the risks of transplantation to a person who has no concept of tissue rejection phenomena, however, may be unusually difficult. Furthermore, potential transplant recipients, even when they know the odds for survival, are most often willing to take the chance rather than continue to live as invalids.

It may be assumed that all key family members will be stressfully affected by organ transplantation. These stresses will be accentuated by the fact that a major investment is being made in the recipient who may, and often does, experience only a relatively short extension of life. This stress is further compounded by the continuous threat of rejection of the transplanted organ. The recipient and his family truly live with an immunological sword of Damocles.

Regarding the recipients and their families, Christopherson and Lunde (3) have found that pretransplant screening and counseling can influence the postoperative psychosocial adjustment of transplant survivors. They found that patients who received unambiguous family support for their decision to undergo transplantation, who were able to discuss their awareness of impending death, and who had specific uses for the "extra time" gained by transplantation, tended to have the best psychosocial adjustment.

The most important and perplexing issues regarding transplant recipients relate to their selection. It is unlikely that the supply of cadaver vital organs will be sufficient to meet the demand in the realistically foreseeable future. Given this situation, the selection of a recipient from among many possible candidates, and the question of who does the selecting and what criteria are used become issues of absolutely critical importance. Subordinate issues regarding maintenance of safeguards and meeting of costs are also important.

More than any other considerations related to organ transplantation, those involved in the selection of recipients most clearly bring to light the fact that transplantation is not the province of any one discipline. Rather, they emphasize the importance of bringing several disciplines together in harmony, and reinforce the argument for the development of special transplant centers. Most clear in the selection procedure is the need for a medical screening process which will evaluate the indications for the transplant as well as the probability of reaching a state of relatively good general health postsurgically. Less clear as a selection adjunct is the value of psychiatric evaluation beyond that required to eliminate individuals with either marked mental deficiency or psychosis unrelated to the condition for which the transplant is to be performed. Finally, we have barely begun to confront the problem of evaluating social worth, and whether or not such a criterion should be a part of the selection process. Sanders and Dukeminier (7) suggest a number of possible methods by which transplant recipients who fulfill medical (including psychiatric) criteria may be selected. These include a) the ability to pay; b) first-come, first-served; c) lottery or random selection; and d) rules announced in advance that are not unconstitutionally discriminatory. No method is without serious defect.

In this report, some of the major psychosocial issues in organ transplantation have been touched on. We may be absolutely sure that psychosocial issues will compound as new techniques widen the range of transplant feasibilities. In a recent satirical writing on organ transplantation Davidson (4) wonders "who" or "what" the recipient will become as various transplant procedures—including that of the brain—develop, and how the demand for new organs will be met. He sees grim possibilities ahead, such as hearse chasers, suicide-assistance squads, organ brokers, transplant supply engineers, and even the development of a tissue-compatible subhuman species with no will to resist being destroyed in order to rejuvenate clients. In that brave new world he postulates, the spirit of innovation will surely not be limited to biological understanding and surgical techniques! Thus, a person with the ingenuity and capacity to acquire the needed fortune, could buy enough organ replacements to achieve immortality!

These conjectures should convince us of the need to confront these problems as soon as possible. We cannot allow ourselves to become complacent about the amount of time left and once again allow technical and scientific advances to do more harm than good for lack of foresight. We must try, *here and now,* today, to resolve foreseeable issues as they are identified and before they must be met in practice. As the ancient proverb tells us, "Where there is no vision—the people perish."

REFERENCES

1. A. Carrell and C. C. Guthrie, "The transplantation of veins and organs," *American Medicine, 10*(27):1101, 1905.

2. L. K. Christopherson and D. T. Lunde, "Experiences with heart transplant donors and their families," *Seminars in Psychiatry, 3*(1), 1971.

3. L. K. Christopherson, and D. T. Lunde, "The selection of cardiac transplant recipients and their subsequent psychosocial adjustment," *Seminars in Psychiatry, 3*(1), 1971.

4. H. A. Davidson, "Transplantation in the brave new world," *Mental Hygiene, 52*(3):467, 1968.

5. J. H. Hall, and D. D. Swenson, *Psychological and social aspects of human tissue transplantation.* U.S. Department of Health, Education and Welfare, Chevy Chase, Maryland, 1968 (Supplement no. 1., 1969).

6. R. R. Lower, and N. E. Shumway, "Studies on orthotopic homotransplantation of the canine heart," *Surgical Forum, 11:*18, 1960.

7. D. Sanders and J. Dukeminier, "Medical Advance and legal lag: Hemodialysis and kidney transplantation," *UCLA Law Review, 15*(267):357, 1968.

8. D. Silverman *et al.,* "Cerebral death and the encephalogram," *Journal of the American Medical Association, 209*(10):1505, 1969.

Chaplain LeRoy G. Kerney

PASTORAL USE OF
"THE SEVEN LAST WORDS"
IN TERMINAL CARE

"The seven last words" is a familiar phrase to those who stand within the Christian tradition. The phrase refers to the sayings attributed by the gospel writers to the Christ figure as he hung on the cross. These sayings are often used in Holy Week and Good Friday worship services.

These sayings bear re-examination, from a pastoral point of view, as a source for understanding the experience of terminally ill people and as a source of wisdom in bringing pastoral care to them. The thesis herein is that these particular word symbols can help expand the insight and sensitivity of the pastor and that they can be used in pastoral conversations to bring insight and comfort to patient and family. No attempt will be made to go into the critical issues of these biblical phrases that rightly concern the biblical scholars.

It is hoped that the reader will sense the direction of thought implied in this examination and will in turn "pick up the ball and run with it" in order to expand his own wisdom and insight and make more effective his work with the terminally ill.

The saying, *Father, forgive them for they know not what they do* (Luke 23:24), points to the experience of being in the midst of people who are ignorant of the meaning of their acts or the moment at hand. It is not clear if the reference is to the soldiers or to Jesus's own people and nation. Perhaps it was toward both. The tragedy was ignorance being pawned off as knowledge.

It is obvious that the terminally ill patient stands in quite a different context from that of a political prisoner being put to death. Nevertheless, both often experience feelings of disappointment, frustration of goals, loneliness, helplessness, and hopelessness that family, staff, and clergy often minimize or miss.

A clergyman, known to the author, had a severe heart attack. In the midst of the acute stage, he found it almost impossible to breathe. He said it felt as if a plastic bag were over his head. He wondered if he could ever get another breath. A nurse came in to tell him that some special equipment was going to be brought in to help him breathe. As she walked out with a very slow gait, he wanted to shout, "Hurry, hurry, don't you know I may die before you even get down to the end of the hall?"

When the patient keeps his thoughts and feelings to himself, is there not an assumption that there is peace when there is no real peace, reconciliation when the family is separated in spirit and attitude? Does he want support and comfort to which we respond with a short visit and a quick prayer? To be aware of the possibility of ignorance of the other person's feeling is the beginning of deeper communication of pastor with patient.

Forgiveness assumes a relationship with something or someone larger than the rift that separates. Trust in a Spirit beyond the human level is the ground on which forgiveness can be expressed. However, it can come only after there is an awareness and acknowledgment of the gulf of understanding between the parties. To see life from the viewpoint of the ill person is to see life differently than from a healthy, up-right posture.

Verily I say unto thee, today shalt thou be with me in Paradise (Luke 23:43). This saying is a response to a conversation that has taken place between three men. Crucified on either side of Jesus were two men who most likely were not common criminals but Zealots who had been caught in acts of violence against Rome. The first one hurled insults at Jesus, taunting him to save them if he was what he claimed to be. The second malefactor, also sensing their dire situation, called out, "Jesus, remember me when you come into your kingly power." Jesus replied that he would be with him in paradise.

Here is the cry of men who sense their missions are ending in failure. Here is the plea to be remembered. The dying person wonders if he will be remembered, or will he be buried and quickly forgotten? And, if he is remembered, how will he be remembered?

In the research hospital setting, patients are often heard to say, "If they cannot help me, perhaps it will enable them to help someone else." Patients are looking for immortality. They wish to have a place in the advance of mankind as well as in the memories of loved ones. It is human to wish to be remembered. It has been pointed out that the greatest sin is the sin of indifference, and this can apply to the dead as well as to the living. Is it not this desire to be remembered that accounts for tombstones and grave markers with names, dates, and inscriptions?

Jesus's response of the promise of a place in the heavenly kingdom is the symbol that needs to be extended pastorally to the dying person. Even the casual words such as, "I shall never forget your courage, or your faith," is a way of assuring this deep cry to be remembered by the terminally ill person.

Woman, behold thy son, behold thy mother (John 19:27). Here is indicated the concern of Jesus for the ongoing welfare of his mother. As the oldest son, with Joseph his father no longer in the home, he felt a responsibility for her future. He took positive action and indicated to his mother and to his cousin, John, that he wished them to form a new bond of love that would sustain their spirits.

One of the chief concerns of dying patients is for their families. Patients often continue to live until a child is a certain age, or has graduated from school, or has been married. These concerns may be expressed in the writing of a will, the setting up of financial trusts, and other explicit instructions concerning family and finances.

There was a patient who, knowing she had only a short time to live, found herself in a panic about her family. She was divorced and had children. There was no one in her family to whom she felt she could turn, and she had no money that could be used to care for the children. She had turned away from her church, but at this stage the pastor of the church was brought back into the picture. He began by saying the church could find a cemetery plot for her. Soon several families in the church indicated a desire to adopt the boy. The mother of a girl friend said the girl could stay with her. A social worker helped the girl get into a beauty school and find a work career. In a few months the woman died in peace knowing her family was cared for.

Good pastoral care of the dying patient concerns itself with family arrangements. This does not mean that the clergyman always has to work out the details. Rather, he needs to seek out information concerning such arrangements from the patient and his family, and if they have not been made, to help find a way to work out the details.

My God, my God, why hast thou forsaken me? (Matthew 27:46; Mark 15:34). Was this cry of dereliction uttered by Jesus, or was it a quotation from the 22nd Psalm ascribed to him by the early church? Could the Christ figure experience abandonment by his Heavenly Father, or was this more of an expression of loneliness, perplexity over his betrayal and desertion by the disciples, and by the tortures of the cross?

Experience in ministering to the dying would suggest that it is human to experience all these feelings. Scripture can become the vehicle to express deep personal feelings. This is a very familiar verse to many patients and has often been shared by them in pastoral conversations.

Perhaps the clue to these questions lies in the structure and movement of the 22nd Psalm itself. The Psalm gives expression to alternating views or moods. Once the psalmist has given expression to being deserted, he goes on to affirm that God is holy. Soon comes the convulsion of horror as he sees himself as a worm, not a man, scorned by men, and despised by the people. This gives way to the expression of remembrance of being safely kept as a child at his mother's breast. Still again comes the convulsive sensation of being poured out like water, feeling his bones are out of joint, seeing himself as lying in the dust of death. After this comes the responsive expression of the call to fear the Lord and praise Him. The psalm continues on this level and concludes on an affirmative note.

Here is the poetic expression of the process of speaking the unspeakable which allows the affirmation of life to break through. To articulate the negative brings relief and release from the terrorizing grip of these overwhelming emotions and allows the individual to find a foundation on which to stand.

To ask the terminally ill what they think Jesus was experiencing on the cross when he gave expression to being forsaken is a pastoral method that allows the person to focus on another person's problems that parallel his own. The author has pointed out at times that if Jesus who was called the "Son of God" could give expression to the anguish of being forsaken, then who are we to think that feelings of abandonment, fear, anger, and disappointment are forbidden? The author has urged the dying to share these emotions and experiences with someone they trust so that they may be lead to a new strength and comfort.

I thirst (John 19:28). Was the Christ figure really human and did he have physical needs such as being thirsty? Is it hard in this day and age to see the threat of gnosticism that underlay this saying with its viewpoint that spirit was good and matter was evil? Today there is a tendency to deny the spirit side of man rather than the material aspects of his being.

And yet, in a strange way, the threat of gnosticism is still with us. It is the nature of a healthy person not to think about his health. To become self-conscious about one's state of health is to move toward illness. When things go well, bodily concerns are taken for granted and pushed out of consciousness. When illness or pain strikes or fatal illness threatens, a person becomes acutely aware of muscles, cells, tissues, and body functions.

Too often sick people are reluctant to seek medical relief of pain. They feel that they should "tough it out" and not give in to accepting a pain pill or tranquilizer. On the other side are medical personnel who, it would appear, are too strict in helping to provide the means for relieving pain and suffering.

Still another aspect of this problem is that of the patients who are so heavily drugged that they are unaware of the seriousness of their situation or are unable to think clearly and communicate their concerns about their possible death. Does a patient have the right to die, and to die his own death?

Because the clergyman is often viewed on the side of the spirit with either a disregard of, or a turning away from, the physical side of life, it is important to articulate the goodness of the body and its important role in the whole economy of God. There is a need to be reminded that the creation story describes the creation of the world as "good," and the creation of man from the dust of the earth as "very good." Man does not have a body or a soul. Rather, man is a body or he is a soul depending on the perspective at the moment from which he is viewed. "I thirst" is a reminder of the physical side of life to both patient and pastor.

It is finished (John 19:30). The end had come. Everything for which the Christ had toiled and sacrificed appeared to be ending in nothing. All that was left was a group of broken hearts who had loved him and a small handful of men who fled at the time of his death. This was the end. But the saying stresses the word "finished" rather than "ended." To state that his work was finished implied a completion of his mission. The Christ figure died trusting God and believing that his work was complete.

As this paper was being written, the author was interrupted by the tragic death of a college girl in a highway accident. Her family waited in the emergency room for a pastor to give comfort and to help them through the "valley of the shadows." Suddenly, a lovely and wonderful girl with much to live for was dead. Life had quickly ebbed away, and she was no longer with us. Life on this earth was at an end. Was it "finished?" In what sense was there a completeness to her life?

Father, into thy hands I commit my spirit (Luke 23:46). Jesus died with a prayer on his lips. The words come from Psalm 31:5. To these words is added the word, "Father." The verse from the 31st Psalm was the first prayer every Jewish mother taught her child to say at bedtime. It was the "Now I lay me down to sleep" of his day. The gospel writer ends the life of Jesus with a childhood prayer on his lips, picturing him as a child falling asleep in his father's arms.

I have always been impressed with the return of early memories, words of wisdom, learned prayers, scriptural verses when people become sick. I recall visiting an old grandmother who was dying. The family requested me to come and asked me to read some scripture and to say a prayer. They told me she had not spoken to any of them for several hours.

They did not think she had the strength nor the capacity to be aware of them or to talk with them. As I sat beside the bed, I took her hand and quietly started to repeat the 23rd Psalm. After saying the first few verses, I noticed that her lips started to move, and with a barely audible voice she spoke the Psalm with me to the end.

Early childhood memories and training, which may seem to have been forgotten or replaced by more sophisticated and different religious points of view, often come flooding back at the time of death. Some of the prayers, and concepts, may appear to be shallow, or inadequate, or naive. But more important than the content itself is the return of the memory of trust and warmth in which they were first learned when life was young and simple.

Summary

An attempt has been made to re-examine, from a pastoral point of view, the sayings of the Christ figure on the cross as a source of understanding the experience of terminally ill people and as a source of wisdom for the pastoral care of dying persons. The writer will count his efforts successful if the reader has been stimulated to find his own meanings in these words, expand upon them, use them in his pastoral ministry to the terminally ill.

Appendix

EDUCATION WORKSHOP

Reported by

AUSTIN HERSCHBERGER

Contemporary American culture is in an era of over-denial which has become hardened to death, with a corresponding over-emphasis upon youth and life. We have abandoned the mourning customs of the past and have lost the ability to handle grief and bereavement. Current sophistication has all but destroyed former rituals which legitimately allowed the expression of anger, the expression of guilt, the expression of loss, and the reintegration of residual infantile feelings reawakened at the time of loss. Society has turned the problem over to professional death handlers, the morticians and funeral homes; and children as well as adults, instead of being allowed to experience and assimilate the phenomena of death, are shielded, even over-protected. Children who do suffer loss, separation, and for whom mourning is cut short often move to delinquency; adults, when there is no mourning, evidence an increase in psychiatric and physiological disorders.

To thanatology, then, will accrue many burdens as mourning practices continue to be lost. What concrete proposals can be made to correct such conditions? What other kinds of intervention are there when ritual is no longer available? Are there preventive measures which will allow the individual to integrate the experience of death positively? Should death as a natural phenomenon be introduced in education at the high school level, at the college level? If so, how would one structure such an attempt? These are but some of the questions to which thanatology must address itself, and since the process of mourning is not yet clearly understood, one suggested line of research is a comparative study of orthodox versus nonorthodox cultural groups and their reactions to death.

Contemporary American culture has a profound impact upon the practicing physician. In addition to its emphasis upon youth and denial of death, there are the added problems of humanism versus individualism and technology. Cure—life—is much more important than comfort and care. Cure equals success. Death equals failure. Technology equals specialization and subsequent remoteness. Too often the physician is unaware of his symbolic importance and thus overlooks or misses the therapeutic effect of care and comfort. Yet, are we not asking the physician to give up a great deal when we ask him to hold hands? Does the physician turn from the terminal patient because of his own fear of death or does he retreat because he feels he would be of better use elsewhere. Medically, "terminal" indicates that no more can be done. It may be that the physician feels his skills are no longer needed. It could be not just fear of death, but also fear of making a mistake, of guilt over causing death. He may feel he has no expertise in psychosocial matters, and that perhaps since such issues are not very important he should turn the terminal patient over to others. A central problem, then, is the lack of involvement in the terminal patient by the professional.

But, is it not dangerous to become too involved with the patient? The answer involves the difference between identification and empathy. Although the line between identification and empathy is never completely and sharply demarked, it should not be necessary to close oneself off in order to maintain integrity. There will always be times when one identifies, but hopefully these instances will be recognized so that they can be handled. There will be some patients with whom identification will occur, and others with whom it will not occur; the problem is not one of identification, but of bringing the identification into consciousness so that it can be handled. Once one has come to grips with death, one can then help the patient live while he still lives, assuring him that the life still left to him need not be meaningless. Ideally, those who are now practicing as well as those who are preparing should look upon curing and helping as a continuous personal growth process. The question is, "Am I going to interact, become involved, and thus enable both the patient and myself to grow personally, or am I going to cut myself off and manipulate just to cure?"

Medical, nursing, and dental students during training certainly express more dissatisfaction with the manner in which death is treated than do faculty. If it is handled at all, it is a hit-or-miss situation and is seldom integrated into the curriculum. The faculty tends to avoid areas in which they feel inadequate, and thus ignores the subject. Too often the attitude is expressed as "you are on your own" with no support coming from the faculty when the medical student or the student nurse has to face the death of a patient. Too often the faculty tends to see the end-product rather than the process toward the end. Medical students uniformly report intense anxiety as the result of their first experience with a cadaver, anxiety which not only colors one's death fears, but which if not handled properly tends to perpetuate those feelings, precluding any adequate treatment later of the terminal patient.

Students have suggested that small groups be formed so that their feelings could be discussed, even though some might be ashamed to discuss these feelings and others might refuse to enter such a discussion. Comparing the first- and second-year medical student with the third- and fourth-year student, the trend is from initial optimism to increasing insensitivity, with the student becoming more and more the narrow, laboratory-oriented, impersonal individual. Likewise with student nurses, the first year is crucial in blocking or opening up the student to the experience of death, and they feel that the nursing faculty is unresponsive to the problem.

It would seem, then, that if one is not supported in these early experiences, the net effect is withdrawal. Both medical students and student nurses need an opportunity to deal early in their training with prior and current negative experiences with respect to death. They must be allowed to feel helpless and to be aided in handling these feelings. A consultant should be available for both medical students and student nurses for all psychosocial problems, especially while he or she is in the early stages of clinical training. As soon as students find that just one of the faculty is willing to talk about these problems, that faculty member immediately finds himself being sought out.

In view of these problems, how does one start teaching death, introducing the subject of thanatology? One must first learn about himself before he can learn about death. Yet, one cannot wait until he has complete self-understanding, since this is a continuous process which ends only with death. Any teacher in this area, since there are no unequivocal answers, must be able to be open with his students, and to deal with individual reactions. Until we can honestly recognize our own anxieties when working with the patient and the family, we cannot help the medical student, and even then the instructor will find himself in an uncomfortable position if he is the single teacher who tries to handle the problem of death.

Death as a formal subject, of course, would be most inappropriate. Death should and must be related to the entire care of the patient, the living, the dying, and those who remain. Because of high initial resistance on the part of present faculties, in introducing thanatology one takes whatever time he can. First one hour, then two hours, and in a very short time students will begin to demand a list of consultants. Whatever teaching does occur must be dramatic, participatory, and nondidactic. Instead of a special death teacher, multiteaching, multidiscipline instruction should be established. Seminars should be formed to assist both students and faculty, as it should be a simultaneous examination of the experiences of both. Death as a natural phenomenon can and should become integrated into the process of living.

MEDICAL CARE WORKSHOP

Reported by
ARNOLDUS GOUDSMIT

For quite a few generations it has been traditional to declare that doctors are practicing the science and the art of medicine. More often than not just exactly which part of their performance constitutes science and which art is left almost exclusively to the imagination of the audience. If the science of medicine takes in all of the area currently referred to as biomedical, it appears to encompass the major share of the visible curriculum of our medical schools. The art, still undefined, is left to be learned without the benefit of a specifically recognized faculty, curriculum, textbook, or undergraduate and graduate slice of assigned or elected training time. Once the biomedical is largely identified as the "hardware" of medicine, the art becomes equated with the "software" of the health professions, a province to which most of the psychosocial aspects of terminal care (PSAOTC) are relegated.

Many existing problems in the field of PSAOTC are tied up intimately with motivations (conscious and unconscious), moods, identifications, sensitivities, and cognitive and communicative capabilities of the minds of all concerned. When these psychological factors operating in patients, doctors, relatives, friends, and allied health professionals remain unidentified, processes of sound and realistic decisionmaking are jeopardized. They add to the feelings of frustration of many health professionals and to the suffering and grief of patients and relatives. They also appear to contribute to the overemphasis of whatever differences may exist between the strictly biomedical and the exclusively psychosocial considerations of terminal care. Needless to say, what constitutes the time of onset of terminal illness depends on subjective points of view; some diseases are more terminal (viz. fatal) than others; and the terminality of some diseases becomes evident only by hindsight. To add to the lack of definition, the bulk of terminal care considerations appears to refer by silent assent to cancer and allied diseases, and to blot out many conditions equally progressive, threatening, incapacitating, expensive, or painful.

At the Veterans Administration Hospital, Allen Park, Michigan, staff members in the areas of nursing, oncology, psychology, religion, and social work have been persuaded that the gap between the biomedical and the psychosocial may be both narrowed and bridged through improved communications. They engage in scheduled weekly multidisciplinary meetings where they discuss patient problems, as well as study the broad existential predicaments facing all who deal with death and dying on the one hand and with cancer on the other. As these sessions progress, the participants gain insights and abilities to communicate in depth and in truth with each other, with their patients, and with their patients' families. In a terminal stage of an illness a situation sometimes arises involving a regular "pandemonium of futile, last-minute heroics." In the process many artifices may be brought to bear on the dying patient substituting for and complementing his own failing functions. Later they may lead to agonizing decisionmakings as to when to "pull the plug." At this Veterans Administration Hospital, the staff has not had to deal with this type of difficulty, a blessing for which credit is due, at least in part, to the results of multidisciplinary exercises.

There are many cases reported which illustrate the tragedy that can be involved in medical care of the patient with a terminal illness. For example, a neighborhood merchant had his life's savings of approximately $60,000 wiped out as a result of his wife's terminal episode of six weeks duration spent at a hospital. No amount of post-mortem reasoning, including the necessity of having adequate medical insurance, was thought likely to alleviate this man's profound resentments about our present health care delivery system. This experience is in contrast to that of a corporation executive who after a similarly critical and expensive hospitalization was able to return to his home and work, cured, with almost all of his bills covered by his fringe benefit package.

Another tragedy was that of a man about fifty, who had been referred to a consulting urologist with a cancer of the penis. He had been assured that an amputation of the organ would almost certainly result in a cure; nevertheless, he had not seen fit to accept the advice. Subsequently, he was treated with a new anti-cancer antibiotic and died from its toxicity and the complications thereof. No psychiatric consultation had been obtained prior to embarking on the management selected; this simple device might well have prevented the catastrophic ending.

Some health care workers express serious misgivings about their involvement with patients whose management differs from their own best professional judgments. There is no doubt that such attitudes are not calculated to contribute to maximally effective services to patients. The institution of some sort of interdisciplinary dialogue among health professionals of various plumage would appear to offer opportunity to open vistas and clear channels which could result in better patient care.

There are many aspects to health care: psychosocial, biomedical, economical, geographic, cultural, religious and personal-idiosyncratic, to name only the more obvious ones. Some of these factorial considerations may be mutually contradictory or partially incompatible. Wherever this occurs, they deserve to be resolved through orderly processes of consultation, involving reasonable value judgments and priority assignments. Thus, in balanced compromise the patient may be provided with the best possible comprehensive terminal care.

PEDIATRIC WORKSHOP

Reported by
JERRY M. WIENER

Scientific inquiry into the area of a child's death and dying is difficult because of the conflicts and anxiety generated in physicians and the families. The pre-school child, five years old, asks questions about his own illness and the possibility of death. How should such questions be answered, and what might be the meaning of such questions? The primary concerns at this age have to do with separation anxiety, the need for parental involvement and support, and the child's fears of loss and abandonment. The meaning of the concepts of death and dying to the pre-school child, and the importance of responding in a way appropriate to the child's developmental level, cognitive understanding, and developmental anxieties are areas of serious concern.

A major effort must be made by the managing physician to sustain involvement, communication, and support with the parents of a dying child. One must be honest, direct, and forthright with the parents, and honest, receptive, and responsive to the child's concerns and questions. What does one tell a child if he asks directly, for example, if he is going to die? There is some disagreement as to how acceptable it is to actually answer such a question directly. One must first find out what anxiety in the child the question might be reflecting, and one must also clarify what the parents have told the child before answering. Much communication among the various members of the hospital staff and health care team is important in order to insure that there is a consistency of understandings among the various members of the hospital staff and health care team and thereby a consistency in the communication to the child. Child psychiatry personnel are generally more in favor of open and straightforward communication with the child as an indicated and perhaps a therapeutic response for the child than are personnel from pediatrics. Different cultural attitudes toward death and the attitude of the physician himself are important, as well as the reactions of physicians, nurses, and other members on the health care team as a result of the stress involved in the management of fatally ill children. Honest and truthful communication with the parents and among the siblings is necessary in a family faced with the management of fatal illness in a child. Particular attention must and should be given to the feelings of the nurses and various nurse reactions which occur during the management of a fatally ill child and particularly after the death of the child.

Rooming-in of the pre-school child's mother should be a routine procedure for the child's first or second night of hospitalization; therefore, it is advisable to have the mother considerably available during this period. However, evidence of anxiety and distress are the normal reactions of the pre-school child on separation from the mother, particularly under these circumstances. The absence of such evidence of distress or anxiety may be evidence of some previous disturbance in the mother-child relationship.

It is also important to help the siblings of the fatally ill child, particularly from the point of view of preventing disturbance and conflict in the siblings. The siblings feel resentment, anger, guilt, jealousy, and rejection. The best way to prevent pathological reactions in the siblings would be honest and sustained communication between parents and siblings and often between the physician and siblings.

RADIATION THERAPY WORKSHOP

Reported by
RICHARD J. TORPIE

It is an important semantic issue to define "dying" and to address discussion and potential solutions to appropriate situations. The word "terminal" also seems too vague. It therefore becomes necessary to identify the patient with a manifest terminal potential (establishment of a cancer diagnosis in an otherwise symptom-free individual) from one with a progressive terminal course (symptoms, failure in curative attempts, and decompensation) or one in terminal extremes (the deathbed).

The radiation therapist must deal with cancer in its initial presentation and/or in any of its progressive stages, often over a protracted period. The concepts of "time and sensitivity" are an ideal goal and certainly reflect the considerate empathy so important in working with the cancer patient and his family. Clinical awareness of working with *all* the physical symptoms of the patient as well as with his anxiety is essential.

Most physicians not in oncological practice may see very few cases of cancer in a year, and they are very uncomfortable working with the disease. In the face of advancing cancer they often deny small complaints, and offer only minimal therapy for major symptoms. Their own denial, together with the medieval attitudes of the family, is the source of lies to the patient. The patient is eventually "referred away" to the radiation therapist, surrounded by this conspiracy of silence, lacking knowledge of his diagnosis, and experiencing increasing loss of interpersonal relationship with his overly protective family. Furthermore, the radiation therapist, through the insistence of the patient's family and physician, may be forced to share in this farce.

Most persons realize the significance of radiation therapy referral and of course are angry at this deception. Often patients will adopt a stoical martyr-like stance rather than offend in this case a rather tenuous patient-physician relationship or chance further isolation from the family. Anger is often the result, and in a hospital situation it is often turned toward nurses and paramedical personnel since direct confrontation with the physician might jeopardize the patient's most dependent status. Therefore, the nurse and the physician are often seeing separate façades of the patient, which of course is frustrating to the nurse who may rightly feel that the physician is neither realistic nor meeting his responsibilities. Resistance to the patient's distress may also take the form of a total condescending comfort which allows no opportunity for the patient to vent his rage.

Another area of difference between nurse and radiation therapist lies in the concept of "let the dying die." The therapist may undertake a course of palliative x-ray therapy with limited goal objectives to relieve the most miserable of the advanced patient's many symptoms. These may include skin ulceration, disfigurement, massive edema, severe pain, or marked neurologic deficit. In instances of success, a burdensome nursing task may be ameliorated; with failure or advancement of another severe symptom the effort seems hardly worthwhile. In the nurse's mind the patient was made to suffer unnecessary distress even with the mere effort of daily transportation to the therapy center. In effect, there may be a thin judicious line between palliation and heroics, and the line may be blurred by the emotionalism of all parties involved.

Several important suggestions may be made concerning the care of the dying patient:

1. There is the evident need for training of all those who will have contact with the dying patient. If he or she isn't born with the knack of compassion, it should be instilled and given every chance to develop. In the large medical center the lack of interpersonal contact leads to role frustration. This may be minimized by a "take the bull by the horns" approach to enforce contact and performance of the group.

2. Referring physicians, if they are uncomfortable in dealing with the realities of cancer, should allow the clinical oncologist full responsibility for the total care and truthful guidance of the patient for the period that the cancer is the most imminent medical threat to that patient. Otherwise, we will continue to foster suspicion, isolation, and even jeopar-

dize the proper therapeutic management of the patient. In this context, at no time should the referring physician use prior radiation treatments as a reason to explain away new symptoms of cancer or other medical difficulties, since this will cause mistrust and uncooperativeness whereby the patient will neglect future radiation therapy when it is most indicated.

3. The patient's psychological defenses against his disease should be respected. It is important to be truthful, but it is also necessary that the truth not be overwhelming. With advancing cancer, hope may be balanced with the capriciousness of the disease and the attainment of immediate therapeutic goals, whether cure, control, or comfort.

4. The renascent interest in thanatology points to the success of the medical profession in prolonging the course and quality of existence of patients with terminal disease, but it also indicates the profession's failure to provide for the total continuity of care in this age of specialization. Physicians can only reflect the pressures of society. It is evident that our cultural attitudes toward death require new humanistic values, and that the economical distress of catastrophic disease and dying be shared by all, so that at least none of us will feel burdensome or disruptive. It is evident that dying must be made a meaningful part of our lives, to be ennobled with those we love and with those who care for us.

PSYCHOPHARMACOLOGY
WORKSHOP

Reported by
IVAN K. GOLDBERG

At least six research areas relating to the dying patient and the bereaved are of dominant interest in terms of psychopharmacology: 1)
pain and its management; 2) emotional problems other than pain, that
is, anxiety and depression; 3) interactions between pain and emotional
states; 4) physical debility and fatigue, and inability to relate with the
environment; 5) the possible role of LSD in altering patients' perceptions
and of THC in reducing nausea and stimulating the appetite; the possible
use of CNS stimulants and anabolic steroids; 6) the role of psychoactive
agents, including phenothiazines, narcotics, anti-anxiety agents, and the
antidepressant group in the prophylactic and therapeutic management of
anticipatory grief, the experience of dying, recovery from bereavement,
and the prophylactic and/or therapeutic management of bereavement.

Of relevance would be a study of the interaction between the patient,
the staff, and prescribed treatments. Projects investigating the attitudes
of patients—particularly among teen-agers and the elderly—toward
their treatment with psychoactive compounds might be fruitful. Of great
interest would be a study of the effects of psychoactive drugs upon the
patient's interactions with hospital staff as well as the specific events
which lead up to the introduction of use of psychoactive compounds.

Some of the public health aspects of bereavement could be clarified
by a prospective study involving individuals with a high risk of becoming bereaved. A large group of subjects in their 40s could be followed
until they began to lose significant family members, probably parents.
The longitudinal study of such a group would make it possible to identify the factors which determine the nature of the grief process. Perhaps

such a study could be set up with the cooperation of either a large industrial union or through a large group practice, such as the Kaiser Plan in California.

Another significant study might indicate the role of antidepressants in preventing grief reactions from progressing into clinically serious depression. The ethics of a placebo study involving the bereaved might legitimately be questioned as it has not been established as yet that antidepressants effectively prevent the bereaved individual from developing a depression. However, any study involving the bereaved should concern itself with both the acute bereavement period and a longer follow-up period during which the grief process resolves.

The problem of which group, the dying or the bereaved, should be given priority in contemplated studies raises other ethical considerations. Some professionals feel that available money and manpower should be devoted to the living (the family of the terminal patient) rather than to the patient himself. Others argue that since death comes to all men, anything that could make dying more comfortable and dignified should be given the highest priority.

GERIATRICS WORKSHOP

Reported by
DORIS K. MILLER

The fundamental question, "Do we really want old people to stay alive?," taps such a spectrum of religious, interpersonal, political, and cultural bias that professionals express as wide a range of responses as would any group of thoughtful laymen. Levels of agreement are not higher within than among professional disciplines.

Ours is a culture dominated by middle-aged power. Both Youth and the Aged serve society primarily as consumers: the former, of goods; the latter, of services. Neither group enjoys opportunities for productive roles. Because the aged pose a less audible and physical challenge to the political status quo, they are assigned a lower priority in public programs and services. They are more superfluous than youth, whose life-styles are attractive to many of the middle-aged. The historical role of the elderly as transmitters of culture and wisdom has been rejected by younger generations and by the advertising media.

Personal descriptions of affection, respect, and inclusion of the infirm-aged in family-life somewhat offset the depressing effects of the general observations, but do not advance a social program for reversing the prevailing social negativism toward the infirm-aged. One concrete suggestion is that within institutions for care of the aged schedules should be arranged and personnel deployed to simulate attentive family-living.

Perhaps the most revealing particular of the professional's attitude toward death is discussion of death in the third person. One professional declared that he had never seen death accepted, equating apparent acceptance with depression susceptible to psychological intervention. However, depression need not be a pathological response, and perhaps death is welcomed not only by many aged-ill, but also by some non-aged terminally ill.

Sharp disagreement exists with respect to "premature" death. Distinctions can be made between the slowly expiring and moribund patient; between the patient with social, emotional, and financial resources, and the one who is essentially abandoned; between the patient who, informed of his deteriorating condition while still physically and mentally able to decide his own fate, would opt for suicide, and the one who would not.

Several persons consider biological survival, even in the absence of emotional and intellectual life, a criterion for exercising heroic efforts to prevent death. Among opponents of this view, the opinion prevails that the professional should keep the patient comfortable, but not actively prolong biological life. A few others express as much discomfort with identifying the medical "point of no return" as with surrendering heroic efforts. However, life decisions for and with patients are made every day on such issues as sterilization and abortion, and reluctance to permit biological death reflects a subjective attitude toward death. The professional might actually gain satisfaction in assisting those terminal patients who request help in choosing burial clothing, and other activities in preparation for death. And, "permissive," rather than "premature," death can confirm the professional's respect for the dignity of the patient and compassion for his survivors, with no real violation of useful data collection.

Some professionals avow their personal attitudes toward death as an event not to be feared, but to be wooed as an attractive alternative to a vegetative existence, an attitude they are certain would be labeled "denial" by dissenters. A diversity of concerns, both self- and patient-directed, emerges in the professional's role-perception. One internist states that the helping professions are charged with satisfying the patient's needs, but these are frequently a social-political issue and not readily definable. A psychiatrist comments that the problems of the aged threaten the professional's sense of mastery and often evoke a retreat from the patient. A young nurse describes feeling uneasy when asked, "Why are you taking care of old people who are going to die anyway?," as though her interest in the aged was a squandering of her professional skills. A student nurse asks, "How can I afford emotionally to care about the dying patient? Who will give me support when he goes?"

Beyond these attitudes toward caring for the aged, again the question arises about decisionmaking and death: hindering it, letting it happen, or speeding it. No one wants to play God; a decision to "permit" death is the outcome of many tacit and explicit cues from participants in the patient's life, and almost never the physician's alone. There is no consensus that "permitting" death is also part of helping.

Questions can be raised about prolonging life for the aged in a social-political system so antagonistic to nonproducing consumers of diminishing resources, such as food and space. Concentration on individual death-prevention often obscures the overwhelming problem of preventing mass death through wars, or the certain mass deaths each year by automobile and driver failure, or the living deaths promised by malnutrition and other consequences of poverty. These issues are not raised as repudiations of the task at hand, but to sharpen two issues: the professionals' attitudes toward mass as well as individual death; and the pernicious sociopolitical context within which one tends the dying patient. The helping professions must engage in political action and provide social leadership to create a feasible environment for rendering terminal care.

The professional's own anxiety with respect to professional role, decisionmaking, and attitude toward death, and his own imperfect formulations of effective programs for treating the infirm-aged, cut across sex, age, and discipline membership, with less and more experienced members contributing equal and different wisdom. Geriatric specialty is sorely needed for all helping professionals caring for the aged; and the public must be a partner in the social planning for this group.

ORAL CARE WORKSHOP

Reported by
AUSTIN H. KUTSCHER

Certain aspects of the oral care of the dying patient should be examined in an attempt to redefine the state of the art and to establish points of departure for future efforts.

1. Although the need for definitions is imperative, there are as yet, regrettably, no definitive descriptions of terminal care nor of terminal status. Definitions vary with the disease, the patient, the service, and the doctor.

2. Of primary consideration in the oral care of the patient who is dying are the meanings of the word "care." How can the patient be made comfortable so that he knows somebody *cares* for him in relation to his mouth? The basic *care* is different for the patient with terminal disease. For the patient whose life may be measured only by days reasonable comfort may be achieved by methods different from those utilized when the patient's life expectancy can be measured in months. Does the same mandate exist to press concepts of rehabilitation or therapy beyond specific immediate procedures for the terminal patient as it does for the medically dischargeable patient?

3. A crucial factor is the person's own psychological status. He is entitled to an adequate oral examination while in the hospital, but what results from the determinations of this examination is another matter. He should, preferably, show a need and express a desire for treatment, whether rational or irrational; and *he must be allowed the choice between active therapy or beneficent and benign neglect* so long as he exhibits no signs of oral discomfort.

People's motivations are different, as are their levels of maturity: their concerns toward their own death differ as do their attitudes toward oral care—which may not coincide with those of their doctors. There are some patients for whom mouth care is an evidence of concern, love, and humane treatment; and there are some for whom mouth care is an invasion of privacy. The patient's whole dental history, his life style, his current request, his current expectations, and his family's expectations must all be considered by those who care for him.

4. One of the most tragic failures in motivating all disciplines toward more complete care for the dying patient is the lack of communication, particularly among the dental department and the rest of the medical and paramedical staff. When dentists, nurses, and other disciplines are motivated, no matter what the motivation is, they perform satisfactorily. However, they may not be motivated to care for the terminal patient and, therefore, may not be prepared to undertake this responsibility.

Patient-oriented therapy is the key to motivation for all the disciplines involved.

5. The administrative and medical personnel in most hospitals are not basically aware of the dentist's capabilities, nor do they realize that their patients have preoccupations with the mouth. For example, because the mouth is one of the most psychologically sensitive areas of the body, the ramifications of an oral cancer extend far beyond those of many other potentially fatal diseases. Frequently, the available hospital and general office facilities are deficient. The problem becomes an institutional one. General dentistry services are urgently needed in our hospitals. However, the problem of establishing such services is not as great as the problem of delivering the immediate and necessary service to the patient. This requires education of both the patient and those responsible for his care. Doctors may shy away from this, but nurses cannot. However, there is no place where a nurse can acquire this education. The attitude of the medical and nursing care services in terms of the roles the dentist and dental hygienists can play and how they should perform in the care of the patient may be responsible for the failure of these services to seek advice and follow-up oral care for the terminal patient. The dentist also fails to provide adequate dental care; he does not address himself to all dental problems, and he is afraid to treat many types of patients. Many dentists are terrified at the thought of caring for the terminal patient. The profession evinces more interest in pedodontics and other specialties than it does in geriatric dentistry. Den-

tists, therefore, do not generally care for, let alone *adequately* care for, the dying patient. The solution lies in his clinical and psychological (even psychiatric) education and the provision of a psychosocial platform from which he can operate with reasonable equanimity.

6. The past lack of emphasis on the mouth in the living patient, as well as in the dying one, has led to our failure to understand how important the mouth is as an organ of pleasure and satisfaction. However, this picture seems to be changing. Medical and nursing students and newly graduated physicians are beginning to acknowledge the importance of the mouth and its manifold functions (eating, tasting, digestion, swallowing; *communications*—speech; expression—love, anger, hate, attack; and so on) in relationship to necessary care of the total person. Established physicians must be exposed to the inclusion of oral care in their ministrations to terminal patients. Dental schools must institute an adequate educational campaign, through suitable additions to the curriculum, aimed at making the profession aware of its responsible role, as well as making professionals emotionally secure, in caring for the chronically ill and terminal patient.

ORGAN TRANSPLANTATION WORKSHOP

Reported by
JOSEPH A. BUDA

Most experience with the psychological, ethical, moral, legal, and social problems of terminal care arising in the relatively new field of organ transplantation has been with kidney transplantation, and, therefore, concerns patients on chronic dialysis or patients receiving renal transplants either from a living, related donor or from a cadaver. The discussion of the psychosocial problems and issues concerning donors raises many questions, including those of: (a) coercive pressures on donors, (b) who contacts or finds donors; and (c) the meaning donating a kidney has for the donor.

Transplantation is a way of preserving life. However, since the procedures of chronic dialysis and kidney transplant are not always effective in saving a life, at times the coercion placed upon potential living-related donors may be too great and may cause too stressful and too disruptive influences upon a family. Also, the physicians concerned may exert undue pressure or coercion upon a potential donor who may be unwilling. By stressing the possible gain and minimizing the possible hazards, the physicians may bring to bear unresistible pressures upon a reluctant donor.

The question of who finds and approaches potential donors is answered by the potential recipient, and by the physician. For the most part, it is the patient who must broach the issue to members of his family in an attempt to seek out family members who will agree to be considered as donor candidates.

The donation of a kidney to a family member who is dying of renal disease has been adjudged to be an act of great significance, of deep satisfaction, and a most meaningful experience. The giving of a kidney to a family member who is terminally ill and who may live is an act that may give a new meaning to the life of the donor. Patients receiving chronic hemodialysis or renal transplants can live productive and worthwhile lives; many return to their pre-illness activities.

Concerning cadaver donors—the passage of the Uniform Anatomical Gifts Act permits an individual to expressly will what he wants done with his body or with any of his organs. In the setting of a dying patient, considered to be a potential cadaver donor, the criteria for "brain death" are used by a committee which consists of physicians not involved in the transplantation effort. In most institutions this committee sees that the criteria for "brain death" are met, that the family members are informed, and that informed consent is obtained.

Regarding recipient related issues, patients who are accepted for dialysis or transplantation are those in whom medical management is no longer effective in the problem of uremia and its implications. These patients are indeed terminal and are treated either with hemodialysis or are given a renal transplant; they are functioning beyond the point of terminal care. This is a situation that is quite unique in medical care. In effect, these patients have been given a new life, and with this, new problems. The problems include a feeling of being on borrowed time, a great dependency on the transplantation and dialysis team, and a reluctance to resume pre-illness activities and responsibilities. These patients require a great deal of emotional support and must be given realistic hope so that they may adapt to their "new" life and live in a manner that is satisfying to them and to their families.

PASTORAL CARE WORKSHOP

Reported by

J. WILLIAM WORDEN

The chaplain who ministers to the dying deals primarily with three groups—the dying, the bereaved, and with those members of the hospital staff who are concerned in the care of the dying. With each of these groups the chaplain may play one or more different types of roles. First, there is the personal role, in which he is involved in interpersonal relationships, dealing as a man with other men. The second role is that of a professional, in which he is involved in relating to persons as a pastor. In the third, or sacramental, role the chaplain is involved in dispensing the sacraments and providing other sacerdotal functions. The fourth role of the chaplain is that of theologian, where it is his task to theologize about such important issues as pain, evil, dying, and other human experiences. In all of these roles his main goal is to help preserve the quality of life, even for the dying patient.

When the chaplain ministers to the dying patient, certain issues emerge. What is the place of fear and hope in the life of the dying patient? Most patients are more afraid of the process of dying than they are afraid of the actual fact of being dead, and most of this apprehension centers around the issue of pain management. Many chaplains feel that pain should be kept to a minimum, as in Saint Christopher's Hospice in England; however, others feel that if patients are too well taken care of in such a place as the hospice, they may be prevented from dealing effectively with certain of their feelings about dying, especially feelings of anger.

Another issue centering around patient care involves the regressive nature of terminal illness and the dependency that it engenders. Dependency and trust are seen as issues at the beginning of life, as Erickson indicates, and at the end. Such a place as the hospice handles this issue well by challenging the dying to give and to help other dying patients. Not only does this give the dying person a purpose but also, in giving oneself as a living sacrifice, one is working out a Christian fulfillment of life. The dependency associated with a terminal illness need not be regressive, but can be accepted in a mature way.

As a person ages he sustains a number of personal losses which he needs to integrate into his personality. When the dying patient begins to turn his back on the significant others in his life this need not be seen as a regressive action but as a necessity, just as a child learns that he must say good-bye to his parents when he is growing up. Theilhard is quoted as saying that it is psychologically expanding to accept full separations and grief as real. The acceptance of death and the process of dying does not necessarily negate hope.

It is generally believed that one's conceptualization of death is important in the process of dying, whether death is seen as peaceful sleep or as an afterlife. Children sometimes see death as being mutilative, a concept which can be disturbing to a dying child. The chaplain can help people with their misconceptions.

The second group to whom the chaplain ministers is that of the bereaved. Special problem areas include ministering to families in which there was the death of a child, where there were sudden or violent deaths, and where there was a lingering death, with the family's having done most of its grieving prior to the member's demise and feeling guilty for emotional withdrawal after the death. The question arises of how much the chaplain feels that as a part of his role he must justify a death. He may be the recipient of anger that people want to place on God, or he may help the bereaved by silent consolation that some events in life are mysterious and can remain uninterpreted. In any case, the chaplain can offer the gift of presence, which is most important.

With regard to the third group, members of the hospital community, a team approach to the dying is very important without buck-passing or excessive specialization. Since death is not a medical problem but a problem of living and humanness, it needs an interdisciplinary approach. One cannot really deal with dying without an adequate view of man. By adequate is meant seeing man as a whole rather than as a triparty of body, mind, and spirit.

One of the areas where chaplains can make a major contribution in an interdisciplinary setting is in defining ethical issues which arise surrounding organ transplants, euthanasia, and suicide. Just as there is a committee that considers suitability for hemodialysis, boards might be established whereby prolonging life could be considered for a given patient. The chaplain could play a major role in helping families and physicians find courage to do what they ought and fear to do.

NURSING WORKSHOP

Reported by
MARY X. BRITTEN

One must define the study population of the dying group, since it will make a difference in the application of the principles of grief and mourning. Much depends upon the age of the patient, strength of family ties, and the cultural heritage. The terminal illness of a child evokes a different response and requires different handling from that of an elderly, debilitated patient. The age of those involved has implications and ramifications for the care that is given and received.

The type of illness is another consideration. Certain illnesses immediately convey to the patient, family, and staff feelings of despair, pain, hopelessness, and death. Stereotyped thinking about the certainty of death due to specific illnesses may or may not be justified. Although other illnesses may be equally relentless in their downhill progression for the patient, the patient may not be labeled as dying or terminal—as for example, the patient with emphysema. The location of the terminal patient—in his home, in a general hospital, or in a hospital dealing only with dying patients—influences the care that is given him.

Many patients whom the nurse encounters are not informed of the nature of their illnesses or that they are dying. Perhaps her task is easier when she deals with those who do know. Superimposed on all the above are the cultural, social, personal, and religious mores of the person who is terminally ill and his family. Included here are the stereotypes of how a person accepts death, including those of the nurse administering care. The patient may have accepted death, but the hospital medical system prohibits this and prevents nurses from accepting it. Denial or noninvolvement with the patient and family to the point of avoidance except for essential nursing care is a common way of handling the dying patient. In contrast, there is the nursing staff that has defined and acts upon the challenge and reward of providing support and care to those with terminal illnesses and to their families.

It is important to determine and explore the nursing components from the standpoint of the individual nurse, the practice of nursing, and the educational elements. For the individual nurse, a system can be structured to provide support for professional, job-related problems. This would help the nurse cope with her feelings, be they satisfaction or frustration, and in addition would be a resource toward the improvement of patient care. With respect to practice, the nurse has much to offer through continuity of patient care. In addition, the nurse must be cognizant of the philosophy of the institution she works for, as well as critically evaluate her own feelings and philosophy about caring for patients who are terminally ill. Continuity of care for the dying patient is extremely important, and effective multidisciplinary team effort is essential.

Students must be educated in caring for the dying patient. They must be introduced to growth and development and its implications for nursing care. They must be familiarized with the ways patients handle death, and should be introduced to sociological and cultural patterns which will influence and determine their nursing care. As students they should be assigned to terminally ill patients and be given the opportunity to show their feelings and receive support from their faculty. Nursing students should be taught to appreciate the need to allow for grief and mourning on the part of the patient and family.

It is not sufficient to educate only the nursing student and in professional disciplines alone. The nursing profession has the obligation to take an active role in the education of the general public. They must teach and permit the family to anticipate and work through grief. By educating the public, nursing educators might in the future generate a climate which is healthier for all concerned and more conducive to support and strength during a crisis everyone must face. This type of education should not be delayed until a time of terminal illness; rather, the elementary and secondary school system may be the place to start instituting discussion. It is definite that the nursing profession has a profound responsibility to develop a course of action in this too often neglected area.

PSYCHOTHERAPY WORKSHOP

Reported by

DAVID PERETZ

The issues related to the therapeutic approaches to the dying patient and his family include the following:

1) the value of psychotherapy;

2) toward whom should psychotherapy be directed?;

3) defining goals of psychotherapy with the dying person and the family;

4) specific psychotherapeutic techniques;

5) special emotional problems for the psychotherapist working with the dying and their families.

The question of whether, with our limited psychiatric and psychotherapeutic resources, it is worthwhile to invest in the psychotherapeutic approach to the dying is often raised. The answer should be a clear "yes," in recognition of the experience of dying as a critical life experience for the three million persons who die each year and also of the far-reaching impact of these deaths on family members and others, with preventive and public health consequences of considerable magnitude. It is useful to distinguish between the more traditional psychotherapy and psychologically beneficial therapies. The latter are seen to be a broad group of approaches to the dying person or his family, ranging from the interest evidenced by staff in the patient's well-being and comfort to the creation of an atmosphere in which sick patients share with one another in group settings things as simple as meals or as complex as their feelings.

Identification of the high-risk family is an important phase in determining the need for psychosocial intervention. Those who treat terminally ill children often find themselves dealing more with the parents than with the child. The "psychosocial" therapist, therefore, is someone trying to help primary, secondary, and tertiary patients, performing not only a direct individual service but also a preventive one by lessening the likelihood of maladaptation effecting others in the "community." Thus, it is clear that at various times the "patient" approached therapeutically may be the dying person, his family members, or even staff and other patients in the setting.

In attempting to define the goals of therapy, some differences of opinion emerge. Those convinced that the central issue to be dealt with is the dying person's sense of valuelessness, burdensomeness, or failure see the goal of psychotherapy as trying to convey to the dying person that he always remains of value as a human being. Yet, it can be said that the problem is also a consequence of the fact that someone of value to others is being lost. The pain and strain produced and the defensive reactions to these are part of a process which involved many problems (including guilt on the part of the patient, family member, withdrawal, consequent depression, and more). In the experience of many therapists, the bereaved—particularly the spouse over sixty-five years of age—may be found to experience an increased sense of his own valuelessness, failure, and self-condemnation.

In defining goals of therapy, it should be clear that the therapist works within an institution with value systems which can at times be contrary to the goals he would like to set. The therapist serves as a model for identification in the usual psychotherapy, and this has an important place in his work with the dying patient. He can help the patient to become a useful model for his children and others in their approach to dying. Telling patients this can give them a conscious goal to work toward, and an indication that the last days and hours of living, as well as the prior life, do remain in the mind and memory of persons close to the patient, effecting their lives.

Another goal, similar to the latter and also a therapeutic technique, involves enlisting the patient's help in dealing with the family. This can provide the sense of continuity and value referred to above as crucial. It would also be therapeutic for the family, which would be working together at the time of dying as it had in the course of living.

Turning to specific psychotherapeutic techniques used with the dying person, differences of emphasis emerge. It has been noted that a principle in the psychotherapy of the dying patient is that the "here and now" be dealt with as much as possible. Fear of dying expresses fear of being abandoned, deserted, pushed off in a back room and left to die alone. The dying person is seen as afraid of pain and of being a burden to the family. This, then, is not a time to engage in analysis and, indeed, the patient's emphasis on past failures is seen as something that could distract from present concerns. When fear in the present is reduced, the patient may freely, without the therapist's intervention, review his past. Families are often seen to operate in the same way. In the opinion of some therapists, the dying person, in reassessing his life, can be led to depression by his unhappiness about failures and unfulfilled potential. It should be acknowledged that the traditional reason for focusing on the past in psychotherapy is to discover patterns of behavior that will be useful in planning the future. For the dying person, the fact of the therapist's being interested in his past might be of special value, and might prove to be a route through which the patient could sense the therapist's value of and fascination with him as a person. In this respect, it would be quite different from a resistance.

The importance of helping the patient to live as he would normally do, without providing false reassurance or rewarding denial, is seen as a vital therapeutic factor. The risk of excessive support is that it infantilizes the patient and reduces self-respect. It is recognized that the balance between shielding the patient and giving respect is a difficult one to maintain.

Several other techniques or approaches for the therapist are:

1) to help the patient come to value the quality of companionship and close relationship, not for the length of its duration but for the quality of inner experience;

2) to attend dressing changes by the surgeon as he cares for patients who are being "eaten away" by their disease, thus smelling and accepting the patient's odors as a reality and not repugnant experiences to be avoided;

3) to concentrate with the patient on the positive in addition to the approaches described above. This means the "living," the "doing," and includes allowing that there are still possibilities for life and helping the patient to discover them, such as extra flowers, a book, someone to talk to, extra company, knowing who is coming to visit;

4) to set up a therapeutic atmosphere in the ward or room (patients seem to do better when they eat in a common room, when one patient brings in a tray to the bedside of another, when reasonable human demands are made upon a patient by the staff rather than allowing him to retreat).

The family needs help often in dealing with their revulsion with the patient, which is provocative of guilt. They may not want to be near, see, and touch the patient, yet they are forced by circumstances to do so. In these instances, the opportunity to talk out their feelings with a therapist can be helpful. Families, too, particularly with sick children, need to be helped not to "give up everything," such normal pleasures as parties, theatre, sex, and others.

A broadened concept of who the therapist is flows from a broadened concept of what therapy is. Attendant, student, nurse, social worker, clergyman, family, fellow patient—all can contribute, perhaps with help and encouragement, perhaps on their own, to a therapeutic effect.

A number of problems face those who would do therapy with the dying person and his family. At times the therapist may feel that the dying patient *is* without value and *is* a failure, although the therapist may deny this feeling. It is important to admit how "tough" this work is and that not everybody can be expected to do it. Because of the fear and guilt associated with dying, there is a greater likelihood of the therapist's making "mistakes." His own fear of loss of control may be mobilized by the patient's loss of control. It may be necessary for the therapist to "gear up" before entering the room each time, and fight whatever it is he is afraid of in the work. This raises questions about how to resolve feelings so that genuine psychotherapy can be done; how to deal with staff who want to avoid the patient; how to create an atmosphere of living in a setting where there is a greater possibility of dying. Another issue of concern is that of the "payoff" for the therapist. The need for a payoff should be acknowledged, yet that payoff can come in the pleasure of helping, in the acknowledgment of the fact that offering of the self is the supreme gift, that some people can do it more readily than others, and that there can be pleasure in the effort itself, as opposed to the effect of the effort.

CARE OF THE FAMILY OF THE PATIENT WORKSHOP

Reported by

NOHMIE MYERS

Many professionals recognize the need to conceptualize the process of anticipatory grief and to individualize the grieving family and the relationship to the dying patient around such factors as age, role, religious and cultural background, among others. Members of these professions —psychiatry, general medicine, theology, social work, psychology, sociology, nursing—raise several important questions: How much is denial or rejection involved in anticipatory grief? Is time predictable? Who should be told the truth—the patient and/or the family? For how long is the grieving process? Is the denial of grief a healthy way of coping? Must there be guilt?

It is necessary for the hospital staff and the family to be "in tune" or together emotionally with the dying patient; and both grief and anger are important components in the mourning process. A process of "no grief" often leads to severe emotional disturbances for family members of the patient. Rituals are needed, as well as anger for both the living and the dying. However, when the elderly die in hospitals or nursing homes, less of the family is involved because the patient is often already detached from them.

The occurrence of guilt, neglect, over-involvement, symbiotic ties, and rage, all sometimes occurring together, is exemplified in anticipatory mourning of parents for children dying of leukemia. There are five different phases of the mourning process: acknowledgment (before diagnosis of the illness); experience of grief (emotional impact of the anticipated loss); reconciliation (significance of the child's illness and death in harmony with personal values, goals, and life styles); detachment (withdrawal of emotional investment from the child as a growing, living being with a real future); and image fixation (investment in a final image of child replacing real child). These parents usually do not allow themselves to express relief after the death of their child.

There is "death in life" as well as "life in death." Anticipatory grief, to quote the Fultons, "like so much else, possesses the capacity to enhance our lives and secure our well-being, while possessing at the same time the power to undermine our fragile existence and rupture our tenuous social bonds."

INSTITUTIONAL CARE WORKSHOP

Reported by

M. URSULA BRADY

The group concerned themselves with the following questions in relation to institutional care of the terminally ill: What are the essential characteristics of an institution dedicated to care for the terminally ill; how is such an institution set up; is it desirable to have such an institution at all?

Where can the dying person go for care? Where can he go and be accepted with his illness and be given a place without a "parking meter," a place to remain in and be comforted? In such a place or institution death would be a companion rather than the antagonist. Neither the dying person nor staff would consider death a failure. When life becomes a difficult struggle, this person would feel the comfort of a human hand rather than a metal electrode, or the support of another's arms for a "sip of tea" rather than the immobilization necessary for intravenous infusions.

In contrast to this kind of environment there is the general hospital, whose every purpose is to fight against death, at all costs. A host of measures are initiated in order to prolong life. It is not only an intellectual but an emotional gymnastic feat for the hospital staff to reassess life-oriented goals when ministering to the dying patient. When do the patient and staff make the transition of battling for life to an acceptance of death?

In an institution designed for the terminally ill, the problem has been settled in advance: the goal is *care*. The staff has accepted this goal and the environment provides a constant reminder that comfort is the *raison d'être*. There are no mechanical, life-sustaining devices within the institution. There is no evidence of the life versus death conflict. There now is a community prepared with a set goal, accepted and sustained by the community members. But what are the measures taken to sustain this community? How can the members of the community develop or maintain a psychological internal economy able to withstand repeated emotional involvements and subsequent losses?

First, the recruited staff must have the desire, and be equipped with the knowledge and skills necessary, to deliver the ultimate of comfort and care to the dying patient. They may relieve all pain, reduce all vomiting, and guarantee physiologic comfort. Comfort is their major goal and they are secure in their ability to accomplish their goals by the selection and administration of pharmaceutical preparations, heroin, and alcohol.

Second, the goal is well-defined and the environment and tools necessary are provided to accomplish it.

Third, there is an on-going inservice process within the institution, through group meetings and staff conferences, which provides for some psychological and emotional support.

Fourth, involvement and deep expression of mourning are encouraged. The personnel develop relationships with members of the dying patient's family and the dying patient shares relationships with members of the staff's family, frequently bringing their children into the institution to romp about while the patients are enjoying the garden air.

As the patient nears termination the staff member shares, to some extent, the grieving process with the patient's family. Frequently, the patient is cantankerous and demanding, but every attempt is made to accept this kind of behavior with understanding. At the time of death, the staff member shares in the prayers at the bedside, perhaps even leads the group in prayer. Crying by the staff member is accepted and is considered natural. After the patient's death, the staff member might visit the family members during the "wake" period, or attend the ceremony in the cemetery. The bed that had been occupied by the deceased patient is left empty for a time as an acknowledgment of the staff's loss. This also gives the staff an opportunity to adjust to the acceptance of a new member into the institution.

It is generally agreed that terminally ill patients often need a particular kind of care and these patients have specific psychological needs which are not presently met in the general hospital. Also, the people who care only for the terminally ill patients are unique and special.

However, other questions arise for which agreement is not as universal. Should the terminally ill patient, at this level of illness, be removed
from the general hospital? Is there a need for the staff in the general
hospital to share in the care for this kind of patient? Is this kind of care
necessary for all "caring personnel" to experience to increase their sensitivity to the fears and thoughts and feelings of those who wait for
death? Is such a high degree of institutional specificity necessary for delivery of this kind of medical care service? What are the needs of society for this kind of care, and do these needs differ from community to
community?

CONTRIBUTORS

Ruth Abrams, M.S., Visiting Associate, Laboratory of Community Psychiatry, Harvard Medical School, Boston, Massachusetts; formerly Clinical and Research Social Worker, Massachusetts General Hospital and Harvard School of Public Health, Boston, Massachusetts

Jeanne Quint Benoliel, D.N.S., Associate Professor, School of Nursing, University of Washington, Seattle, Washington

M. Ursula Brady, R.N., Assistant Professor, Department of Nursing, Faculty of Medicine, College of Physicians and Surgeons, Columbia University, New York, New York

Mary X. Britten, R.N., Assistant Professor, Department of Nursing, Faculty of Medicine, College of Physicians and Surgeons, Columbia University, New York, New York

Lester A. Bronheim, M.D., Associate Medical Director, J. B. Roerig Division of Charles Pfizer and Company, New York, New York

Joseph A. Buda, M.D., Associate Professor of Clinical Surgery, College of Physicians and Surgeons, Columbia University, New York, New York

Arthur C. Carr, Ph.D., Professor (Medical Psychology), Department of Psychiatry, College of Physicians and Surgeons, Columbia University, New York, New York; Chairman of the Professional Advisory Board of the Foundation of Thanatology

Ned H. Cassem, M.D., Department of Psychiatry, Massachusetts General Hospital, Harvard Medical School, Boston, Massachusetts

Mary I. Crawford, R.N., Ed. D., Associate Dean, Department of Nursing, Faculty of Medicine, Columbia University, New York, New York; Director of Nursing of the Presbyterian Hospital in the City of New York, Columbia-Presbyterian Medical Center

Douglas Damrosch, M.D., Director of the Columbia-Presbyterian Medical Center, New York, New York

Rose Dobrof, M.S.W., Hunter College School of Social Work, New York, New York

Julie Fulton, M.A., National Institute of Mental Health Fellow, Department of Sociology, University of Minnesota, Minneapolis, Minnesota

Robert Fulton, Ph.D., Professor of Sociology and Director of the Center for Death Education and Research, University of Minnesota, Minneapolis, Minnesota

Edward H. Futterman, M.D., Assistant Professor, Department of Psychiatry, Abraham Lincoln School of Medicine, University of Illinois College of Medicine, Chicago, Illinois

Ivan K. Goldberg, M.D., Department of Psychiatry, College of Physicians and Surgeons, Columbia University, New York, New York

Thomas A. Gonda, M.D., Associate Dean and Professor of Psychiatry, Stanford University School of Medicine and Director, Stanford University Hospital, Palo Alto, California

Arnoldus Goudsmit, M.D., Ph.D., Associate Professor of Oncology, Wayne State University School of Medicine, Detroit, Michigan

Thomas P. Hackett, M.D., Associate in Psychiatry, Department of Psychiatry, Massachusetts General Hospital, Harvard Medical School, Boston, Massachusetts

Henry O. Heinemann, M.D., Associate Professor, Department of Medicine, Cornell University College of Medicine, The New York Hospital-Cornell Medical Center, New York, New York

Edward Henderson, M.D., Head, Leukemia Service, Medicine Branch, National Cancer Institute, National Institutes of Health, Bethesda, Maryland

Austin Herschberger, Ph.D., Chairman, Department of Psychology, Greater Hartford Community College, Hartford, Connecticut

Frederic P. Herter, M.D., Professor of Surgery, College of Physicians and Surgeons, Columbia University, New York, New York

Irwin Hoffman, Ph.D., Instructor in Psychology, University of Illinois College of Medicine, Chicago, Illinois

Robert Kastenbaum, Ph.D., Professor of Psychology, Department of Psychology, Wayne State University, College of Liberal Arts, Detroit, Michigan

Chaplain LeRoy G. Kerney, Chief, Department of Spiritual Ministry, Clinical Center, National Institutes of Health, Bethesda, Maryland

Alfred S. Ketcham, M.D., Chief of Surgery and Director of Clinics, National Cancer Institute, National Institutes of Health, Bethesda, Maryland

Morton M. Kligerman, M.D., Professor and Chairman, Department of Radiology, Yale University College of Medicine, New Haven, Connecticut

Lawrence C. Kolb, M.D., Professor and Chairman, Department of Psychiatry, College of Physicians and Surgeons, Columbia University, New York, New York; Director, New York State Psychiatric Institute, New York, New York

Melvin Krant, M.D., Director, Tufts University-Medical Cancer Unit, Lemuel Shattuck Hospital, Boston, Massachusetts

Austin H. Kutscher, D.D.S., Associate Professor, Director of Psychiatric Institute Dental Service, School of Dental and Oral Surgery, Columbia University, New York, New York; President of the Foundation of Thanatology

Louis Lasagna, M.D., Professor of Pharmacology, School of Medicine and Dentistry, University of Rochester, Rochester, New York

David Maddison, M.D., Professor of Psychiatry, University of Sydney, New South Wales, Australia

Doris K. Miller, Ph.D., Past President, Division of Clinical Psychology, New York State Psychological Association, New York, New York

Robert H. Moser, M.D., Maui Medical Group, Wailuku, Maui, Hawaii

Nohmie Myers, Academy of Certified Social Workers, New York, New York

David Peretz, M.D., Associate, Department of Psychiatry, College of Physicians and Surgeons, Columbia University, New York, New York; Chairman of the Research Committee of the Foundation of Thanatology

Beverley Raphael, M.D., Research Psychiatrist, New South Wales Institute of Psychiatry, Sydney, Australia

W. Dewi Rees, M.D., Wales, United Kingdom

Fred Rosner, M.D., Director of Hematology, The Long Island Jewish Medical Center, Queens Hospital Center Affiliation, Jamaica, New York

Elisabeth K. Ross, M.D., Medical Director, South Cook County Mental Health and Family Service, Chicago, Illinois

Melvin Sabshin, M.D., Department of Psychiatry, Abraham Lincoln School of Medicine, University of Illinois College of Medicine, Chicago, Illinois

Cicely Saunders, M.D., O.B.E., M.A., M.R.C.P., S.R.N., Medical Director, St. Christopher's Hospice, Sydenham, London, England

Bernard Schoenberg, M.D., Associate Clinical Professor, Department of Psychiatry, College of Physicians and Surgeons, Columbia University, New York, New York; Chairman of the Executive Committee of the Foundation of Thanatology

Rudolf Toch, M.D., Instructor in Pediatrics, Harvard Medical School, Boston, Massachusetts

Richard J. Torpie, M.D., Department of Radiotherapy, Hahnemann Medical School, Philadelphia, Pennsylvania

Avery D. Weisman, M.D., Principal Investigator, Project Omega, Department of Psychiatry, Massachusetts General Hospital; Associate Professor of Psychiatry, Massachusetts General Hospital, Harvard Medical School, Boston, Massachusetts

Jerry Wiener, M.D., Director of Child Psychiatry, Emory University School of Medicine, Atlanta, Georgia

J. William Worden, Ph.D., Project Omega, Massachusetts General Hospital, Harvard Medical School, Boston, Massachusetts

INDEX *

* Some entries and page numbers italicized for special emphasis.